EDITION **6**

Being A Homemaker/ Home Health Aide

Elana D. Zucker, RN, MSN

Consultant/Former Director of Nursing
Chief Nursing Officer
Hospital and Emergency Services
Overlook Hospital
Summit, New Jersey

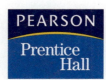

PEARSON
Prentice Hall

Upper Saddle River, New Jersey 07458

Library of Congress Cataloging-in-Publication Data

Being a homemaker/home health aide / [edited by] Elana D. Zucker.—
    6th ed.
        p. ;   cm.
    Includes index.
    ISBN 0-13-170106-1
    1. Home health aides.   2. Home care services.
      [DNLM: 1. Home Care Services.   2. Home Health Aides. WY 115
B422 2005]   I. Zucker, Elana D.
      RA645.3.B45 2005
      610.73'43—dc22

                                                                    2005023231

In memory of Sandra Gustafson who made the whole book possible.

Publisher: Julie Levin Alexander
Executive Assistant: Regina Bruno
Editor-in-Chief: Maura Connor
Executive Editor: Debbie Yarnell
Managing Development Editor: Marilyn Meserve
Development Editor: Sheba Jalaluddin
Supplements Editor: Michael Giacobbe
Director of Manufacturing and Production: Bruce Johnson
Managing Production Editor: Patrick Walsh
Production Liaison: Mary C. Treacy
Production Editor: Karen Ettinger, TechBooks/GTS
Manufacturing Manager: Ilene Sanford
Manufacturing Buyer: Pat Brown
Director of Marketing: Karen Allman
Marketing Manager: Francisco Del Castillo
Marketing Coordinator: Michael Sirinides
Marketing Assistant: Patricia Linard
Media Product Manager: John J. Jordan
Media Production Manager: Amy Peltier
Media Project Manager: Tina Rudowski
Senior Design Coordinator: Maria Guglielmo-Walsh
Interior Design: Patricia McDermond
Cover Design: Wanda España
Composition: TechBooks/GTS York, PA Campus
Printer/Binder: Banta/Menasha
Cover Printer: Phoenix Color

Printed in the United States of America

Pearson Education LTD.
Pearson Education Australia PTY, Limited
Pearson Education Singapore, Pte. Ltd
Pearson Education North Asia Ltd
Pearson Education, Canada, Ltd
Pearson Educación de Mexico, S.A. de C.V.
Pearson Education—Japan
Pearson Education Malaysia, Pte. Ltd
Pearson Education, Upper Saddle River, New Jersey

NOTICE

It is the intent of the author and publishers that this textbook be used as part of a formal Homemaker/Home Health Aide course taught by a qualified instructor. The procedures presented here represent accepted practices in the United States. They are not offered as a standard of care. Home health care is to be performed under the authority and guidance of qualified supervisory personnel. It is the reader's responsibility to know and follow local care protocols as provided by the medical advisers directing the system to which he or she belongs. Also, it is the reader's responsibility to stay informed of home health care procedure changes.

The material in this textbook contains the most current information available at the time of publication. However, federal, state, and local guidelines concerning clinical practices, including without limitation those governing infection control and standard precautions, change rapidly. The reader should note, therefore, that new regulations may require changes in some procedures.

It is the responsibility of the reader to familiarize himself or herself with policies and procedures set by federal, state, and local agencies, as well as the institution or agency where the reader is employed. The authors and publishers of this textbook, and the supplements written to accompany it, disclaim any liability, loss, or risk resulting directly or indirectly from the suggested procedures and theory, from any undetected errors, or from the reader's misunderstanding of the text. It is the reader's responsibility to stay informed of any new changes or recommendations made by any federal, state, and local agency as well as by his or her employing health care institution or agency.

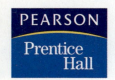
PEARSON
Prentice
Hall

10 9

ISBN 0-13-170106-1

About the Author

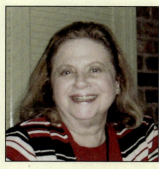

Elana D. Zucker

Elana Zucker has been an active contributor to the nursing and health care professions for 40 years. As a graduate nurse she worked in the community in New York, Washington DC, and New Jersey. She has written both federal and state legislation, testified before Congress, and advised lawmakers as they fashioned programs. She has taught at Fairleigh Dickinson University in the graduate nursing program and has been a frequent guest speaker at both national and state events. In her capacity as administrator of a federal grant to the Home Health Agency of New Jersey, she was the guiding force in training thousands of Homemaker/Home Health Aides. In this capacity she was instrumental in regulating the curriculum within the state and in establishing a system for regulating and credentialing the Homemaker/Home Health Aides within the state. Ms. Zucker has held positions at Overlook Hospital, New Jersey, as director of community health services, director of nursing, and as chief nursing officer. She now focuses her energies on consulting, writing, volunteer work with the local medical day care program, and working as an expert witness.

HOW TO USE THIS BOOK

Case Study

The beginning of each chapter presents a photograph of a client and a realistic situation, allowing you to visualize the home care setting and anticipate issues you might encounter on the job. Clients of different ages and cultures are portrayed.

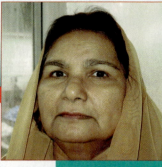

CHAPTER **11**

Basic Body Movement and Positions

CASE STUDY

Mrs. Mahamoud suffered a broken hip in a fall in her kitchen. She was trying to retrieve a dish from a high shelf and slipped off a stool. Her sons are young adults and are in college and working. Prior to her fall, Mrs. Mahamoud was active in her neighborhood religious activities, but she is unable to drive now. Her husband works six days a week and spends his free time with his elderly father living nearby with his also elderly aunt. Mrs. Mahamoud exercises when she is reminded and when you are there to assist her, but she does not initiate the exercises. She remains in bed until everyone has left the house in the morning and then gets up using her own procedures. Her husband communicates with the doctor and the therapists via telephone. Mrs. Mahamoud manages to keep the house tidy and cook simple meals. She seldom eats with the family, preferring to eat after everyone is finished at the table. Shopping for food poses a serious problem as Mrs. Mahamoud cannot go herself and does not want to ask her family for help.

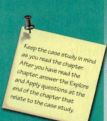

Keep the case study in mind as you read the chapter. After you have read the chapter, answer the Explore and Apply questions at the end of the chapter that relate to the case study.

Certification Exam Review

Five multiple choice questions in each chapter allow you to test your knowledge and practice for the certification exam.

Certification Exam Review Questions

Choose the best answer for each question or statement.

1. **Good body mechanics means**
   a. taking into account only how your body works.
   b. taking into account only the proper position of the client's body.
   c. using the proper muscles to move a client or an object.
   d. using only the proper muscles when you are working.

2. **A client's ability to move**
   a. is always the same regardless of the time of day.
   b. varies with the time of day.
   c. is prescribed by the physician.
   d. is delegated to you by the physical therapist.

3. **The client's position in bed**
   a. is always prescribed by the physician.
   b. is always prescribed by the physical therapist.
   c. is a combination of the client preferences, client safety, and the client's medical condition.
   d. should always be the same so the client becomes used to it.

4. **Client's position should be changed and toileting and water offered**
   a. when you think the client needs the change.
   b. at the minimum every two hours.
   c. before you leave the client.
   d. when you arrive in the house.

5. **Restraints**
   a. should be used whenever you think the client will hurt himself.
   b. should be put on by the family and left until you can take them off.
   c. are used when all other avenues of calming and protecting the client have failed.
   d. should be used before you try other avenues as it is the safest and most time-efficient method of calming the client.

Guidelines

Important principles, ideas and methods are highlighted throughout the text to guide you on the job.

+ GUIDELINES

Using Elastic Support Stockings

■ Always use clean, dry stockings that have been prescribed for the client. Do not switch stockings with anyone else.

■ Ask when the client should wear the stockings. Should they be left on when he sleeps, is in bed, walking?

■ Always remove stockings before bathing.

■ Remove stockings at least twice a day to check the skin and toes for reddened areas or edema of the feet and/or ankle.

■ Check the client's entire leg frequently to be sure stockings are not twisted or bunched up. This can hurt and cause decreased circulation.

■ Always put on stockings before the client leaves the bed.

■ Be sure the client's leg is dry before putting on the stockings.

■ Never roll the stocking down or wear a garter to hold it up. This drastically decreases circulation to the limb.

■ Wash and dry stockings according to manufacturer directions. Do not use bleach.

Procedures

Step-by-step approaches to your assigned tasks or duties are carefully explained. When performing client care procedures, it is important to do every step correctly. That's why you will find brightly colored procedure boxes throughout that clearly outline each procedure, from beginning to end, step by step, so you are sure to get it right every time.

PROCEDURE 2

Sterilizing Bottles

RATIONALE: Removing bacteria from baby bottles is a major factor in decreasing the possibility of infection and disease in an infant.

1. Assemble your equipment:
   Bottles
   Nipples, caps, and jar
   Bottle brush
   Dish detergent
   Hot water from the tap
   Large pot with cover or a special sterilizing pot for baby bottles
   Small towel
   Tap water
   Stove or heat source for cooking
   Timer, watch, or clock
   Tongs

2. Wash your hands.

3. Scrub bottles, nipples, and caps with hot soapy water. Use the bottle brush to clean inside the bottles. Always squirt hot soapy water through the holes in the nipples to clean out any dried-on formula.

4. Rinse thoroughly with hot water.

5. Fold the small towel to fit in the bottom of the pot and lay it there. This will prevent the bottles from breaking. (This is done when you do not have a bottle rack.)

6. Stand the washed bottles on the towel in a circle around the inside of the pot.

7. Place the caps and nipples into the clean, empty jar. Place into the pot at the center of the bottles.

8. Pour water into and around the bottles and into the jar with the nipples until two-thirds of each bottle is under water (Figure 5.7 ■).

9. Cover the pot.

10. Place the pot on the stove burner and turn on the burner to the high or full setting.

11. When the water comes to a full boil, begin timing. Allow the water to remain at a full boil for 25 minutes.

12. Remove the jar with the nipples and caps 10 to 15 minutes after the full boil begins. With the nipples still inside the jar, stand the jar on the table to cool.

13. Turn off the burner.

14. Take the cover off the pot and allow it to cool.

15. Remove the sterile bottles from the pot with sterile tongs.

16. Empty the water out of the pot. The pot is now sterilized, so you can use it for mixing the formula.

17. Wash your hands.

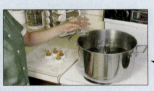

FIGURE 5.7 ■

SAMPLE CHARTING: 11/5/05 12:30 P.M. Mrs. Dow sterilized 8 bottles as per procedure and filled them with formula. Left in refrigerator. Sally Bowles H/HHA

NEW! Rationale

An explanation that lets you know the reason for the procedure and the importance of adhering to its principles.

Illustrations

Photographs and art show you key steps in the procedures.

NEW! Sample Charting

Each procedure is followed by a sample that shows you what kinds of care to document and how to document it.

Clinical ALERT

Cleaning Thermometers
Wash all thermometers with warm soapy water before use. If you think a thermometer was used to take a rectal temperature, do not use it for an oral temperature, no matter how you wash it. Digital thermometers must also be cleaned after each use and after they have stayed in a drawer for awhile.

NEW! Clinical Alerts

Important facts and concepts that impact on practice and safety of the homemaker/home health aide.

Preface

Being a Homemaker/Home Health Aide has been compiled by a multidisciplinary team of practicing home health care professionals. It is formulated to teach homemakers/home health aides to be efficient, sensitive, caring members of the health-care team, and to make decisions based on objective observation, critical thinking skills, and timely reporting to supervisors.

Information is presented as a homemaker/home health aide would use it within the context of home and community. All material is designed to assist students in developing their role within the home health care system and alerting them to their responsibility to observe, report, and act responsibly in many situations and cultural settings. All activities are geared toward encouraging and creating an atmosphere of client safety and independence while helping the aide achieve maximum level of job satisfaction. The activities are also intended to build confidence in the homemaker/home health aide to model appropriate behaviors so that clients attain their maximum level of independent functioning and the homemaker/home health aide achieves maximum job satisfaction.

The authors, reviewers, and numerous advisers who contributed to this book have endeavored to produce a comprehensive, thorough, yet enjoyable text for the fastest-growing segment of the home care industry—the homemaker/home health aide.

New and Expanded Topics

- *Children Under Stress,* both as clients and as family members affected by the illness of others. The homemaker/home health aide's role in observing & reporting is emphasized.
- *Geriatric Clients,* in both home and community with their special needs of socialization, sex, and fullfillment; the role of culture is highlighted throughout.
- *Terminally Ill Clients,* discussing not only the client's physical and emotional needs but those of family and friends as well; the role of palliative care and advanced directives are highlighted.
- *The Physically and Mentally Disabled* as clients and family members, effects on the family, and the homemaker/home health aide's role in relating to them.
- *Rehabilitation in the Home,* stressing the relearning process and helping a client learn ways to function with a disability.
- *Diseases Common in Clients* and the role of the homemaker/home health aide in assisting the client to live with the disease.
- *Nutritional Information,* including instruction on food allergies and aspects the homemaker/home health aide should consider when caring for clients with food allergies; several recipes (found in Appendix B: Additional Recipes) and reference charts included.
- *Emergency and First Aid Procedures* meet current standards of delivery and content.
- *Communication* principles to enhance the communication between team members, the client, and the homemaker/home health aide.
- *Infection Control* and its role in everyday activity to create a safe environment; the importance of the chain of infection and daily activities to protect all members of the home.

- ***Corporate Compliance*** discussions and the homemaker/home health aide's role are introduced early in the text.
- ***Client Satisfaction*** is incorporated throughout the text, as well as the clients role in his care.
- ***Client Independence*** is a major focus throughout the text. All chapters emphasize the role of the homemaker/home health aide in assisting both family and client in setting and maintaining realistic activities when the aide is no longer in the home.
- ***Cultural Competencies***—Through case studies and additional expanded text, students have opportunities to more fully understand culturally sensitive issues and to become more culturally competent as a home health aide.
- ***Identifying Abuse*** discusses the role of a homemaker/home health aide in abuse cases; gives specific guidelines to follow; and stresses the importance of thinking about the aide's feelings on this subject.
- ***Standard Precautions*** addresses the latest guidelines for infection control throughout the text.
- ***Documentation, Reporting, and Observation Methods*** includes end-of-chapter exercises and references throughout the text. Develops students' decision-making and critical-thinking skills in documenting procedures, reporting findings, and observing their clients.
- ***Decision-Making and Critical-Thinking Skills***—The Chapter Review is designed to provoke thinking and to develop critical-thinking skills that will enhance the student's ability to work in complex family situations in a nonjudgmental way.
- ***Role of the Homemaker/Home Health Aide*** gives students a sound and realistic overview of the multifaceted role they will assume as a homemaker/home health aide professional.

Built-in Study Aids

This manual provides a simple, clear, and ***Concise Framework for Learning.*** It can be used both as a primary learning tool and as a vehicle for future review of procedures, theoretical information, and ideas for teaching families how to cope when the homemaker/home health aide leaves the house.

Step-by-Step Procedures   Each procedure gives a logical, step-by-step approach to tasks performed in the work setting, with detailed illustrations. A rationale introduces each procedure. A task is an assigned duty, something you are expected to do. In this manual, each task has been divided into a logical, orderly series of actions or steps. The full set of steps is a procedure. In health care agencies, procedures are done according to a set method. Although procedures will be somewhat different in different agencies, the underlying principles or ideas are always the same. Only the sequence or style for a task may differ. Be sure you know the methods, policies, and style of the agency where you are working. Usually, however, the way things are done will be very similar to the series of steps given in this manual for a procedure. A Sample Charting completes the procedure.

Guidelines   Guidelines are important basic principles, ideas, and methods that must be remembered for overall client care. In some situations the order in which the tasks are done doesn't matter, and such pieces of information are often presented as guidelines.

Clinical Alerts   Highlight important facts and concepts relating to text.

End-of-Chapter Case Study Exercises   These activities provide a mechanism for exploring students' thoughts about the material presented and its application in realistic situations, and their feelings about their activities. By discussing this with each other and through reflection, the student is able to identify his/her role within the team.

Certification Review Questions   These provide another activity for review and discussion. Answers can be found in Appendix A: Answer Key for Certification Review Questions.

Case Studies   This realistic snapshot of a real client presents a situation that focuses on the material to come. It provides a tool for directing the student to synthesize information and to think critically, and for exploration and for assisting the student to understand the complexity of all human activity.

New Words / Marginal Glossary / Glossary   New words are printed in color and immediately defined in the text and presented in the margin with definition. The glossary, found in the back of the text, lists all new words presented in the text and includes related health care terms and their definitions.

Notes Column   The wide margins allow space for students to make notes or underline the important information on each page.

Anatomy and Physiology   An understanding of anatomy and physiology is presented throughout the text as it relates to the home health setting.

Abbreviations   Provides a list of common abbreviations for specific health care terminology. The Abbreviations chart is found at the end of the text.

Organization of Material   Each chapter is divided into short, manageable sections. To further encourage learning, each section is titled, has a set of objectives, has an introduction, and concludes with topics for discussion.

Objectives   Objectives state what students will learn in each section of the text.

Chapter Introduction   Serves as a general introduction to specific topics covered in the chapter and provides the reasons for each procedure given in the chapter.

Illustrations and Photographs   Visuals integrated throughout the text enhance discussions and make critical visual connections that show the students how a particular action is performed.

To the Student: Tips for Success

Welcome to *Being a Homemaker/Home Health Aide*. You are, or will be, working as part of the home health care team. This team cares for people who need skilled, professional health care in the home for a period of time.

You will work with nurses, doctors, and technicians; speech, physical, and occupational therapists; and nutritionists. You can take pride in your work. The most important person in the health care system is the client. Everyone strives to meet the needs of the client and his family. You will play a pivotal role in helping the client and the client's family learn new skills for meeting and coping with the illness of one of its members. You will learn new skills, too. You will become familiar with different cultures and different coping skills. Just as each client will benefit from your knowledge and skill, so you, too, will benefit from each client and learn something new.

This book has been written to help you do well in your job. The first step is to learn how to use it efficiently so that you get the most out of it. This manual is designed to guide you. It is a learning tool and a reference book, like a dictionary. Use it in classes for taking notes. Look at it whenever you have a chance. Use it at home for studying and reading before class. Use it during your work, to review the procedures. Study the pictures. They will help make things clear. All tasks described in this manual are listed in the table of contents. Use it to find the page number of any procedure you might want to review. Most chapters are divided into sections. This makes it easier for you to learn the many and varied tasks of your job.

Though this occupation is currently held mainly by women, more and more men are entering the home health field. However, for convenience and ease of presentation, the text will normally refer to the supervisor as *she* or *her* and to the clients as *he* or *him*.

Things to Remember

You will be working under the supervision of the nurse, team leader, or therapist. They are not necessarily the same person. We will use the term *supervisor* to refer to the person who supervises you with that particular procedure.

- If you don't know how to do a procedure, ask your supervisor for help. If you are not sure of yourself, tell her. It is better to get help than to do something wrong.
- Use this book. Read the procedures until you remember every step. Check the Glossary for the meanings of words you don't know.

Using Your Text Successfully!

The **Case Studies** will focus you on the complexity of caring for clients. Thinking about the case study and chapter material will help you apply new knowledge, observe changes, and discuss your feelings with your supervisor.

The **Objectives** serve as realistic goals for you to reach as you go through each section. Objectives tell what a successful student can do at the end of the section.

Under the chapter **Introduction** you will find the reasons behind each procedure you will be doing. Knowing why you are doing something will help you to prepare for and carry out the procedures in the best possible way.

New Words are tools for communication. In your work, you will be introduced to medical terminology. You should increase your vocabulary as much as you can so you always understand what the supervisor tells you. Also, it is a personal achievement. Learning new words can help make you more self-confident. When you report to your supervisors, you must make yourself clearly understood. It is important that you accurately communicate information about the client and his or her situation or condition. The text **Marginal Glossary, Glossary,** and **Abbreviations** list will help you understand the meaning of many words and terms used in health care. New words appear in the text in boldface. Those words also appear in the marginal glossary for extra clarity. You can look up other new words in the end-of-book glossary.

Use the blank space on each page to make notes or underline the important information on each page. Writing important points in the **Notes Column** will help you remember them. Keep a pencil in hand as you study. Jot down key words and thought clues. They will come back to you later when you need them. As your instructor goes over each procedure with you, he or she will explain things that are done differently in your setting. Taking notes is a good way to record these differences.

A task is an assigned duty, something you are expected to do. In this manual, each task has been divided into a logical, orderly series of actions or steps. The full set of steps is a **Procedure.** In health-care agencies, procedures are done according to a set method. Procedures differ somewhat in different agencies, but the underlying principles or ideas are always the same. The rationale or reason for the procedure will be the same. It is important to understand why you do the procedure. Be sure you know the methods, the policies, and the style of the agency where you are working. Usually, however, the way things are done will closely resemble the series of steps given in this manual for a procedure. Sample documentation gives you an idea of how to indicate you have successfully completed the procedure.

Often basic principles, ideas, and methods must be remembered for overall client care. These are called **Guidelines** in this text. As an example, you will always treat the client with courtesy, kindness, and sympathy. Such a principle does not make up a full procedure, but it is important for you to remember. In some situations the order in which the tasks are done doesn't matter. Your instructor will tell you this and discuss these guidelines. These are not true procedures and so appear in guideline boxes.

The multiple choice questions will provide another way to practice critical thinking.

Contents

Procedures

The number shown with each procedure gives the page where the procedure begins.

SPECIAL PROCEDURES

Guidelines

The number shown with each guideline gives the page where the guideline begins.

Acknowledgments

Books do not get written without the dedication and work of many people. They read, compose, mail, file, suggest, and review endless pages and pieces of work that ultimately become a book. To all the unseen people, thank you.

- To the homemaker/home health aides who took the time to comment and make suggestions, thank you.
- To my friend Barbara Krawiec for being the person who cajoled and provided the initial focus of this edition.
- To Sheba Jalaluddin who acted as liaison between the production team and myself and worked with me and with the text for endless hours to resolve every tiny detail and issue in the way best for the text.
- To Karen Ettinger who coordinated the production of the book and kept it on schedule.
- To the reviewers who spent hours reading and suggesting changes and additions.
- To Marilyn Meserve, Maura Connor, and Mary Treacy for their faith and creativity in making this the best *Being a Homemaker/Home Health Aide* yet!

And, finally, to my husband, whose love and support makes everything possible.

Elana D. Zucker

Reviewers

Gloria Bizjak, MEd
Instructor, Curriculum
Designer
Maryland Fire and Rescue
Institute
University of Maryland

Cora Lynn Cline, RN
Allied Health and EMS
Coordinator
Pratt Community College
Pratt, Kansas

Paula Ray Hardee, BaP, RN
C.N.A. Program Coordinator
Richmond Community
Hamlet, North Carolina

Medeline Gervase, MSN, CCRN, FNP, RN
Assistant Professor
Union County College
Flemington, New Jersey

Ann M. Larson, RN, BSN, PHN
Instructor
Minneapolis Community
and Technical College
Minneapolis, Minnesota

Vicky Popel, RN
Instructor
Canadian Valley Technology
Center
Mustang, Oklahoma

Rhonda Sanders, LPN II
Pueblo Community College
Pueblo, Colorado

Karen Wiley, RN, BSN
Adjunct Professor
Johnson Community College
Overland Park, Kansas

Shaaron Vogel, RN, MSN
Nursing Instructor
Butte Community College
Oroville, California

Contributors

Joan B. Kane BS, RPT
Registered Physical
Therapist, Private Practice,
New Jersey

Theodosia T. Kelsey OTR
Occupational Therapist,
Private Practice,
New Jersey

Janne Litzelman MS CCC
Speech Pathologist,
Private Practice,
New Jersey

Elaine Muller MA
Private Practice,
New Jersey

Patricia Taboloski RN, MSN
Research Assistant,
University of Rochester
School of Nursing,
New York (Family Health,
Nurse Clinician
Practitioner)

Eleanor Bannon RN
Enterostomal Therapist,
Overlook Hospital,
Summit, New Jersey

Gloria J. Bizjak
Maryland Fire and Rescue
Institute,
University of Maryland

Photo Credits

George Dodson
Mike Gallitelli
R. Logan
Posey Corporation
SENSO by Widex
Johnson & Johnson
Sheba Jalaluddin

CHAPTER 1

Orientation to the Home Care Industry

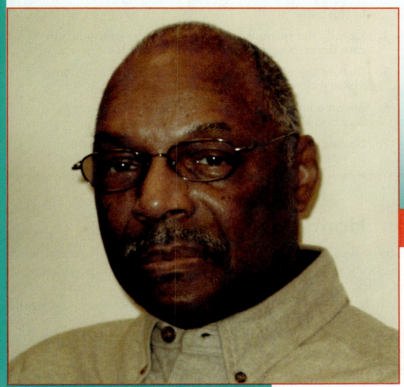

CASE STUDY

Mr. Banks, a middle-aged father of two sons, lives with his eldest son, who is confined to a wheelchair following a car accident. Mr. Banks is the primary caregiver. His son assists with cooking and some cleaning although he has never had a job. Both men have always been independent and seldom ask for help. Mr. Banks has developed arthritis in his hips and now walks with a cane. Physical therapy and medication improved Mr. Bank's range of motion, decreased his pain, and increased his stamina, but he is not sure he will be able to return to work as a customer service representative at the local building supply store.

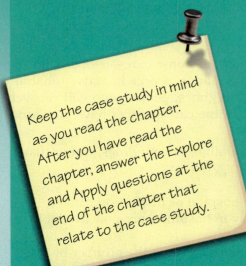

Keep the case study in mind as you read the chapter. After you have read the chapter, answer the Explore and Apply questions at the end of the chapter that relate to the case study.

The Home Health Agency

OBJECTIVES

What You Will Learn to Do

1. Explain the purpose and organization of a home health agency.
2. Become aware of the changes in health care that affect home health care.
3. Discuss the place of customer satisfaction in present health care.
4. Identify the responsibilities of members of the health care team to each other, the client, and the agency.
5. Discuss the ethics associated with working as a home-maker/home health aide.
6. Become familiar with the various agencies and regulatory bodies that credential your agency.
7. Discuss various methods of paying for home care services.

Introduction: Home Health Care

During your orientation period, the agency will give you the names and titles of personnel in key positions in your home health care agency and those agencies with which you will work. A home health care agency delivers care and services to people within their homes. There are many different types of home health care providers. Some agencies mostly deliver services to people; some agencies deliver equipment for home use, some agencies deliver specialized care such as respiratory services or IV therapy. You will come in contact with all types of agencies. Your supervisor will tell you what policies are in effect as you relate to these agencies. It is important to know what you, as a member of the health care team, can expect from each type of agency and what your responsibilities are (Figure 1.1 ■). Approximately 20,000 agencies in the United States give some type of home health care. They see about 7.6 million clients a year.

WHO USES HOME HEALTH CARE?

People of all ages and economic capabilities use home care—people who require both short-term help and long-term assistance, people in active rehabilitation programs and those on maintenance regimes, people who will recover from their illness, and people who will die. Home care services have increased in recent years because:

■ People prefer to be cared for at home in familiar surroundings, rather than in institutions.
■ Hospital stays are becoming shorter.
■ Home care is usually less expensive than hospital or institutional care.
■ Sophisticated services, once available only in hospitals, are now available at home.
■ As people live longer and the elderly population grows, the number of people requiring assistance is increasing.

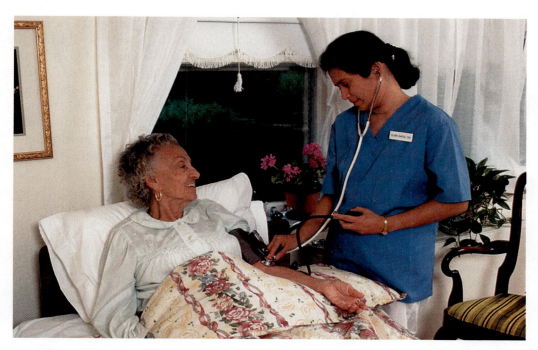

FIGURE 1.1 ■ You will learn when to check vital signs in the home and how to record and report the results to your supervisor.

FUNCTIONS OF HOME CARE AGENCIES

1. Provide care for the ill, disabled, injured, or dying within their homes and communities
2. Become involved in preventive community health care
3. Promote individual and community health
4. Provide health workers with further educational opportunities.
5. Promote research in the health-care professions

CHANGES IN HEALTH CARE

Within recent years, various groups have streamlined and tried to control costs by making changes. These changes have affected how people receive health care, as well as how they use it and pay for it. In addition, different people are now involved in clients' care.

How people receive health care has also changed. In some cases, the insurance/managed care company may have identified doctors, hospitals, and vendors to whom the client is referred for care and equipment. If the client goes anywhere else, his coverage may be less. You are obligated to use the designated vendors so that the client will continue to receive coverage of the needed services. Do not suggest that the client go to another, more familiar doctor or vendor without first consulting your supervisor. Some insurance/managed care companies also designate hospitals and rehabilitation services for use. Only in emergencies can a client go to another facility.

MANAGED CARE

This term describes many of the insurance industry's different payment options. Usually, the client prepays the company providing care a sum of money each month. When care is needed, the company provides the care for the fees already paid and the fees the client has agreed to pay in the coming months. In this way, the managed care company pays your employer for the care you give the client. Each company has clear and strict rules for each insurance option. Assist your client in following these rules. Insurance coverage may depend on these details. If you have questions, call your supervisor or advise the client to call the insurance company directly. Always have the client write down the name of the person with whom he speaks. Be sure to let your agency know if the insurance company calls the client, asks to visit, or sends papers for the client to complete. If an insurance company asks you direct questions, be polite and refer them to your supervisor.

CASE MANAGEMENT

case manager
coordinates care for the client with all caregivers

Insurance/managed care companies and other payors coordinate and organize the care of each client. A **case manager** is employed to review the care provided by all members of the health care team, ensure no duplication of services, and ensure that the client is progressing according to the original plan of care. If changes occur in the client's status, the case manager will change the plan of care. Your supervisor will discuss changes with the case manager. The case manager may or may not visit the client.

CORPORATE COMPLIANCE

corporate compliance
when organizations deliver care according to state and federal laws and regulations

Regulatory agencies such as the federal and state governments, and the Joint Commission Accrediting Hospitals and Organizations inspect several documents throughout the year to be sure the agencies are delivering care according to the law and the regulations. This means that the organization delivers care according to policies and that no one receives special care because of their status either within the community or the organizations, the promise of money, or whom they know. As an example, it would be wrong to deny others care by sending two homemaker/home health aides to a client because he was prominent in the community. However, if a client's health care status required such treatment, it would be appropriate and medically indicated.

CUSTOMER

customer
person receiving a service from another person for a payment

A **customer** is one person who receives a service from another person for payment. Each of us has customers and is a customer to many people. Your health care agency has many customers: the client, the client's family, the doctor, the insurance/managed care company, and you. Each has different expectations of the agency, all of which must be met. Because it is not possible to meet the needs of all customers all of the time, an agency and the people who work there identify their key customers. This way, they can concentrate their efforts on meeting the needs of these customers first. Ask your agency whom it lists as its key customers. If you disagree, discuss it with your supervisor.

CUSTOMER SATISFACTION

customer satisfaction
meeting patients' expectations thus leaving them content

One of the big changes in health care is that the payor and the health-care agency are all interested in what the clients think of their service. This is good business. Agencies will use these scores and comments in their advertising and in planning future programs. All agencies are aware that the public has many choices for health care. Therefore, each agency strives to be the best, give the best care and service, and satisfy its customers. The public assumes that the care will be safe and technically correct. To increase customer satisfaction, the care must be given by competent, pleasant people who demonstrate they care about their work and the client. When that is not the case, the client is not satisfied. A dissatisfied client will not return for future service and will tell many people about his poor experience. People who hear the story may choose to receive their health care from another agency.

Every agency asks its clients what they thought of the service and the people who care for them. By asking and knowing what people think, the agency can make changes, establish procedures, and teach its employees to give excellent care in the way the client wants it. You have a major responsibility to ensure that client satisfaction is high. Most agencies will have a special program to teach employees techniques and behaviors that contribute to high client satisfaction.

PATIENT RIGHTS

Every client has certain rights and expectations of the agencies and people who care for him. Your agency has a published list of these rights. Carry them with you. Share them with the client when you first meet. Although the format and wording may be slightly different, the document will contain at least the following:

- The right to civil and religious liberties
- The right to voice complaints without fear
- The right to refuse care
- The right to have an active part in establishing an individualized, appropriate care plan
- The right to be treated with respect
- The right to be free of physical and mental abuse
- The right to be free of chemical or physical restraints
- The right to privacy
- The right to communication with family, friends, and medical-care providers
- The right to have competent personnel caring for them.

AGENCY CREDENTIALS

All states require health care agencies to conform to standards and submit to periodic inspections and surveys. This process assures the public and the agency's employees that the agency is operating within minimum standards. The documents indicating that the agency has achieved these standards are called **credentials**. As you learn more about the agency, ask for the agency's credentials. The following agency credentials may be displayed:

1. *Licensure.* The agency has met minimum standards set by the state. Some states do not have this procedure, and some require that only certain types of agencies apply and receive a license.
2. *Certification.* All states must certify that Medicare and Medicaid minimum standards have been met so they are eligible for Medicare and Medicaid reimbursement. You will be asked to provide certain documents so that your agency can conform to the standards of certification.
3. *Accreditation.* Several professional organizations will investigate and accredit an agency. This is a voluntary process and indicates that the agency has met the standards of the organization.

credential
a letter or certificate indicating that a right or privilege has been attained or that a position of authority may be exercised

4. *Bonding.* The agency pays a bond, or insurance policy, so that if it is sued due to an employee's actions, any damages can be paid to the consumer.

All regulatory bodies granting credentials survey the agencies before credentials or certifications are given. Agencies prepare extensively for these visits. During these visits, the surveyor will review policies, procedures, and charts to see that they comply with the requirements. They will also speak with employees and clients. It is your responsibility to follow their requirements all the time.

PAYMENT FOR SERVICES

Someone or some insurance/managed care company pays for your services. These charges are collected by the home health agency and eventually make up your salary. Payment for home health care services can come from many sources. Medicare, Medicaid, and private insurance companies are all sources of payment. These payments vary from state to state and from year to year (Table 1.1 ■). Refer all questions to your supervisor.

Your client or his family may pay the agency directly for your service. Your agency has a **protocol** (set of plans or procedures) for deciding the method of payment that clients will use. Payment sources and amounts are arranged by your supervisor and the client before you are assigned to the case. It is not wise

protocol
rules directing the actions of specific people

Table 1.1: Sources of Payment

	Eligibility	Services Covered
Medicare: federally financed health plan	Over 65 years old: disabled more than two years; on dialysis; must be homebound under medical supervision; needs intermittent skilled nursing, physical, occupational, or speech therapy; must obtain services through a certified home health agency	Nursing, PT, OT, ST, MSW, HHA, some supplies and equipment
Medicare hospice: federally financed program providing care to terminally ill patients	Eligible for Medicare, uses certified hospice, relinquishes usual Medicare benefits, six-month prognosis	All necessary services with copayment
Medicaid: state health care for low-income persons	Financial eligibility differs from state to state; services must be provided under MD supervision	Part-time nursing, HHA, medical supplies/ equipment, possible coverage for PT, OT, ST, audiology, personal care, day care, transportation
Health insurance: private	Individually purchased coverage	As per policy
Special	Worker's compensation, auto insurance	As per situation
HMO	Prepayment health	As per plan

to discuss payment with clients. If clients have questions, refer them to your supervisor.

HOME HEALTH AGENCY PERSONNEL

The Homemaker/Home Health Aide: Part of the Team

The goal of the home health-care team is to provide care so the client can function optimally—to help him be the best he can. If he is ill, the team will assist him with recovery. If he is disabled, the team will assist him with adapting his everyday needs so that he can function in society and his home environment. As a homemaker/home health aide, you are an important member of the health-care team (Table 1.2 ■). As part of the team, you will be assigned to care for a specific client in his home. Teamwork means that everyone knows what to do and does it to the best of his or her ability with a spirit of cooperation. Teamwork means that you are concerned about the effect of your actions upon other members of the team.

Table 1.2: Home Health Care Agency Professional Personnel

Community health nurse (public health nurse)	A registered nurse (RN) with a college degree, licensed by the state to practice nursing. She applies her knowledge to the promotion and preservation of health.
Registered nurse	Has a license from the state to practice nursing.
Licensed practical nurse or licensed vocational nurse	Has a license from the state to work under the direction of a registered nurse, physician, or dentist.
Physical therapist	Licensed by the state to practice physical therapy; concerned with restoring function and preventing disability following disease, injury, or loss of a body part.
Occupational therapist	Graduate of an approved occupational therapy curriculum and granted a certificate/license from the state; concerned with patient's ability to perform essential daily living tasks.
Speech pathologist	Graduate of an approved speech pathology program and granted a certificate of clinical competence; treats persons with speech disorders caused by physical defects or mental disorder.
Respiratory therapist	Graduate of an approved respiratory therapy program and granted certificate/license from the state; concerned with evaluating breathing, assisting with prescribed breathing treatments/regimes, and equipment.
Nutritionist	Applies the science of food consumption and utilization to the growth, maintenance, and repair of the human body.
Social worker	Has formal education required to treat individuals, families, groups, or communities with social and/or psychological problems; coordinates community resources to meet client and/or family needs.

The agency that employs you will assign a supervisor to your case. This person may be a professional nurse or another professional member of the health care team. All these people recognize the homemaker/home health aide as a valuable worker and member of the team. Your supervisor will help you learn and understand your job. If you have a question about one of your tasks or something that happens in your client's home, ask the professional member of the team who assigned the job to you.

Your Job as a Homemaker/Home Health Aide

OBJECTIVES

What You Will Learn to Do

1. Become familiar with the concept of delegation so that you can explain it to your client.

2. List behaviors that will help you and the client be more comfortable at your first meeting.

3. Be familiar with qualities desirable in a homemaker/home health aide.

4. Become familiar with activities that contribute to teamwork.

5. Become comfortable with the legal and ethical rules that govern your activities.

6. Discuss activities you will perform to prioritize your work.

Introduction: Tasks, Responsibilities, and Delegation

job description
written document listing the parts of employment, such as the tasks for which one is responsible

responsibilities
those tasks one has to execute and for which one is held accountable

delegation
your supervisor assigns you to complete tasks and activities that remain the responsibility of the supervisor

The tasks and responsibilities expected of you are summarized in your **job description**. This is a document unique to each agency. It is important that you understand this and agree to it, to help prevent later misunderstandings as to what you are expected to do. **Responsibilities** are trusts expected of you. Everyone you work with will have a set of responsibilities and expectations. By being familiar with your responsibilities and the expectations employers, clients, and team members have of you, you will be able to act in the proper manner and feel more comfortable.

There are many parts to client care. Some care must be performed by a specified licensed person. Some can be **delegated** or assigned to others. Although the actual task completion may be assigned to you, the licensed person cannot delegate responsibility for the task and always is accountable to be sure that the task is completed correctly. Your supervisor will discuss with you which activities and task will be delegated to you and for which you will be responsible. Usually you will receive this assignment both verbally and in writing. If you do not understand or are unsure about what is being assigned to you, discuss this at the time you receive the assignment.

Your responsibility is to complete the task correctly, document its completion, and note how the client tolerated the activity. If you cannot complete a task as it is assigned or the client's condition has changed during or as a result

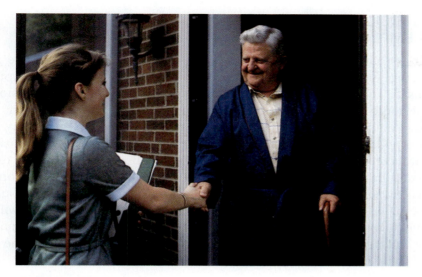

FIGURE 1.2 ■ First impressions set the stage for future interactions.

of the activity, be sure and communicate this to your supervisor, state the reason, and document this. Also document the communication between you and the supervisor.

Your **role** will be slightly different in each house, but your overall function will be spelled out in the job description.

role
one's function

WORKING IN A CLIENT'S HOME

You will be caring for people in their homes. Until they get to know you, you will be considered a stranger. Many people are afraid of strangers and have fears about letting them into their home. They are often afraid you are there to "make order." It will be an important part of your first meeting with the client and his family to assure them that you are in the home to help and to abide by their routine as much as possible (Figure 1.2 ■). Although your agency trusts you and knows you are an honest and considerate person, the client does not—yet. There will be a brief period when you, the client, and his family will get to know each other. Besides relating with the client, you will also relate with the **principal care person**. This is the person in the family designated as "being in charge" of the client's care. Here are some helpful hints to decrease fears clients may have about you as a new person:

principal care person
person in charge of the client's care

- Wear your uniform. Be sure it is neat and clean. It identifies you as a member of the health care team. A uniform indicates that you are focused on the job and on your role as a homemaker/home health aide and separates this role from other roles.
- Wear your name pin and any identification your agency requires. This tells the client you are who you say you are.
- Introduce yourself immediately in a clear, quiet voice. Identify your agency and your job title. Look at the client when you speak. Write down the information if the client asks you to.
- Discuss with the client your responsibilities, tasks, and hours of work. Assure the client you are there to work in his home in a manner that is comfortable for him. You are not there to change everything.
- Ask the client if he has any questions. If you cannot answer his questions, refer him to your supervisor.

RESPONSIBILITIES OF THE HOME CARE AGENCY TO ITS EMPLOYEES

The agency that employs you has many responsibilities. When you are given a job, the employer assumes the responsibilities of paying you for your work, providing a safe and meaningful working environment, providing supervision, providing periodic evaluations of your work, and treating you with respect.

During your orientation period, you will become familiar with many agency personnel policies. These explain what the agency considers *its* responsibilities and what it considers *your* responsibilities. These policies deal with such topics as health examinations, salaries, uniforms, evaluations, documentation, communication, vacations, assignments, and hours of work. It is important that you review and understand these policies, for these are the rules under which you will work.

You will always work under the supervision of a registered professional nurse or other health professional. It is that person's responsibility to plan the client's care and to assign tasks to you in an understandable manner.

EMPLOYEE'S RESPONSIBILITIES

age-competent
caregiver is knowledgeable about needs of specific age group

It is your responsibility to do only those tasks assigned and to do them to the best of your ability. You are expected to care for your clients with thought, consideration, and respect. You are also expected to care for your client as is appropriate for his age. This means you must be **age-competent**. You must know what expectations you may have of the client at a particular age and what behaviors you must exhibit to clients of certain ages. If you do not know a procedure, ask! If a procedure must be adapted to the client's age, discuss this with your supervisor. It is also your responsibility to be a contributing member of the health-care team. Share your ideas, your thoughts, and your knowledge. The clients will benefit, your fellow employees will benefit, and the agency will benefit.

EQUIPMENT

It is always necessary to have the proper supplies and equipment to perform your tasks. When you accept your assignment, ask your supervisor:

- What equipment is needed for the client's care?
- Who will obtain the needed equipment? Will the family buy it? Will the nurse bring it? Will it be delivered?
- Are the necessary tools and equipment available to keep the house clean? Can they be borrowed from neighbors? Will the family purchase the needed equipment?

You may be asked to work with supplies already in the client's home instead of new ones. In many cases you will have to improvise by using an item for a task for which it was not originally designed. An example of an improvisation is the use of a tablecloth as a draw sheet on a bed. It is important to take good care of the client's equipment. Families often judge your attitude toward them by the way you care for their belongings. Respect for their possessions indicates your respect for them as people.

Think through your tasks before you do them. This exercise allows you to note the items you will need for a particular job. In this way, you will be able to assemble all the needed equipment before you start a job and not have to stop in the middle of it to get the required tools. By planning your work and the supplies you need, you save your energy and decrease the number of times you leave the client in the middle of a procedure.

If you find that the supplies needed to care properly for your client and his home are not available, discuss your needs with your supervisor and arrangements will be made.

MOST EFFECTIVE QUALITIES TO SUCCEED

You have decided that you want to be the best! You want to do the best possible job. What kind of person makes a good homemaker/home health aide? Certain behaviors, attitudes, and habits are common in people successful in the health-care field. Some of these traits are built into one's personality. This means you have had them since you were young. Other traits can be learned through practice. Then they become part of one's improved personality.

Read through this list, review those behaviors you have already, and then check those you think you could learn and use in your work and personal life.

- You can be trusted.
- Others can depend on you.
- You enjoy working with others.
- You get along well with others.
- You are sensitive to the feelings and needs of others.
- You are a good listener.
- You try to be courteous.
- You get satisfaction from helping others.
- You show sympathy and patience with others.
- You always try to control your temper.
- You believe you are doing important work.
- You want to improve your skills.
- You try not to let your private life interfere with your work.
- You are comfortable meeting and working with people from cultures different from yours.

Dependability

Your agency is organized to function efficiently when a certain number of people are on the job. If you are not there, a client may be deprived of needed care. Your absence may cause your fellow workers to have an overload of work. It is important that you arrive promptly every day when expected. If you are sick, call your office as you have been instructed by your agency. Your clients can then be assigned to another homemaker/home health aide.

Dependability means more than coming to work every day and coming in on time. It means that your supervisor can rely on you to do things at the proper time and in the proper way.

Accuracy

As part of the health care team, you will be concerned with human lives and feelings. What might appear to you a tiny mistake or oversight could affect the recovery of your client.

It is important for you to follow your supervisor's instructions exactly. Be accurate when you are recording a temperature. Be careful in making a bed. If you make a mistake, report it. If you do not understand something, ask again. Always remember: There is a reason for every step of the client's care.

Following Directions

Everybody follows instructions and goes by rules; otherwise, jobs would never get done. Even supervisors and administrators have rules to follow. These rules—policies and protocols—are made to give everyone guidelines for their work. They are made up with professional, ethical, legal, and practical relationships with in mind. If you do not understand a rule or protocol, ask!

The following good rules can help make you a better homemaker/home health aide and can help you in your relationships with fellow health-care workers.

- Be accurate to the best of your ability.
- Follow carefully your supervisor's instructions.
- If you do not understand something, ask your supervisor.
- Report accidents or errors immediately to your supervisor.
- Keep information about clients to yourself, except when it might affect the client's health.
- Do not waste supplies and equipment.
- Be ready to adjust quickly to new situations.
- Try to finish tasks on time—use a systematic work schedule.
- Report all complaints, no matter how small, to your supervisor.
- Perform all your duties in a spirit of cooperation and teamwork.
- Keep personal problems out of the workplace.

ETHICS

ethics
system of moral behavior
and beliefs

Ethics involve a code of rules set up to govern behavior. These behaviors always consider the feelings and needs of all concerned. These behaviors are based on the respect of individuals and their rights. It is assumed homemaker/home health aides work within an accepted set of rules (Figure 1.3 ■).

- Do your job correctly to the best of your ability. This means you should ask for assistance when you are unable to do an assignment correctly. It is not ethical to accept an assignment without knowing the correct way to do it.
- Be honest with your clients, their families, and your coworkers.
- Respect the rights of clients, their families, and your coworkers.
- Honor the responsibility of the agency that employs you.
- Do not discuss client information with relatives or friends of the client, with fellow workers except when client-related, with your family, or with another client.

LEGAL CONSIDERATIONS

Laws concerning clients and workers in the health-care system are written to protect both the client and the worker. Each state has its own laws governing which procedures a homemaker/home health aide may and may not do. You

---

DO NOT DISCUSS CLIENT INFORMATION WITH

- One client about another client
- Relatives and friends of the client
- Representatives of news media
- Fellow workers, except when in conference
- Your own relatives and friends

DO NOT

- Read a client's personal papers
- Solicit financial information
- Share your opinions with other agencies

FIGURE 1.3 ■ Confidentiality is an important part of client care.

should be familiar with the laws and how they affect you and the clients under your care. Clients must be cared for properly and within the law. When you accept this job, you also accept this responsibility.

The agency that employs you assumes legal responsibility for your actions as long as you work within its guidelines. It is your duty to know what tasks you have been assigned and to carry them out according to instructions. If you have any questions, ask! If you are in doubt as to what to do, report the situation to your supervisor. It then becomes your supervisor's responsibility to interpret the situation and tell you what to do.

Your agency has policies and procedures to guide you and your coworkers in your jobs. They are written to give everyone the same framework for work. When you come to work, you agree to follow these policies and procedures. If you do not agree with them, discuss this with your supervisor, but do not just ignore the rules. If you do not follow the policies, you leave your agency and yourself open for question by the client, the doctor, and, if something unplanned happens, the law.

Negligence is a legal term meaning the failure to give proper care, when you know how to do so, which results in physical or emotional harm to the client. Your agency will discuss with you how to protect yourself from any question of negligence.

INCIDENTS

An incident is an event that does not fit the daily routine of the home or agency where you are working. It may be an accident or an unusual happening. Types of incidents include:

- Client, visitor, or employee accidents
- Accidents that happen to you anytime while you are on the job
- Accidents occurring on the outlying property of the client's home, such as sidewalks, parking lots, or entrances

Whenever an incident occurs, a report must be made (Figure 1.4 ■). Careful, prompt reporting is important to the safety program of the agency and for the

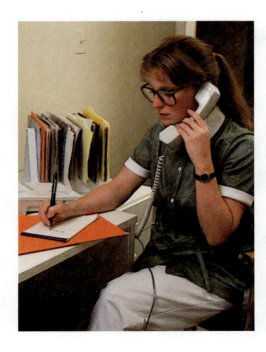

FIGURE 1.4 ■
Reporting incidents protects you, the client, and your employing agency.

protection of all health-care workers. For the agency to be prepared for possible liability suits or damage claims, report promptly all facts related to any incident or accident.

PERSONAL SAFETY

You will never be required to enter or to remain in a setting where you are in danger from the neighbors, the client, or the family. Discuss with your agency their policy about contacting them if you are afraid for your personal safety. Ask for emergency telephone numbers when the agency is closed. Danger could present itself before you meet the client or after you have been in the home for some time. If you are forced to leave the client during your assignment, be sure to call your agency immediately. *Do not hesitate to call for help or assistance.*

PERSONAL PRACTICES

All members of the home health team are teachers by the example they set. They influence each other, their clients, and their families (Figure 1.5 ■). Remember:

- Dress properly and neatly. Follow the dress code of the home health care agency where you work.
- Bathe daily.
- Use an unscented deodorant.
- Keep your mouth and teeth clean and in good condition.
- Keep your hair clean and neat.
- Wear clean clothes every day.
- Wear comfortable low-heeled shoes with nonskid soles and heels that can be wiped clean frequently.
- Repair rips and replace missing buttons on your clothing.
- Do not wear jewelry such as earrings, bracelets, pendants, or large rings.
- You may be asked to remove piercing jewelry from nose, lip, and tongue. Discuss this with your agency.
- Keep your nails short and clean.
- Wear conservative makeup.

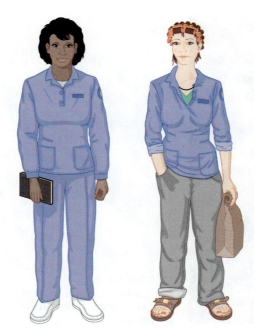

FIGURE 1.5 ■
Taking pride in your appearance says you respect yourself and those with whom you come in contact.

- Do not use perfume, scented sprays, or aftershave lotion.
- Keep yourself in good health by eating properly.
- Get plenty of sleep—be alert when you come to work.
- Polish your shoes—be sure the laces are clean.
- Always wear a wristwatch with a second hand.
- Always carry a pen and a pad of paper.

CREATING A WORK PLAN

When you have received your assignment you will also be told how long you will stay at the client's home. To meet client and supervisor expectations you must **prioritize** your activities. That is, decide in what order you will do things. The following are factors to consider when you prioritize:

- Which activities does your supervisor think are the most important?
- Which activities does your client consider most important?
- Does the client already have routine for accomplishing his care?
- What is the client's physical status?
- Is anything unusual happening today, such as visitors or therapists?
- Which activities take the most time?
- Do you have the proper equipment in the house for all activities?
- Are any activities uncomfortable for the client?
- Do you have time to do everything assigned to you?
- Can anyone else do some of the activities? Can they complete the activities if you start them?
- How often will you see the client? Can any activities wait until your next visit?

It is important to discuss your plan with your client and perhaps his family for his/their agreement. Remember, the client and his family are important parts of the health-care team and should be included in all decisions. If the client is unable to take part in the decision making, his family may have input. Be alert as you work as to how your plan is progressing. Changes may be needed in the middle of the plan of care. A caring, flexible person always reviews a task or activity both as it is being done and after it is completed.

If you cannot complete any delegated task, document this and the reason it was not completed. Also document any communication with your superior about the uncompleted task.

prioritize
to put into an order or schedule that usually lists the most important task first and the least important task last

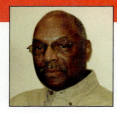

Case Study

Review the case study that appears on the first page of the chapter. Answer questions about the case study contained in the Explore and Apply sections below.

EXPLORE

1. A fellow worker tells you that since her daughter began living with her she gets less sleep. Therefore, she arrives at her first client late. She asks you not to mention this to the agency supervisor. She also tells you that she sleeps on the job at the client's home and, if you want, she will teach you the tricks to do the same thing.

   a. *How do you feel about your coworker telling you about her personal problems?*

   b. *How do you feel about her arriving late to the client and sleeping when there? Why?*

   c. *What will you do with the information you now have?*

2. Your nurse supervisor calls you after she has visited the Banks house. She gives you a list of tasks and activities she is assigning to you. You ask her to hold the phone so you can get a pencil and write down the assignment. She says she is in a hurry and you should remember them. When you return, she goes over the assignment again. You ask for background on the client and family. She says, "There is no need for you to know anything except what I am delegating to you. Just go there and do the assignment."

   a. *How do you feel about being part of the health-care team at this agency?*

   b. *How do you feel about going to care for Mr. Banks tomorrow? As you drive up to Mr. Banks' house, you notice that the wheelchair ramp has no railings, the wood is rotted, and the windows are broken. What do you do? What do you document? Who do you call?*

APPLY

1. Mr. Banks' employer calls to speak with Mr. Banks, but he is resting. You know that Mr. Banks is concerned about the status of his job so you decide to speak with the employer yourself. What do you say to the employer? Why? Do you tell Mr. Banks about the conversation when he wakes up?

2. Mr. Banks wants his son to make dinner for them every night, including the days you are in the home. Your supervisor has assigned you to make dinner according to a low-fat diet. You tell Mr. Banks this, and he says that he doesn't keep a special diet because it is too expensive and it is good for his son to do the cooking because "it keeps him busy." After you discuss your assignment with Mr. Banks, you realize that he wants you to only help him with his physical therapy. He will not allow you to do anything else. He also will not allow his son out of his room when you are there. What do you do with the information about Mr. Banks' lack of compliance to his prescribed diet? Why do you think Mr. Banks treats his son the way he does? What do you do about the discrepancy between your assignment from your supervisor and what Mr. Banks wants done?

Certification Exam Review Questions

Choose the best answer for each question or statement.

1. The people who use home health care are

    a. *all on Medicare.*

    b. *all on Medicaid.*

    c. *all receiving some type of state aid.*

    d. *on Medicare, Medicaid, or pay privately.*

2. The satisfaction of clients who use home health services is important because

    a. *some insurance companies give contracts based on what the client thinks about the service.*

    b. *hearing what the client has to say is part of the therapy.*

    c. *your supervisor's license depends on patient satisfaction.*

    d. *the doctor receives a copy of the client's patient satisfaction survey.*

3. All communication about the client should go through you when you are in the house.

    a. *True because you know best what is going on in the house.*

    b. *False because that violates the patient's right to take an active part in his care.*

    c. *True because you know what the insurance company wants to hear.*

    d. *True because you can protect the client from all his nosey friends.*

4. When a nurse delegates a task to you, she will

    a. *not check to see it is done if she trusts you.*

    b. *assume you have done everything you were assigned unless you report to the contrary.*

    c. *retain responsibility for you and the task.*

    d. *allow you to decide which tasks you do and which ones need not be done.*

5. The principle care person is rarely in the house when you care for the client.

    a. *This shows a lack of interest even though he leaves you notes about the client.*

    b. *A method of communication should be developed between this person, the supervisor, and yourself.*

    c. *The client can be trusted to deliver messages.*

    d. *As long as the bills are paid, there is no need to contact the principle care person.*

CHAPTER 2

Communication Skills

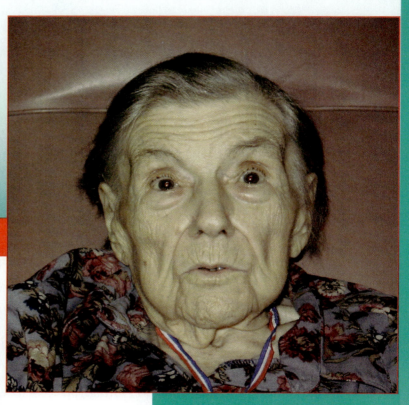

CASE STUDY

Mrs. Cummings has been suffering from leg ulcers and decreasing vision. She has always enjoyed her hobbies of crocheting and going to bingo once a week. Recently, poor vision and pain in her legs have forced her to remain indoors. She spends the days in her chair with the curtains drawn and the radio on. Her daughter and grandchildren visit once a week to bring groceries they think she will need. They stay about 2 hours or until everything is put away. Mrs. Cummings has a friend who calls her each day and visits several times a week. Her friend notices that Mrs. Cummings often is wearing the same clothes and the same food is in the refrigerator as when she left. When Mrs. Cummings has to go to the doctor, she hires a taxi to take her back and forth.

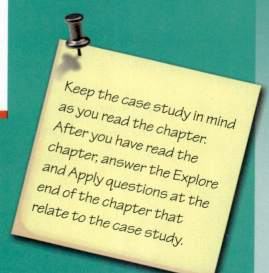

Keep the case study in mind as you read the chapter. After you have read the chapter, answer the Explore and Apply questions at the end of the chapter that relate to the case study.

SECTION 1

How We Communicate

OBJECTIVES

What You Will Learn to Do

1. Know what is meant by communication.
2. Recognize the three basic ways of communicating.
3. Become aware of what we communicate.
4. Become familiar with the basic rules of communication.
5. Be able to discuss the role of culture in communication.
6. Recognize the impact of our communication on others.

Introduction: Communication

Communication means exchanging information with others. We exchange information about feelings, opinions, or facts. People let others know how they feel or what they want all day and even during the night. You can tell if your friend, supervisor, or client is happy, in pain, sad, or bored. They can tell the same about you. You can tell if a sleeping client is in pain or resting comfortably. Communication takes place in several ways: through verbal exchange, written words, and body language or nonverbal methods. Communication is necessary so that people can function together—in other words, so they can "get along" (Figure 2.1 ■). Developing the ability to get along with people—clients, visitors, fellow workers—is an important part of your job. Being a good communicator is essential.

communication
exchange of information

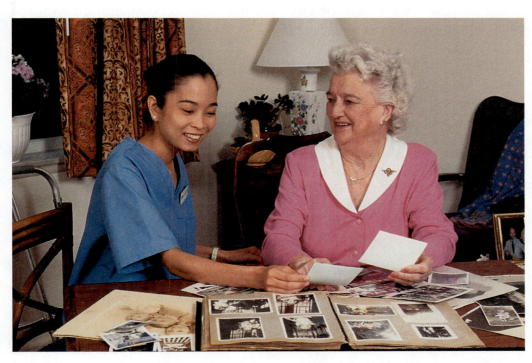

FIGURE 2.1 ■ When you communicate with another person, it is important that you make eye contact with that person.

ethnic diversity
a variety of religions, cultures, and races living within an area

culture
a group's collective shared thoughts, values, beliefs, and behaviors

CULTURE

We are a nation of **ethnic diversity**, and these differences are respected and celebrated. Each group of people has a **culture** of their own. That is, they share values, behaviors, and beliefs. These form the framework of their actions toward themselves and others and influence their health care. When you enter a house, you must be alert and conscious of the culture within that home. You may be familiar with this culture, or you may find it different from your own. Showing respect and asking questions will indicate to the family and the client that you wish to incorporate their culture into the care you give them.

Cultures communicate differently. Some cultures speak softly, others more loudly; some use hand gestures, others do not; some touch people to whom they are speaking, others consider this rude behavior. It is important to know what the client finds acceptable. After understanding how you usually communicate—your tone of voice, the speed at which you speak and your ability to make yourself understood—you can make changes to accommodate the client.

Clients who do not speak English have the right to safe, effective communication. If you speak more than one language, let your agency know so they can assign you accordingly. Clients feel safer when their caregivers speak their language.

- If you do not speak the same language as the client, do not assume he does not understand your language. Do not say anything you would not want the client or his family to understand.
- Maintain the level of formality in the house comfortable to them.
- Speak in appropriate tones. Do not shout. Repeat yourself when necessary.

You can use an interpreter to communicate with the client. Be sure the client approves of the interpreter and wants to share information with the person. You must be sure that having the interpreter does not violate the client's confidentiality. Discuss with your supervisor the best way to communicate with the client and the interpreter.

VERBAL COMMUNICATION

Verbal communication is the exchange of ideas or information through the spoken word. When your supervisor tells you about an assignment, or you say, "Good morning" to your client, that is verbal communication. The tone of your voice, the speed at which you speak, your inflection, and your actual choice of words are all part of the verbal picture you paint as you speak. Many cultures traditionally communicate different pieces of information to different family members. For example, in some cultures, finances are always discussed with the eldest male and intimate health-related information is always discussed with the eldest female. Determining whom to talk to about specific information will save time and misunderstandings later.

WRITTEN COMMUNICATION

Any time you write or draw, you communicate through writing. Each time a nurse leaves instructions for you in a home, or you write a note describing your activities with a client, you exchange facts. The way in which you write tells a great deal about you and how you feel about the subject and your activity. The neatness, legibility, choice of words, and how you give the written work to the reader sets the scene for how it is received.

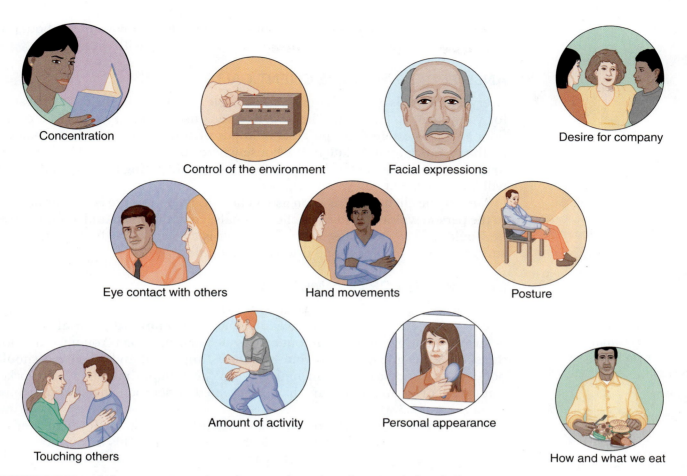

Concentration

Control of the environment

Facial expressions

Desire for company

Eye contact with others

Hand movements

Posture

Touching others

Amount of activity

Personal appearance

How and what we eat

FIGURE 2.2 ■ Body language gives silent clues to others about how you feel and what you want other people to do.

NONVERBAL COMMUNICATION

People have many ways of telling each other how they feel, that is, if they are happy or sad to be in a certain place or if they are doing a task willingly or unwillingly. One way is by saying what we feel. The other way is with our body. This is called **body language** (Figure 2.2 ■). No words are spoken, but the message is given and received by others. Pay attention to the way your body language will be received within the client's culture. People in some cultures do not appreciate being touched unnecessarily. Some take it as a sign of caring. Some people expect you to address them by their last name, some do not care. It is always wise to discuss these fine points with your supervisor or even with the client. "How would you like me to address you? Would you rather I call you Mrs. Davis, or would Anne be more comfortable for you?" Body language includes:

■ The way we do or do not look at people
■ The way we stand—with hands in pockets, on hips, or at our sides
■ Where we stand—close to the person or far away
■ What else we may be doing at the time—reading, folding laundry, or talking on the phone

As a homemaker/home health aide, you will notice clues and other signals that tell how a client feels. These signs will tell you a great deal about the client and the care you are giving. Report your observations accurately to your supervisor so that she can help you interpret them and plan the client's care accordingly.

body language
gestures that function as a form of communication

Be alert to your body language! Your client will know how you feel about giving him care by the way you carry yourself and interact with him.

ANSWERING WHEN THE CLIENT CALLS

Every client needs a way to signal other people. You will have to devise a system for your client to call you. A hand bell, a stick used to bang on the bed or the floor, or a voice signal are possible methods of communication. Use whatever method is most appropriate in the house where you are working. Having a way to call for assistance helps the client feel he is participating in his own care. He will know he is not alone and helpless.

Answer the client's call as soon as you hear it. Every minute is very important to the person waiting. When the client signals, go to the client and ask him what he would like. Do what he asks as long as it is correct and safe. If you are not sure, call your supervisor and discuss the situation.

BASIC RULES FOR COMMUNICATING

Be a Nonjudgmental Observer and Listener

nonjudgmental
accepting communication without stating a personal opinion

It is important to learn to receive information in a **nonjudgmental** way; that is, in an accepting manner without expressing your opinions. You must develop the skill of recognizing when your opinion is important and when you should not express it and be nonjudgmental. Often, a client, family member, or coworker wants to express an opinion and have it accepted rather than have it commented upon (Figure 2.3 ■).

When you work in people's homes, they often ask your opinion. If you are unsure or think your opinion will upset the client, you might say, "This is your house and here it is more important how you feel about this situation than how I feel."

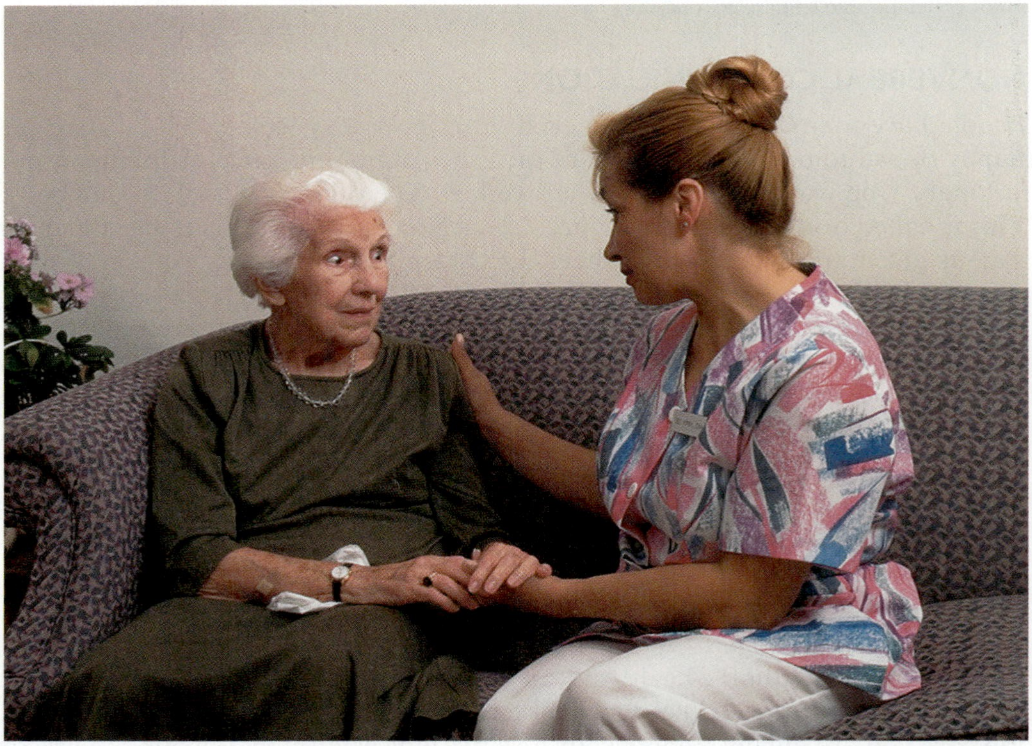

FIGURE 2.3 ■ Present your ideas in a nonjudgmental way so as not to offend your client.

Be a Careful Listener

Always listen when someone speaks to you. Listen to what the person says. Listen to what information is left out of the conversation. Listen for the speaker's tone of voice and breathing pattern. Is it fast? Is it slow and slurred? Do the words make sense? Is it appropriate to ask questions? Listen to what the speaker says, not what you think he or she says. Pay special attention when a client makes a complaint or brings up a problem.

Sometimes it is helpful to write down important information as you hear it. Do not always trust your memory.

Be Sensitive

Sometimes the client does not want to talk. Respect his moods. Saying nothing may have more meaning than any words or facial expressions on your part. Sometimes, a pat on the shoulder or hand means more to a client than anything you could say. Simply being near the client in a moment of trouble may be the most comforting message of all.

Be Courteous and Tactful

Courtesy means being polite. Tact means being considerate of others. You should be courteous and tactful at all times. Never be critical or impolite in your contacts with others. If you feel like being impolite, try to understand why you are feeling or acting the way you are. By reviewing the situation, you may be able to prevent it from happening again. Both courtesy and tact are important in your relationships with your fellow workers. Your supervisor and instructors will be giving you advice and directions. Your coworkers and clients will be sharing information with you. Show them you are willing to hear what they have to say and then reply in a thoughtful manner.

If you are not clear as to what you have heard, you can summarize what you think you heard and ask the speaker if that is so. For example, "I heard you say that John was going to the store, then coming home and fixing you dinner before he went to the doctor's. Is that correct?"

When the speaker is talking and you have nothing to add, but you think the speaker is not communicating clearly, try a technique called *reflection*. This allows the client to know what you understand and provides an opportunity for him to clarify it. For example, "You seem in pain today." "I'm not, but it is cold in here."

EMOTIONAL CONTROL

Sometimes a client or a visitor can upset you. You feel like making a rude or nasty remark. Don't do it! Remember that the client is worried about himself, his illness, his family, or his job.

A client may be rude or difficult at times. Often, the client is unable to determine exactly what is causing him to feel bad and act in a difficult or unpleasant manner. Tell him you know that he has many things on his mind. Offer to listen to him or bring another member of the health care team to listen to his problem.

Client or family stress levels may affect their ability to communicate and listen. Be sensitive to this. Speak in simple terms. Do not be upset if you have to repeat yourself several times. Be understanding if the client or family member repeats himself, too.

Learn to take constructive criticism and accept suggestions from your supervisor and coworkers. You may feel angry when somebody tells you that you are wrong, but remember, your supervisor and your coworkers want to help you

tact

knowing the proper thing to say; a sensitive skill in dealing with people

give the best possible care. If you do not agree with what is said to you, answer in a polite, courteous manner. Discuss the criticism, not the person giving it.

Be as tactful as you can. **Tact** means doing and saying the right thing at the right time. Before you make a remark to a client or his family, think! Is this the right time? Is this the right word to use? What is the best way to express the idea to this person? Do not speak within hearing distance of the client if you do not want him to hear you, even if you think he is asleep, under the influence of medication, or unconscious.

Using the Telephone

The telephone is one way most people communicate with others not in the immediate vicinity. This may take the form of a cell phone or a "land line" attached to the house. Either way, you must remember that the phone is in the client's house for their use and your emergency use, not for your personal calls. Never ask to use it unless for a client-related issue you must communicate to your office, or you have a real personal emergency. Never charge personal long-distance calls to the client. Remember, the time you spend on the phone is taken away from client care. You are in the house to do a job. This is not the appropriate time to take care of personal issues.

If you wear or carry a cell phone, put it on "silent" mode while you care for the client. If you receive a personal call, you can answer it after you leave the house. Never speak on your cell phone pertaining to personal issues while you are caring

---

PROCEDURE 1

Talking on the Telephone

RATIONALE: Speaking politely and clearly shows respect for the caller. It also presents a caring impression to the caller and provides an atmosphere in which information can be exchanged accurately.

1. Answer the phone as soon as you can get to it, making sure that the client is safe when you do.

2. Identify the house you are in and yourself. "Hello, this is the Smith's residence, Sally McNamara home health aide speaking."

3. Speak slowly, clearly, and courteously. Remember, your voice can display anger, patience, and acceptance to name a few emotions. You do not want the caller to think it is too much trouble to answer the telephone.

4. Ask the caller's name, "Who is calling please?" If you do not understand the caller, ask him or her to please spell it.

5. Answer the caller's questions as best you can. If you cannot give the caller all the information, take a message, write the time of the call, the caller, the message, and what you

want the next person to do. Should they call the caller, or wait for the caller to call back? Example: 6/24/05 10:15 a.m. Mrs. Dwyer called to ask if Mother and you could attend her luncheon next week at her church. I told her you would call her back to discuss it. She said you have her phone number." Alexandra Fisher H/HHA

6. If the caller asks for information you should not share, tell the caller politely that this is not information you are comfortable sharing, and they should speak with the family. Leave this as a message for the family.

7. End the conversation politely, saying "Thank you for calling," "Good-bye," or "Is there anything else I can help you with?"

8. Let the caller hang up first.

9. Leave the message in an appropriate place.

SAMPLE CHARTING: This is unnecessary unless the call relates to client care, in which case note the date, time, caller, and message content in the chart. Note follow-up, if any.

for the client. Never take a client's picture with your camera phone or discuss one client while at another's home. This is an unacceptable invasion of privacy. Remember that a client's answering machine is considered private, and you should not listen to the messages unless you are asked to do so.

When you first arrive at the house, determine with the client and the family if they wish you to answer the phone, let it ring, or if messages will go to an answering machine.

RELATIONSHIPS WITH CLIENTS

You are important to the client and his family. You may spend more time with the client than any other member of the health care team. You perform necessary personal tasks that permit the client to remain at home in a safe, comfortable, clean environment. Clients and their families come to depend on you and share their feelings and thoughts. Often, you are the only person a client will see all day.

The client may ask you a question about his doctor or his diagnosis. Do not lie to the client! Do not tell him you do not know when you should be aware of the information. If you lie, the client may find out and never trust you again. It is no shame to say you do not have the information readily at hand. But if you say you do not know, you close the conversation. Tell the client you will find him an answer. Then call and talk to your supervisor. Plan an answer with her. When you promise to find an answer for a client, do it! Do not go back on your word!

Family and Visitors

Visitors are often the highlight of the day for clients who must remain at home. A client usually feels better when he knows his family and friends are concerned and make the effort to see him.

Visitors may be worried and upset over your client's illness. They, too, need kindness and patience. Pleasant comments, privacy, and polite, efficient manners will make them feel at ease.

If it appears that visitors are upsetting or tiring your client, you may have to tactfully suggest that the client rest. Remember, you are in the house to care for the client, not to wait on or socialize with the visitors. If they leave a mess or dirty dishes and expect you to clean up, speak to your supervisor. The two of you can find ways to deal with this situation.

You will find the following hints helpful to remember:

- Listen to visitors and family members. Whether it is a suggestion, a complaint, or "passing the time of day," listen. Suggestions by visitors can be helpful. Some complaints may be valid, others not. When a complaint is first presented, you will need more information. You might ask, "Where did this happen?" or "What did you do?" Offer to report the problem to your supervisor, and then do so.
- Try not to become involved in family affairs. Never take sides in a family quarrel.
- If visitors have questions about your client and you are not sure you should answer, tell them you will find the information. Then contact your supervisor. You also may discuss these questions with your client to be sure he wants the information given to his visitors.
- If a visitor or family member asks how he or she may help, give suggestions.
- Visitors may arrive at the house and give you orders: "While I'm here to watch Mama, you clean the bathroom." Be open about your responsibilities. Explain that your supervisor sets up the plan of care and that you will discuss all changes with her.

Clinical ALERT

Personal Safety
Always strive to keep yourself safe. This includes dressing properly for your job, taking the safest transportation, and feeling comfortable in a house while you are working. If you do not feel comfortable, identify the reason. If you can change the situation yourself in a tactful manner, do so. But in any case, speak with your supervisor immediately. If you can identify others who are unsafe, mention this also. You will do a good job for your client only if you are comfortable. You are not expected to stay in an unsafe situation.

- It is important to use the talents and energy of family and friends in setting up a plan of care. Often, these family members must assume the client's care when you are out of the house. Therefore, the more comfortable they feel with the care and the more they know, the better your client will feel when you are gone.
- Report the roles family and visitors play in the life of your client. Report changes in family functions, relationships, and roles both as you observe them and as the client relates them.

SECTION 2

Client Observation, Recording, and Reporting

OBJECTIVES

What You Will Learn to Do

1. Use your senses of sight, touch, hearing, and smell to observe your clients.
2. List observations you will make and when you will report them.
3. Demonstrate the difference between subjective and objective reporting.
4. Discuss the importance of reporting your observations.
5. Record your observations accurately and meaningfully.

Introduction: Observing, Reporting, and Recording Your Observations

observation
gathering information about a client

Get into the habit of observing the client during all of your contacts with him. These contacts include bathing, bed making, mealtimes, and any other time when you are with a client. Client observation is a continuous process. Observing begins the first time you see a client. **Observation** means more than just careful watching. It includes listening to the client, talking to him, and asking questions. Be extra alert to anything unusual when you are with a client. Changes in the client's condition or appearance are most important. Watch also for changes in the client's attitude or moods and the way in which he interacts with other people. Pay attention to complaints of pain or discomfort and to complaints that seem to have no reason. Be alert when the client relates events that took place in your absence. Observation of the client's family and friends is also important and may have great implications for the client's future care.

You are the health-care team worker who will spend the most time with the client. You will often be the first to notice a change in the client's condition. This change may be for the better, or it may indicate a worsening of his condition. Observations are useful only if they contribute to the total care of the client. Therefore, it is an important part of your job to report these changes to your supervisor. Then the client's total care plan can be revised.

METHODS OF OBSERVATION

Use all of your senses when making observations:

- You can see some signs of change in a client's condition. By using your eyes, for example, you can observe a skin rash or swelling of the feet.

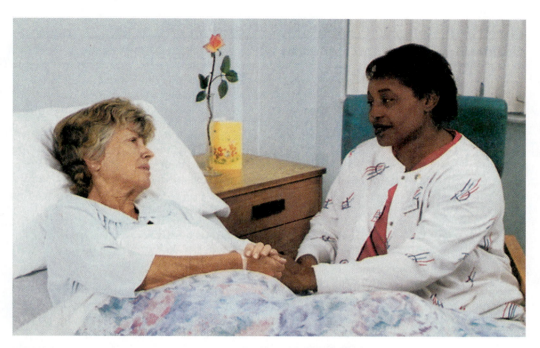

FIGURE 2.4 ■ Use all your senses as you observe and report your client's condition.

■ You can feel some signs with your finger—a change in the client's pulse rate, puffiness in the skin, skin temperature.
■ You can hear some signs, such as a cough or wheezing sounds when the client breathes.
■ You can smell some signs, such as an odor in the client's urine.
■ Listen to the client talking to hear other changes in his condition. Some changes only the client can feel and describe. Examples are pain, nausea, dizziness, a ringing in the ears, or a headache.

Making useful observations is one of the most important things you will have in your work. Learning how to make useful observations will give you great satisfaction (Figure 2.4 ■).

Table 2.1 ■ on the following page is a summary of general observations you will make every day with every client. The method of recording and reporting of these observations varies from agency to agency. It is your responsibility to be familiar with the recording and reporting system in use in your agency.

SUBJECTIVE AND OBJECTIVE REPORTING

Subjective reporting means giving your opinion about something or stating what you think. You might report, for example, what you think is the cause of a change in a client's condition or what might be the proper treatment. When you report your opinion to your supervisor, be sure you say it is your opinion. Your opinion could be important to the care of your client. An example of subjective reporting would be "Yesterday, Mrs. C. and her landlady were talking in loud voices. I think they were fighting."

Objective reporting means reporting exactly what you observe—that is, reporting what you see, hear, feel, or smell. The homemaker/home health aide must always use objective reporting unless it is clear that the information is an opinion.

subjective reporting
giving your opinion about what you have observed

objective reporting
reporting exactly what you observe

Table 2.1: **General Client Observations**

Concern	Observations
General appearance	Has it changed? If so, in what way? Is there a noticeable odor or smell in the client's room? Does he always complain about the heat or cold?
General mood	Describe the client's actions rather than your interpretation of them. ("The client threw a shoe at his daughter" rather than "The client was angry at his daughter"). Has it changed? Does he talk a lot or little? Does he make sense? Can he report things to you accurately? Does he hallucinate (see or hear things)? Is he oriented (know where he is, who he is, and who you are)? Is he anxious, calm, excited, or worried? Does he talk about pain? Does he speak rapidly or slowly? Does he look at you when he speaks? Can he be understood when he speaks? Can he remember? Is he confused or forgetful?
Sleeping habits	Have these changed? Is he a quiet or restless sleeper? Does he complain about lack of sleep? Does his report agree with your observations? How many pillows does he sleep with? How much does he sleep?
Pain	Where is the pain? How long does the client say he has had it? Is it new pain? How does he describe it? Is it constant? Does it come and go? Is it sharp, dull, or aching? Has he had medicine for the pain? Does the client say that the medicine relieves the pain? Is there any activity that brings on the pain?
Daily activities	Does the client dress himself? Does the client walk with or without help? What kind of help?
Personal care	Can the client bathe himself? Can the client brush his teeth, comb his hair, go to the bathroom, or wash his face? Does he ask for assistance?
Movements	Does the client limp?
Skeletal system	Pain; limited movement; swelling in joints; warm, tender joints; unusual positioning of any body part; redness in joints.
Muscular system	Painful movement, swelling, limited movement, color of skin over painful areas. Does he lie still? Does he change position frequently? What is his favorite position?
Skin	Temperature, texture, moisture, bruises, healing of bruises, incision appearance, mouth condition. Has it changed? Is the client's skin unusually pale (pallor)? Is it flushed (red)? Are his lips or fingernails turning blue (cyanotic)? Is there noticeable swelling (edema)? Any reddened or tender areas? Where are they? Is the skin shiny? Any puffiness?
Circulatory system	Chest pain; swelling of fingers, toes, feet, ankles, around the eyes; pulse rate and quality; color of lips, nails, fingers, toes; headaches; pain in legs when walking.
Respiratory system	Pain while breathing, rate and quality of respirations, cough, sputum (color and consistency), wheezing, shortness of breath, color of fingers and toes.

Table 2.1:   **General Client Observations** (*continued*)

Concern	Observations
Digestive system	Pain; appetite; flatus; vomiting (color of vomitus); feces (color, amount, frequency, odor); discomfort before or after eating. Can he control his bowels? Have his eating habits changed? Does he complain he has no appetite? Does he dislike his food? What and how much does he eat? Is he always thirsty? Does he seldom ask for fluids? Is it difficult for him to eat or swallow?
Nervous system	Painful areas of body, twitching, involuntary movement, inability to move, inability to feel stimuli.
Urinary system	Pain during urination; ability to control his urine; urine color, odor, amount, frequency; blood in urine; pain in kidney area.
Eyes	Pain, discharge, redness, sensitivity to light, vision change.
Ears	Pain, discharge, hearing change.
Nose	Pain, discharge, bleeding, change in sense of smell.
Female genitalia	Menstrual periods (frequency, amount of flow, pain); vaginal discharge (color, odor, amount); breasts (lumps); discharge; soreness; parasites; draining sores.
Male genitalia	Pain, discharge, parasites, draining sores.

Here are examples of objective reporting:

1. Mrs. Smith's breathing has changed since yesterday. She is breathing 20 times a minute and complaining of chest pain. Yesterday, she had no pain and her respirations were 12 per minute.
2. Cindy Jones says that she has a pain in her right upper abdomen.
3. Every time John takes the pain pill, he gets very quiet and then says that he sees horses on the ceiling.

HOW DO YOU REPORT?

Each agency has a protocol for homemaker/home health care aides to communicate with their supervisor. It is your responsibility to be familiar with this protocol and use it (Figure 2.5 ■).

Is it by telephone? By calling the correct phone number and asking for the correct person, you will save time for yourself, the client, and the person in the agency. Is it by mail? By sending the correct information to the right person, you will save time and postage. You may be expected to make specific observations at a specific time of day. Be sure you know what to do with the information you collect.

WHEN DO YOU REPORT?

It is important to know when your supervisor expects to hear from you and when your agency expects you to report to them. Some agencies may have a dedicated call-in time. Others may want you to call after each client or at the end of the day. Your supervisor may want you to call with a specific piece of information. Be sure you know when you are expected to communicate.

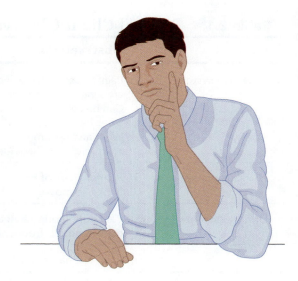

- Is there a special time for me to call the office?
- Is there a special telephone number to call to reach my supervisor?
- If my supervisor is not in the office, who can help me?
- Can I call from the client's home? If not, where is the nearest telephone?
- What information does the agency give by telephone, and what is given in writing?

FIGURE 2.5 ■ Know what to report, when to report, and to whom to report.

GUIDELINES

Reporting and Recording

When you take an assignment, be sure that you know (see Figure 2.5):

■ To whom you report.

■ When to report.

■ Any specific observations that members of the health care team need.

■ The basic observations you should always be aware of as you interact with the client.

■ What types of information must be written and what should be reported verbally.

■ Details about the client's condition.

Although each client is different, and you will report different observations, certain basic guidelines to all your reporting and recording.

■ Be sure of your information.

■ Obtain complete information.

■ Report objectively. When reporting subjectively, say so.

■ Reporting and recording objective observations are important to protect the client and enable the health care team to deliver the best care possible.

■ Reporting and recording objective observations protect you from being held responsible for a possible mistake.

■ Report all changes in a client's condition.

■ Report events in the order in which they occur. Include persons present at the event. You may find it helpful to indicate exact times for clarity.

■ When reporting, report the condition of both sides of the body—"the left leg is cooler than the right leg."

■ Report and record quietly and calmly.

■ Report and record soon after the event. You will forget details if you do not write them down.

WHAT DO YOU REPORT?

The importance of reporting the proper information at the proper time cannot be overemphasized. Each agency has a policy as to what a homemaker/home health care aide reports in writing and what is reported verbally. There are two types of client information:

1. General observations: observations and information about visitors, family, and changes in the environment. This also includes subjective information.

    EXAMPLE: Mrs. Jones's sister came to visit for the first time. Her sister had an opinion about everything we and the client did. Mrs. Jones couldn't explain why we had set up the routine the way we had. Mrs. Jones started to cry. Before leaving, her sister promised to come back with another doctor's opinion. Mrs. Jones said she always takes over and tries to change things. I have never seen the client in this state. Mrs. Jones's sister made Mrs. Jones very uncomfortable.

2. Specific information: Observations of particular client behavior or changes. The supervisor will discuss this type of observation with you. She will explain to you what information is needed and when.

    EXAMPLE: When I changed Mrs. Brown's nightgown, I noticed some blood on the sleeve. I asked her where this came from, and she said, "Oh, you know how it is, I hit my hand." Then she pulled her hand away and said, "I don't think you have to report this." This was the first time this happened. She seemed upset. I can't figure out why.

With one client, the reaction to medication may be important; with another client, mental alertness may be the most important observation. Ask your supervisor if any particular observations are important for you to note. In addition to any specific information, you will always report the total client picture.

WHERE DO YOU DOCUMENT YOUR REPORT?

It's important to communicate orally when you are expected to do so. It is just as important to be sure where you should write your observations. Some agencies have a special part of the client record in which you document your activities and observations. You should also indicate what you reported to your supervisor or anyone else. These notes should be dated, timed, and signed with your full name and title. If there is a reason to check back as to what was done for the client or what you observed and reported, there will be a record. These notes are made at the time you give the care.

SECTION 3

Teaching Your Clients

OBJECTIVES

What You Will Learn to Do

1. List five reasons for differences in the way people learn.
2. Recognize the differences between an adult learner and a child learner.
3. Become familiar with your role in the teaching process.

Introduction: Teaching Clients

Teaching clients is an important part of your job. You will teach clients by example, by discussion, or by taking part in activities with the client. You will teach them new skills, help them relearn old skills, and help them gain independence in as many activities as possible. Everybody learns differently; therefore, you must have a teaching plan individualized to each client. Some people learn by reading, some by listening, and some by observing. It is necessary for you to be familiar with the teaching plan that your supervisor has established for your client that should be based on the client's preference. If you are not sure about your role, ask!

REASONS FOR DIFFERENCES IN LEARNING

As your supervisor individualizes the client's teaching plan, the following factors will be taken into consideration:

- Life experiences
- Disease process
- Motivation for learning
- Family dynamics
- Language skills
- Past experiences with learning
- General abilities
- Teaching skills of teacher
- Age
- Culture

Your supervisor will also teach children differently from adults. Adults can often read material and then discuss it. They can practice skills on their own. They can also often clearly relate learning a skill to achieving a certain outcome. For example, an adult who understands the reasons for keeping or maintaining a special diet will learn how to shop for and prepare special foods, because he can understand that if he fails to follow this diet, he will become ill. A child, however, may not be able to think about the future and relate the activity of eating to the deterioration of his general physical condition. So, even though the outcome will be the same—learning the diet—the teaching method will be different.

Clients who are not fluent in English may need to learn with the help of a family member. When this occurs, be sure you confirm that involving another person is acceptable to the client and the translator. Also, be sensitive to the information you discuss as you may have to review personal information and activities (Figure 2.6 ■).

POINTS TO REMEMBER WHEN TEACHING A CLIENT

- Be sure the client is paying attention and is not distracted by television, a visitor, or other activities (Figure 2.7 ■).
- Be sure the client wants to learn.
- Be sure you are familiar with the material you will teach him. Do not try to teach something you do not understand.
- Relate the teaching to the client. For example, do not tell him the skill will help him become a faster runner if he has no interest in running.
- Speak slowly and clearly—not baby talk, but in words the client can understand.
- Tell the client the reasons you are doing each step. This will help him understand that it is important to follow your example. It will also assure him that you are not wasting energy or time.

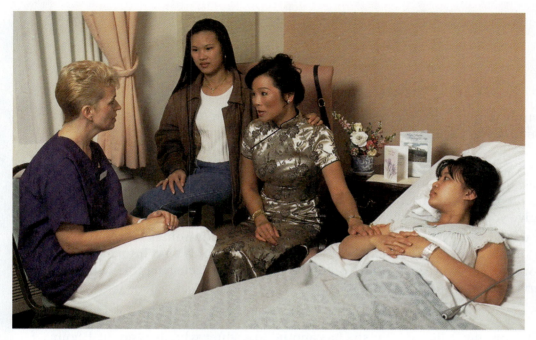

FIGURE 2.6 ■ Teaching a non-English-speaking client may involve a translator or material written in the native language.

■ Do not try to teach too much at once. Everyone has a different attention span. People who are ill or who are taking certain medication often find it hard to concentrate for long periods. Plan your teaching in small sections.

■ Teach at the time of day most convenient for the client. Some people learn better in the morning, some in the afternoon. Whenever possible, ask the client which he prefers.

■ Use written material so the client will have something to refer to when you are gone.

■ Do not lose patience when you must repeat yourself or show him an activity many times. When the client demonstrates the skill to you, praise him and discuss the positive part of the demonstration before you show him the corrections.

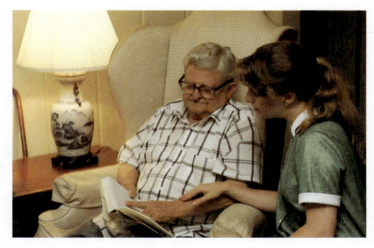

FIGURE 2.7 ■ A quiet comfortable atmosphere is best for you to teach and for the client to learn.

CHAPTER REVIEW

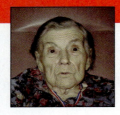

Case Study

Review the case study that appears on the first page of the chapter. Answer questions about the case study contained in the Explore and Apply sections below.

EXPLORE

1. Review the picture shown in Figure 2.7 and share with the class what you see happening in the picture. Be prepared to report both subjectively and objectively and give your reasons for why you made the decisions.

2. How would you gather more information about the Cummings family if you were unfamiliar with their culture? How would you apply that information as you organized your care? How would you feel about discussing this with your supervisor?

APPLY

1. Mrs. Cummings tells you that she has another daughter who lives about 1 hour away but does not come to visit because she does not get along with her sister. Mrs. Cummings shows you gifts she has received from the second daughter but states she is afraid to wear them or use them because Rose, the daughter who visits each week, will be angry.

   a. Is it your role to interfere in this relationship?

   b. How would you discuss this with your client?

   c. What would you document?

2. Mrs. Cummings has visited the doctor since your last visit. She seems more forgetful and has not eaten this morning. She is still in the same clothes she was wearing two days ago.

   a. Identify the subjective and objective information you would collect before you discuss this with your supervisor.

   b. How would you apply the information you have learned about the family's cultural background to this situation?

Certification Exam Review Questions

Choose the best answer for each question or statement.

1. **Communication consists of**

   a. *verbal communication.*

   b. *body language.*

   c. *written communication.*

   d. *only those messages you receive from your supervisor.*

2. **The culture of the client**

   a. *is not important because he is in the United States now.*

   b. *is important because it will affect his care.*

   c. *should be noted, but only the family need be concerned.*

   d. *will change as soon as you can explain to him that your way of looking at health is the better way.*

3. **When you relate to clients,**

   a. *you are entitled to your moods since you are human, too.*

   b. *your needs should be discussed with the family before the care starts.*

   c. *you should be a careful and sensitive listener but need not document all the information.*

   d. *you should document information even if you are not sure it will affect the client's care.*

4. **When documenting,**

   a. *it is important to write in short notes that include the date and time of the entry, but calling your supervisor is not necessary because she will eventually read the note.*

   b. *it is important to write down anything unusual that occurs concerning the client.*

   c. *it is important to write down if the client tells you that something unusual happened when you were not there.*

   d. *it is important to write down subjective things.*

5. **Your documentation**

   a. *is for only your supervisor to read.*

   b. *proves that you were in the house so you can get paid.*

   c. *is a legal document and will be saved with the client's record.*

   d. *can be written in pencil.*

CHAPTER 3

Working with People

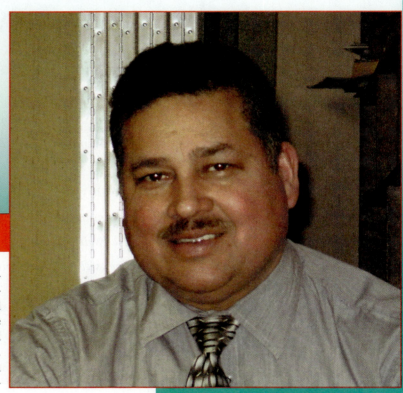

CASE STUDY

Mr. Ricardo has been in this country 20 years. He worked in the flower business and until recently owned a small flower store in a strip mall, which he closed when a large chain store moved into the mall. He is outgoing, likes people, and speaks English well. His four children are all grown and live far away with families of their own. His wife of 35 years recently went back to their native country to care for her father. She hopes to return in three months. The house he has owned 25 years is in a changing neighborhood. Most of his former neighbors have moved out and younger people with small children have moved in. The house is far from town center, and he must drive to the grocery store. Mr. Ricardo, a smoker since age 15, has difficulty breathing and pain in his legs. He has not told anyone about his discomfort, but he walks more slowly each week and his legs hurt him even though he rubs liniment on them.

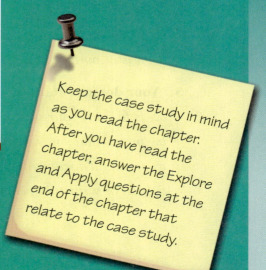

Keep the case study in mind as you read the chapter. After you have read the chapter, answer the Explore and Apply questions at the end of the chapter that relate to the case study.

Basic Human Needs

OBJECTIVES		
What You Will Learn to Do	**1.**	List the physical needs shared by all human beings.
	2.	List the psychological needs shared by all human beings.
	3.	Distinguish between needs of the client, the family, and the caregiver.
	4.	Become aware of behavior that results when basic human needs are unmet.
	5.	Describe your role in helping to manage patient pain.

Introduction: Basic Needs

Every person has certain basic needs that must be met to survive. A **need** is a requirement for survival. Sometimes an individual can satisfy her own needs, and sometimes she requires help. A person becomes your client when he is unable to satisfy all his needs himself. For example, a person may need help with meals or to meet his need for nourishment. As a homemaker/home health aide, you will help your client meet basic needs until he can meet them without your help.

> **need**
> a requirement for survival

It is important—and often difficult—to be sure health care team actions are meeting the client's needs. Your knowledge of these needs and your objective observations will help your supervisor determine whether the plan of care meets all needs in a particular home.

BASIC PHYSICAL AND PSYCHOLOGICAL NEEDS

Not all needs must be met completely each day, but the more each person's needs are fulfilled, the better the quality of life (Figure 3.1 ■).

Psychological needs also must be satisfied to have a healthy emotional and social outlook. As with physical needs, these do not have to be met totally each day. However, the more completely each need is met, the better the person's emotional state will be. Needs can be met by family, by oneself, or by someone not a family member but available on an intermittent basis.

BALANCING NEEDS

Children's needs are usually met by family members. During adult years, most people are expected to meet some or most of their own needs. These physical and psychological needs overlap and affect each other. Each person determines his or her particular balance. When one need is out of balance due to illness, the other needs are also affected. For example, when a person is ill and requires more rest, food intake must meet this change in activity. Clothing will change. Weight may change, and moods may alter. The client is often the one who knows how to restore balance. In such a case, the client might determine when to eat and what foods to decrease so that he does not gain weight. By consulting the client, you will more likely meet actual needs and not guess what they are. Needs can change, so be alert.

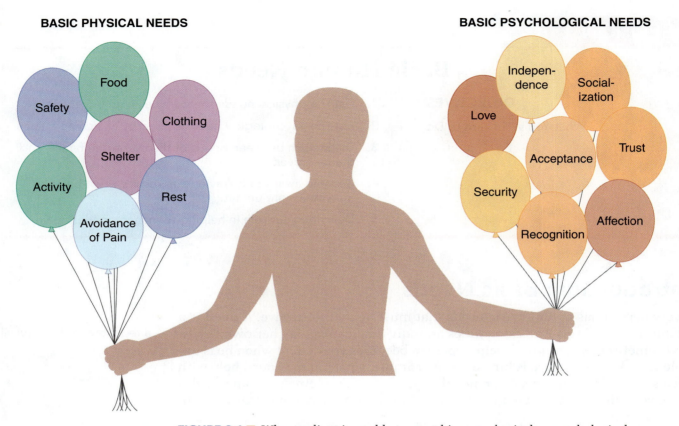

BASIC PHYSICAL NEEDS

Safety
Food
Clothing
Shelter
Activity
Rest
Avoidance of Pain

BASIC PSYCHOLOGICAL NEEDS

Independence
Socialization
Love
Trust
Acceptance
Security
Affection
Recognition

FIGURE 3.1 ■ When a client is unable to meet his own physical or psychological needs, it is your role to assist him.

Several factors affect the way in which we balance a client's needs:

- client knowledge
- disease state
- family support
- mental state
- age
- available resources
- culture
- financial resources

The way in which these elements interact will determine how the client's needs are met and how all other family member needs are satisfied. Many things can change a client's behavior and attitude during an illness. The client may be frightened, angry, or sad.

FAMILY NEEDS

If your client is part of a family unit, his change in status will affect all other members of the family. Remember that, although you are in the home primarily to meet the needs of the client, your observations about the family are important. The family unit will continue support when you are no longer there. Every member of the family has a set of basic needs and these needs must continue to be met even though one of its members, your client, now has a changed status. Balancing all these requirements is difficult. Discuss this with your supervisor so a plan of care can be established that will be useful for the family and your client.

YOUR NEEDS AS A HOMEMAKER/HOME HEALTH AIDE

Homemaker/home health aides have the same basic needs as their clients. It is important that your needs be met, too, but not at the expense of your client's. Many times your needs will have to be put aside until you leave the client. Discuss with your supervisor both your client's needs and yours. Then a plan will be made so that the needs of the client will be satisfied and you will not feel slighted. Caregivers must be alert to the reasons they do and say things. As you care for your clients, be alert and identify what basic need you are satisfying and whose it is. Ask yourself these questions:

- Are you acting because the client's needs must be met or because your needs must be met? For example: Are you giving the client a bath because he will feel better or because you will feel better having done it?
- Do you perform a procedure with the client because he enjoys having you help him and shows improvement or because you feel that you must do it?
- Does helping a client become independent and no longer need your help make you feel good or useless?

UNMET NEEDS

When basic needs are not met, human beings react. If a physical need is not met, the reaction is usually obvious; for example, if the need for food is not met, the person might become irritable or weak. If an emotional need is not met, a person's reactions may be feelings of anxiety, depression, aggression, or anger or else a physical ailment without apparent cause.

You will not always be able to decide why a client behaves in a certain manner. That is all right. It is necessary, however, for you to report these actions to your supervisor. Often, by reviewing client's actions, your supervisor can determine if a need is unmet. Then, by altering the plan of care, the need will be fulfilled and the behavior changed.

PAIN

The word *pain* means different things to different people. What is painful to one person may not be to another. It is important to find out how your client reacts to pain and how his family views pain. Many people think that pain is normal and must be tolerated; some believe it is a punishment; some do not want to complain; some people are afraid of medications; and some are afraid that, if they complain their caregivers will leave them. Some people are afraid to discuss their pain with their physicians because they believe that if a physician could relieve the pain, she would do so without being asked.

Clients in pain often cannot participate in their care, relate to their families, or expend energy on the healing process. Clients in pain cannot have a good quality of life.

Pain causes many reactions. Some you can see, and some you cannot see. A client in pain may

- Have a rapid pulse, shallow and rapid breathing
- Have increased fatigue
- Have increased anxiety
- Have increased stress
- Withdraw and decrease communication
- Decrease food and fluid intake
- Make faces and make gestures with his hands

■ Moan and talk in baby talk and cry
■ Demonstrate angry behavior

Different cultures treat pain in different ways. People of various cultures may hang a charm near the bed, say special prayers, burn candles, or dress the client in special clothes. If these actions help the client, support them even though they may seem unusual to you. Some people do not want to take medication. They are afraid they will become addicted, be questioned by the authorities, or bring shame to their family and to themselves. Encourage your client to take medication as prescribed. If it does not have the expected result, report this immediately to your supervisor.

Health care teams are becoming more and more aware of the many things that contribute to an individual's response to pain. Medication is becoming more and more acceptable and available to clients at home who are in pain. When it is prescribed by a physician and given as prescribed, no one should be afraid to take it.

Your Role as a Homemaker/Home Health Aide

Your role as a homemaker/home health aide is to help the client and his family manage the pain. This can be done in many ways:

■ Ask the client what usually decreases his pain. Do not change his routine!
■ Talk to the client. Explain what you will do and how he may help.
■ Allow the client to move at his own pace. Do not rush him.
■ Support the medication schedule. Encourage the client to take medication before the pain becomes severe.
■ Encourage the family to support the client as he deals with pain.
■ Observe the client for any increase of pain. Alter your care accordingly.
■ Report to your supervisor if the client's pain changes or if he does not respond to his medication.
■ Encourage the client to share his feelings about his pain.
■ Encourage the family to share their feelings about the client's pain, his reaction to it, and its effect on them.

SECTION 2

Family

OBJECTIVES

What You Will Learn to Do

1. Define *family*.
2. List the functions of a family.
3. Recognize reasons that family structure and function are changing in today's society.
4. Become aware of your role working within a family unit.
5. Discuss the role of culture on the client and your care.
6. Discuss the place of family in decision making.

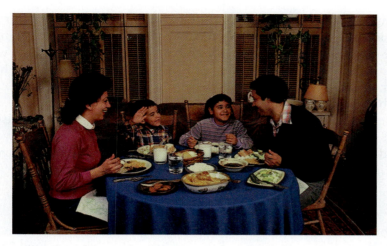

FIGURE 3.2 ■ Families provide stability, transmit culture, meet members' individual needs, protect, and teach self-sufficiency.

INTRODUCTION: FAMILY

Most human beings live in some sort of family. It may be an extended family with several generations in the same house. It may be a single-parent family. It may be a unit made up of friends who live together and regard themselves as a family. Different cultures define family in different ways. In the broadest sense, a family is a unit bound together by common interests and working to maintain the well-being, and meet the needs, of all members (Figure 3.2 ■).

CHANGING FAMILY

About 75 years ago, families made up of several generations were common. Grandparents, maiden aunts, and orphaned children returned to the extended family home and were incorporated into the functioning family. Families were also bigger, with many more children. With all these members, necessary tasks were divided and everyone benefited. For example, a grandmother might care for the young children and fold all laundry. She would also tell family stories and transmit the family's culture to the younger generation. The mother would cook, clean, and discipline the older children. She would teach the girls to sew and cook. Older children would care for and play with younger ones and assist with household chores and caring for the sick. The boys worked outside and learned a trade from their father. The father worked and earned money for the family and provided leadership and protection.

Today, families have changed in many ways and for many reasons.

■ Families are smaller.
■ Women go to work.
■ Roles are not as carefully prescribed.
■ Family members do not always live near each other.
■ People live longer.
■ The sick can be cared for in institutions.
■ Society now assumes some of the care of the sick and elderly.

Each family has needs and rules of its own. As you enter a family to care for one of its members, you become aware of how that family operates. Do they care for one another? Do they punish their members with violence? Do they speak lovingly to each other? Do they stop speaking to one member when they are angry? Do they tease members? As well as you can, it is your responsibility to work and care for your client within the framework of his family. If you change the client substantially and bring in too many new ideas, you will not be welcome and the client will no longer be welcome as a member of his family. Remember, when you leave, the client remains in his family and might have difficulty with changes you taught him.

You are encouraged to discuss your observations with your supervisor so that the plan of care can reflect the family's values. If there are activities you do not understand or that make you uncomfortable or that you consider dangerous, report them immediately to your agency.

CULTURE AND THE FAMILY

Many factors influence family function: size, economic resources, needs of each member, culture of members and of the country in which they live. Sometimes, a family functions within the rules of their native country but lives in the United States. This may cause conflict between family member roles and the relationship and expectations of the health care team. In some families the senior male makes decisions; in others, the mother-in-law makes the decisions. In some families, children are important, educated, and cared for; in others, they enter the work force at a young age. The family culture has a great impact on its structure; decision-making pattern; and members' reactions to illness, pain, and healing. You must be sensitive to these issues as they will affect your client. If you do not understand certain actions or decisions or believe actions are not helping your client, discuss this with your supervisor.

Health care workers must be **culturally competent**, which means have basic knowledge and understanding about the culture of their client and the family. If the family is multicultural (more than one culture) the homemaker/home health aide and the supervisor must take all the cultures into consideration when planning and carrying out the care.

Understanding a culture means understanding its members' basic ideas about themselves, their relationship to their family members, and their ideas about health care. Learning new skills and information is accomplished in different ways in different cultures. It is important that you are aware of how each person learns and obtains new knowledge.

FAMILY MEMBERS AND THEIR ROLES

A **role** is the part a person has in his family or situation. Each member of a family has many roles. Sometimes these roles are learned from older members of the family; sometimes, if there is no role model, the role must be shaped to the best of the person's ability. Family members each have several roles; for example, a woman may be a mother, daughter, wife, and grandmother. Each role demands different behavior and a different set of responsibilities. The important point is to balance these roles so none conflict with the others. This is difficult and often impossible. Family members who have difficulty balancing roles may need professional help to accomplish this task.

GENERATION IN THE MIDDLE

In many homes, you may find a family member in "the generation in the middle." This often is a woman about 45 to 50 years old who cares for her mother or father, 70 to 75 years old, and mothers her own children, often teenagers.

culturally competent
familiar with basic understanding of the client's culture and function within the family group and greater community

role
a person's place(s) within their culture, family, and community

Clinical ALERT

Cultural and Ethnic Diversity
We live in a country that expects and welcomes people from all over the world. These people view health care, illness, and others as taught in their culture. Exploring their feelings and beliefs will help you provide more complete care, allow clients an active part in their care, and provide a forum for discussion. Remember, part of recovering from illness or learning to live with chronic illness are beliefs and cultural support. Knowing what those beliefs are allows us to support, respect, and incorporate them into care.

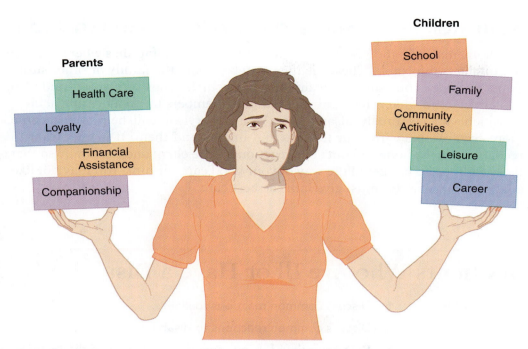

FIGURE 3.3 ■ Women often find themselves in several roles and balancing several sets of demands on their time and emotions.

She may also work and have a husband. This generation is often in need of special understanding and assistance, for its members must always balance the needs of others in addition to trying to meet their own needs. In this special situation, as in others, it is important to understand family dynamics and work to maintain them so all members can survive without hurting one another (Figure 3.3 ■).

In another scenario you find a person who has raised a family and now cares for a parent. This requires an adjustment of resources, time, family responsibilities, and outlook. Your understanding of this process and ability to help the primary caregiver, family, and client meet their needs is your most important role. It is necessary to be nonjudgmental as family members learn new roles and readjust the ways in which their basic needs will be met.

ECONOMICS

All families have some money, which they spend according to their own rules and beliefs based on family history, family needs, culture, and state of the client's disease. Many families will spend on things of which you personally do not approve. You will often find yourself being asked by one family member or another to comment on how their money is spent. For example: "Do you think my son should have bought that car?" or "How could my daughter pay so much for that dress?"

It is most important to act in a nonjudgmental way and not to inflict your opinions about money on the client or his family. All that you need to say is "I'm not really in a position to comment on this situation. I suggest that you discuss your feelings with your son." If you believe that money is being spent in such a way as to injure a family member or cause danger to the family, report your observations to your supervisor immediately.

Your Role as a Homemaker/Home Health Aide

As a homemaker/home health aide, you may be sent into families where you are not totally comfortable. These feelings may be due to the family or other situations. Speak to your supervisor and discuss your feelings. Are you afraid? Do you understand what is happening? Do family members have values and actions of which you personally disapprove? Your supervisor will help you become more comfortable with your feelings and understand them. It is important to recognize and be honest about your reactions to the client and his family so that these feelings do not get in the way of your good care for him. You may not like a person, but you still must give him the best care.

SECTION 3

Working with Clients Who Are Ill or Have a Disability

OBJECTIVES

What You Will Learn to Do

1. Discuss common reactions to illness.
2. Discuss common reactions to disabilities.
3. Recognize your feelings concerning illness and disability.
4. List broad goals of caring for clients who are ill or have a disability.
5. Learn to recognize family support systems and their effect on the client.

Introduction: Reactions to Being Ill and Dependent

Every person reacts to illness, being disabled, and being dependent in a different way. Individual reactions are determined by age, family, culture, emotional health, and all the other parts that make up a particular person. Even though there are individual reactions, there are also certain common ways in which most people react to being ill or having a disability. As a homemaker/home health aide, you must be aware of common behaviors so that you will know what to expect while caring for your clients.

It is important to remember that you bring certain feelings about illness with you when you care for a client. These feelings are part of you. Sometimes these feelings are helpful to you and your client. Sometimes they are not. The important thing is to identify these feelings and not let them get in the way of your work.

The most useful action you can take as a homemaker/home health aide is to involve the client and his family in the plan of care. Remember, you will leave, but they will all remain in the home. By establishing a routine in which they take part, they can continue care of the client after you are gone. Everyone, young and old, regardless of illness or disability, has a right to take part in his care if they want. They also have a right not to take part.

The Difference Between Illness and Disability

An **illness** is the absence of good health. An illness usually has pain and discomfort associated with it. This absence of health may be acute or it may be chronic. An **acute** illness starts suddenly and does not last long. A **chronic** illness continues for a long time.

illness
deviation from the healthy state

acute
state of illness that comes on suddenly and may be of short duration

chronic
state of disease that lasts a long time

A **disability** is a condition that produces a physical or mental limitation that may or may not respond to adaptive aids. Usually, a body function that we take for granted is impaired. A disability may be produced by an accident, an illness, or a birth defect. A chronic illness may cause a disability. For example, diabetes, a chronic illness, may cause a person to have poor eyesight. A disability may or may not be painful or cause discomfort. The most important thing to remember about a disability is that it is usually permanent.

The National Organization on Disability estimates that at least 49 million Americans of all ages have a disability. Some use wheelchairs, canes, walkers, hearing aids, or glasses to assist them in their daily activities. The way in which you interact with people with disabilities will indicate the understanding and respect you have for them.

Remember . . .

disability
partial or complete loss of the use of a body part or parts

- Ask before you help a person. The person may not want or need your assistance. Do not assume that all people with disabilities require assistance.
- Speak directly to a person with a disability, not to their companion or sign-language interpreter.
- Do not speak as though the person was not present.
- Be sensitive about physical contact. Some people require all their limbs for balance, and touching one limb may cause them to fall.
- Do not touch a person's assistive device. These devices are considered part of the person's personal space.
- Do not ask personal questions. Children may ask questions or act curious. Most people with disabilities do not mind this. But be sensitive to perceptions of rudeness.
- Do not lean over a client in a wheelchair to speak to or shake someone else's hand.
- Sit on a chair, whenever possible, when speaking to a person in a wheelchair. If this is impossible, stand a short distance away so she does not hurt her neck looking up at you.

REACTIONS TO ILLNESS AND DISABILITY

Reactions of families to illness, disability, and crisis vary (Figure 3.4 ■). The unique way in which all members of a family function is called **family dynamics**.

family dynamics
the ways in which family members interact and get along with each other

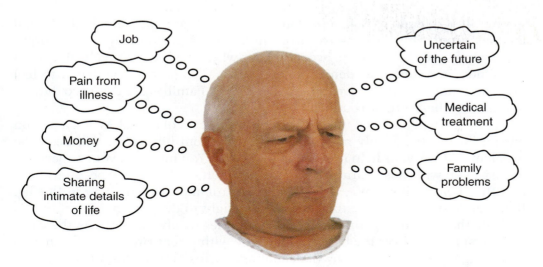

FIGURE 3.4 ■ Illness and disability cause clients to worry about many temporary and permanent changes in their lives.

support systems
arrangements that give
aid and comfort to a
person

Clinical ALERT

People and Disabilities
Some people are born
with disabilities and others acquire them as a re-
sult of illness, surgery, or
accidents. Disabilities
may be permanent or
temporary. People with
disabilities expect to be
treated as a whole, func-
tioning person much as
they would be treated
without the disabilities.
Always provide a safe
and accepting environ-
ment. Respect the per-
son and his or her wishes
for assistance. If you disagree with an activity,
discuss it with the client
and your supervisor.

This method of functioning has been shaped over many years. **Support systems** are people or actions that help a person adjust to a new or difficult situation. Families may be able to make the necessary adjustments in their functions and rally to the short-term crisis or acute illness but fail to adjust if the illness is a long-term or chronic situation. Other families make long-term adjustments. Still others fail to make any changes in their structure and fail to cope with any illness or disability.

Ideally, a family chooses support systems that allow them to continue functioning—even in time of crisis. You will recognize many kinds of support systems:

- *Informal systems:* people help one another because they want to—church groups, neighbors, and friends.
- *Formal systems:* people help because they are paid to do so and/or they have a particular knowledge necessary and/or an outside agency or government says they must do so—visiting nurses, homemaker/home health aides, caseworkers.
- *Support groups:* people gather, usually with a leader or facilitator, to discuss and share similar problems, help each other, and gain knowledge from each other.

Your supervisor, along with the family, the physician, and the client, will work to set up an acceptable support system for the situation. As a sensitive member of the team, your observations as to "what works and what doesn't" are important. Be sure to share your observations with your supervisor.

Often, when the proper help is offered, a family in crisis can make necessary changes to cope with illness or disability. Remember, the family unit has set up patterns of coping over a long period of time. You must work with these patterns and help establish a support system that makes the family and patient secure and comfortable. If you are not comfortable with the support system or do not believe it will meet the client's needs, discuss this with your supervisor. You will not be asked to take part in any system that puts you or your client at risk.

DENIAL

denial
refusal to believe or
accept reality

Denial is used by some people when people meet a situation with which they cannot cope at the time. They simply say, "This doesn't really exist, nothing is wrong". It is difficult to help a person who denies that a problem exists. Denial is a way people shield themselves from situations. A person may deny an event or situation and then come to accept it later when she is emotionally able to do so. Almost everyone uses denial at some time. Clients may use denial to feel more acceptable to themselves and their families. Families use denial so they do not have to change their routines.

Often, you will be asked to take part in this process of denial. When a person has an illness, the family may wish to keep it from him. They will deny the problem and ask your help in keeping the secret. You must ask your supervisor to assist you with this charade. It is most difficult, and you may become angry that the client or his family is denying the truth and involving you in this lie. Remember, the family and the client have a right to deny a situation if that is their method of coping and the client is not negatively affected. As the caregiver, you must deliver the best possible care within that situation. The important thing to remember is why the client and/or his family find it necessary to deny the situation.

ABUSIVE WORDS AND DIFFICULT BEHAVIOR

Many clients can be impatient. A client may show his impatience to one member of the family or only to you. It is important to remain calm and not take the client's words as a personal insult. Often, he is angry at the situation, not at you, but you are the closest person to whom he can react. A client may complain that the medicine isn't working, that the exercises aren't working, and that he isn't getting better fast enough. He may complain that you are doing too much or not enough. He may become irritable due to pain, the general situation, or his feeling of helplessness. Remember, remain calm and put the client's actions and words into perspective. If you have difficulty doing this, speak to your supervisor.

Clients may say things to you that they would not say to their relatives. They may use unpleasant or nasty, **abusive** words. Why? You are not a family member and, therefore, you do not have all the years of family relationship behind you. Because you are paid to care for the client, he may think that you will return even if he isn't nice because it is "your job." A visiting family member does not have to care for the client, and if the client is unpleasant, the family member may not return. Some clients may say and do things to test you and the limits of the situation. Often, clients will be nice to you but not to their families. This is to make families jealous and show them that the clients are still in control of the situation. Clients may do or say unpleasant things but are not aware that their behavior is a problem to anyone. If you tell a client that something he does makes you uncomfortable, he often will stop it.

Working with an unpleasant client is difficult. Remember that there is a reason for such behavior. Discuss the entire situation with your supervisor, and she will assist you in dealing with it. Abusive words may indicate many things about the family dynamics. It is important to explore these. Do not assume this behavior is temporary or done only when you are present. If you are really uncomfortable, you may be transferred to another case.

→ **abusive**
insulting or mistreating

GOALS TO KEEP IN MIND AS YOU CARE FOR YOUR CLIENT

All clients, whether they are ill, disabled, have a chronic condition, or are having an acute attack, will have a plan of care. As the homemaker/home health aide, you will be asked to follow this plan of care. A plan is carefully made up by the professional nurse, a supervisor, and therapists who care for the client. This plan is formulated to meet both short- and long-term client needs. Your maintenance of this routine is most important. Your careful observation and reporting to your supervisor are also important.

The goal of the client's care plan will be established by the professionals and the client. It is essential that the client and his caregivers share the same goals. Then they all work toward the same end. Although each client has his individual care plan, certain broad goals are present in all care plans:

- Promote self-care
- Promote self-respect
- Promote behavior appropriate to the client's condition and age
- Promote a safe, clean environment

Advance Directives for Health Care

Each client has the right to determine the kind of health care he wants if and when he cannot actively make the decision. This document, often called a *living will*, indicates to others the client's wishes concerning heroic measures, accepting or refusing treatment, and/or withdrawing life support. It is always a good idea to discuss the presence or absence of a living will before you accept an assignment. The contents of this living will influence the plan of care and your activities in the home. If a client tells you that he is interested in making a living will, contact your supervisor so that the appropriate person can be called.

Mental Health and Mental Disability

OBJECTIVES

What You Will Learn to Do

1. Identify characteristics of good mental health.
2. Identify misconceptions about mental disabilities.
3. Describe your role as a homemaker/home health aide when caring for a client who is mentally disabled.

Introduction: Mental Health/Mental Disability

mental health
the ability to function satisfactorily in a society; a sense of well-being

Mental health is the ability to function effectively and satisfactorily in a certain society. Mental health is a condition of the whole person. It reflects how a person deals with daily life and crises. Our mental health is the basis for our behavior and relationships with others.

Mental health is also a matter of degree. At times, everyone shows behavior that may be judged unusual. The difference between a mentally healthy person and one with a mental disability is that the person who is mentally disabled adopts characteristics or behaviors that no longer enable him to function within society.

Mentally healthy people can:

- Adapt to change
- Give and receive affection and love
- Tolerate stress to varying degrees
- Accept responsibility for their own feelings and actions
- Distinguish between reality and unreality
- Form and keep relationships with people

MENTAL DISABILITY

mental disability
the temporary or permanent disruption in the ability of a person to function satisfactorily in society

contagious
readily transmitted by direct or indirect contact

Not long ago, **mental disability** was thought to be a punishment or a curse. Many people thought mental disabilities were **contagious** and could be spread. People who were mentally disabled were put into institutions so that the rest of society would not catch their disease. We now know that mental illnesses are not contagious and that there are many different causes for mental disabilities and socially unacceptable behavior. Not all mental disability is permanent. With treatment and medication, many people recover and lead productive lives.

Mental disabilities often start slowly, and people cannot tell you when the problem started. They can, however, say when the behavior became no longer acceptable. There are many levels of mental dysfunction. Do not try to label a client. Just treat him with respect, support him and his family, see to his safety, and follow the plan of care.

Common causes of mental disability are:

- Isolation
- Medication
- High fevers
- Family and interpersonal relationships
- Environment
- Chronic stress
- Alcohol/substance abuse
- Specific traumatic event
- Heredity
- Circulatory diseases

Besides reacting to illness and disability in physical ways, people also have mental and emotional reactions. Some people become mentally disabled as a result of a physical ailment. In these cases, caring for the client's mental disability will be an added component to caring for his physical condition.

People show their disability in different ways. One classic symptom is a marked change in behavior patterns. If you notice any change in your client's behavior or his family tells you that his behavior is changed, report it to your supervisor immediately. After a careful assessment, your supervisor may change the client's plan of care to reflect his mental needs.

Other symptoms of mental disability are

- Hallucinations
- Sleeplessness
- Fears
- Decreased memory
- Disorientation
- Forgetfulness
- Withdrawal
- Mood swings

Defense Mechanisms

A person who experiences stress reacts with certain defenses. This is normal. When **defense mechanisms** are used to such an extent that a person loses touch with reality, he is said to be mentally disabled. The most common defense mechanisms are:

- *Denial*—"It's not happening."
- *Depression*—"It's no use. It's hopeless."
- *Regression*—acting like a child or becoming very dependent.
- *Repression*—forgetting about the situation, putting it out of the mind.
- *Projection*—"It's not my fault but the fault of the medical people."
- *Rationalization*—explaining how one's behavior is acceptable even though it isn't.
- *Aggression* —behavior that attacks everyone regardless of cause.
- *Overdependence* —taking no responsibility for personal decisions; relying on others for all needs.

You will care for clients with many combinations of mental disabilities. Two of the most common ones you will see are depression and overdependence.

Depression

Depression may be an illness, a way in which a person deals with illness, the result of an illness, or a side effect of medication. The primary sign of depression

defense mechanism
a thought used unconsciously to protect oneself against painful or unpleasant feelings

depression ,
low spirits that may or may not cause a change of activity

is lack of interest in the present situation and environment. Other signs of depression are:

- Poor appetite
- Disinterest in people and things previously of interest
- Statements like "I'm not up to that" and "What does it matter anyway?"
- Being overappreciative of help
- Lack of activity or social interaction
- Lack of expression in face or voice

Allow the client to take part in as much of his care as he wants and is able to. Point out the decisions he can make. Consult the client whenever you can. Encourage his decisions and opinions. Try to establish routines that are good for the client and have a high rate of success. For example, it may be more convenient for you to help the client exercise before his bath. But the client may want to do his exercises after his bath, and he does them better at that time. It would then be appropriate for you to alter your schedule and do the exercises when the client feels they are most helpful. You must remember that some clients will remain depressed no matter what you do. Do not become discouraged. Continue to try to interest them in meaningful activities.

Overdependence

Some people adopt this type of behavior because they have learned it brings them rewards. Some cannot function any other way.

When people realize they are no longer in total charge of their situation, as with the new diagnosis of a chronic disease, they may fail to adjust to this change. Instead, they become totally dependent on others and take no responsibility for their care. When a client refuses the responsibility he is able to take, he is said to be overdependent. It is important to assist the client in assuming, at his own pace, the role of being somewhat dependent, while continuing to be responsible for himself when possible. No matter how ill he is, a client still may take some part in his care. Remember, though, clients will assume their independence when they are ready to meet their own needs. Until then, it is your responsibility to assume the care.

Your Role as a Homemaker/Home Health Aide

As society recognizes the causes of and develops better treatments for mental disability, more and more people are being returned to the community after hospitalization. Communities have set up clinics, foster homes, day care programs, and halfway houses to help these former institutionalized patients adjust to community life.

You may be assigned to a client with a mental disability or you may be in a home where a family member is disabled. Be sure you understand your responsibility to the person. Your plan of care will be your guide to both the physical and emotional care of the person. Care of the client who is mentally disabled is like care of any other client. One of the important parts of your care will be to support the client's family. Encourage family members to discuss their feelings and concerns with the client's doctor. For the client to reach his maximum ability, he needs an accepting environment. Remember:

- Your observations of the client and family are important.
- Report your observations objectively.

- Your friendly, understanding manner will show how you feel about the client. It will encourage others to feel positively about the client.
- Be aware of your body language.
- Encourage the client to take part in his own care as is appropriate.
- Speak to the client in simple sentences. Do not shout or talk baby talk to him.

Substance Abuse

OBJECTIVES		
What You Will Learn to Do	**1.**	Understand what is meant by substance abuse.
	2.	Identify misconceptions about substance abuse.
	3.	Describe your role as a homemaker/home health aide when a substance abuser is in the home where you work.
	4.	Describe your role as a homemaker/home health aide when you are caring for a client who is a recovering substance abuser.

Introduction: Substance Abuse

The definition of **substance abuse** is the continued use of a substance despite adverse consequences that impact major life areas and alter the ability to interact in society. There are many types of substance abuse. A person can abuse drugs, alcohol, or a combination. The drugs may be prescription or illegal. Substance abuse is seen in all ages and in all economic levels. Abuse may be obvious or subtle. Some people think altering the way they feel through the use of alcohol or drugs is a way of escaping their problems; some people do it because their friends do it; others start out using drugs to help them with an illness and then are unable to stop; still others start out using alcohol slowly and do not realize they are in trouble until it is too late. The term *substance abuse* means that a person uses a drug or alcohol to excess and that his or her behavior alters due to the abuse. In the past, most people believed that no one could help substance abusers. We know now that is not the case. Many receive treatment and return to living useful and productive lives. The treatment is not easy and it takes a long time, but those who continue treatment may well accomplish a complete cure.

substance abuse
the use of anything, usually alcohol or drugs, to excess and to the detriment of the person

GENERAL MISCONCEPTIONS ABOUT SUBSTANCE ABUSE

"Everyone does it."

This is not true. We read a great many stories in the newspapers about famous people who use drugs, and we read about everyday people who try them. This leads some readers to believe that everyone is doing it. Actually, nobody knows how many people really use drugs and abuse alcohol, and although the number certainly seems to be growing, not "everyone" does it!

"I can control it."

Wrong! The body becomes used to drugs and alcohol and then no longer reacts to the usual amount that is taken. Therefore, the person must increase the "dose" to achieve the same feeling. As the dose increases, so does the price.

There has never been an addicted person who could control it. Sooner or later, the habit controls the person.

"No one will know."

Wrong! It is entirely possible that when the user starts, no one will know. But as the body accustoms itself to the foreign substance, there are definite changes in behavior. Soon, employers know. Families can no longer deny the problem. Finally, somebody must confront the user.

"It makes me feel good."

A person who starts to use drugs or alcohol may do so to get "high." But this state does not last long. Some people may enjoy this feeling because they feel they are avoiding their real problems. When they are no longer high, however, they do not feel good, and their problems are still present.

GENERAL SIGNALS OF SUBSTANCE ABUSE

Many signs are associated with abuse of specific substances (Figure 3.5 ■). The most important sign is a change in the person's behavior. Some general signals are:

1. Personality changes, such as mood swings, bizarre activities, or change of friends; disinterest in familiar activities
2. Change in the way money is spent
3. Change in employment or in the relationship with present employer
4. Change in school habits
5. Alteration in physical appearance, such as weight gain or loss, reddened eyes, dilated pupils, nausea/vomiting
6. Change in eating habits or consumption of fluids
7. Change in sleep habits
8. Liquor missing
9. Unusual breath odor, unusual smell on clothing

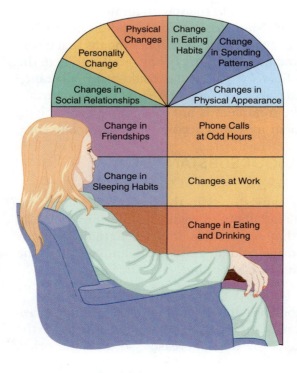

FIGURE 3.5 ■ Be alert to subtle changes in behavior of both clients and family members.

10. Change in gait; change in sense of smell, vision, or hearing
11. Change in breathing pattern
12. Continued discussion about drugs or alcohol
13. Phone calls at odd hours

Your Role as a Homemaker/Home Health Aide

You may be assigned to care for a client who is in a house with a drug user or an alcoholic. First, you must be sure your client is in no danger and that the abuser cannot harm your client—or you. Discuss the situation with your supervisor so that a plan can be made to offer help to the abuser. Do not try to obtain help on your own. Offering help to a long-time abuser can be a complicated affair and must be carefully planned. It is important that the correct help be offered and that the most appropriate community resource be used. Your supervisor will know how to plan this.

Do not tell the abuser he must stop. The chances are he would if he could but is unable to do so without help.

Do not make family members feel guilty that they have permitted the situation to continue. They may not know what to do. With your help and support and that of your supervisor, a plan can be made. Families of abusers need a great deal of support. Your understanding and demonstration of nonjudgmental behavior will be important in this household.

If you are assigned to a client who is presently under treatment for having been an abuser, you should act in the manner we have already discussed. You must be observant to detect if the client has reverted back to previous habits of abuse. Report to your supervisor any actions that suggest the client is not drug- or alcohol-free. Follow the care plan carefully and support the client. Recovery from drug abuse or alcoholism is not easy. With your presence and support, it can be made easier.

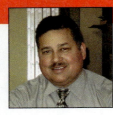

Case Study

Review the case study that appears on the first page of the chapter. Answer the questions contained in the Explore and Apply sections below.

EXPLORE

1. What questions might you ask your supervisor as you receive the assignment to care for Mr. Ricardo? Remember, the questions should relate to your role as a homemaker/home health aide and the information should be useful to you as you work with your supervisor to help establish the plan of care.

2. One of the neighbors, a young woman with three children, often asks Mr. Ricardo if she can buy him anything at the market. She also has offered to take him when she does her weekly shopping. He always refuses. One of the children, Mark, is always at Mr. Ricardo's house when you come. He is 8 years old. When you suggest he goes home, he says, "I like it here. It is quiet and I can think. I even have my own toys here." And he shows you his pile of small cars. What is your reaction to the fact that Mr. Ricardo refuses his neighbor's assistance? How do you respond to Mark when he answers you? What objective information do you gather before you call your supervisor? When do you call your supervisor?

APPLY

1. You have been assigned to assist Mr. Ricardo with his cooking. There is food in the house and small covered dishes in the refrigerator. Mr. Ricardo says his friend with whom he plays cards brings him food when he comes to visit. How would you approach Mr. Ricardo so that you could make a plan of care he would support? Where would you find recipes that might entice Mr. Ricardo to eat?

2. You notice that Mr. Ricardo's garden is dying and that all the plants in the house need attention. Mr. Ricardo walks a little, but his legs hurt and he has been "resting" them. He reluctantly shows you his feet when you ask to see them. One foot is slightly darker than the other.

   a. What information do you gather?

   b. What do you do with the information?

Certification Exam Review Questions

Choose the best answer for each question or statement.

1. **Basic human needs**

   a. are different in all cultures.

   b. must be met by the family so that you can care for the client.

   c. are the same in all cultures.

   d. must be met every day or the person will not be well.

2. **Although people from different countries live in the United States,**

   a. they should all be treated alike since that is the law.

   b. their families should care for them because they know how to do it best.

   c. caregivers should take different cultures into consideration when caring for people.

   d. people should be cared for according to American standards since they are living in this country.

3. **When caring for people who are ill, it is**

   a. a good techniques to share your personal experience with them so they know you care.

   b. important to be tough and have high expectations so they strive to succeed.

   c. important to remember that everyone reacts differently to being ill and disabled.

   d. wise to use a plan of care that worked for one individual on another individual.

4. **A person who is mentally ill**

   a. can appear perfectly normal and be productive when taking medication.

   b. must live alone to develop independence.

   c. does not have to see a doctor as long as he takes his medication.

   d. should be kept away from small children.

5. **People who abuse drugs and/or alcohol**

   a. all become mentally retarded.

   b. never become productive members of society.

   c. always become productive members of society.

   d. sometimes become productive members of society.

CHAPTER 4

Caring for a Geriatric Client

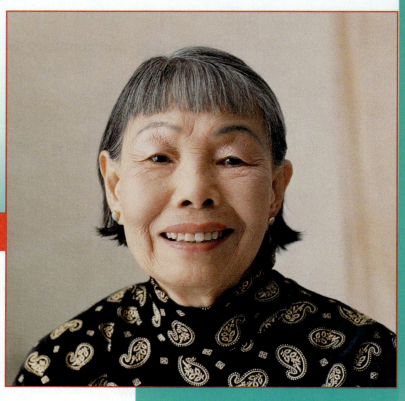

CASE STUDY

Mrs. Lee lives in a small apartment in the center of town with her daughter, Ms. Lee, an engineer. Mrs. Lee speaks no English. Ms. Lee maintains her professional dress and is used to giving directions and working with Americans. She works six days a week and is seldom home before 10 p.m. She attends church, but her mother does not join her. Mrs. Lee continues to wear her native dress and cook her native foods and continually chastises her daughter for not doing the same. While Ms. Lee works, her mother cleans the apartment, cooks the meals, and does all the laundry. There are no visitors to the apartment, and the two women do not take part in any local activities together. When Mrs. Lee must visit the doctor, her daughter takes time off from work. They also consult a native herbalist who prescribes teas, which Mrs. Lee prefers to her Western medication.

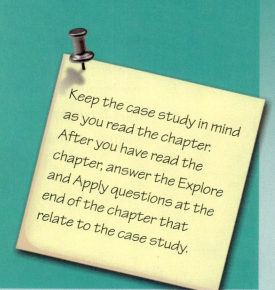

Keep the case study in mind as you read the chapter. After you have read the chapter, answer the Explore and Apply questions at the end of the chapter that relate to the case study.

SECTION 1

Aging

OBJECTIVES	
What You Will Learn to Do	1. Describe the general aging process.
	2. List common problems facing the aged.
	3. Discuss your feelings about aging.
	4. Become familiar with your role as a homemaker/home health aide caring for an elderly client.

Introduction: The Aged

The elderly population is growing faster than any other segment of our society. Here are some interesting facts:

- About 65 million people in America are more than 65 years old.
- The fastest-growing segment of the elderly population is the over-85 age group.
- One of the main sources of income for the elderly is Social Security.
- More than 8 million elderly live at the poverty level.
- Women live longer than men and outnumber them 3 to 2.
- Half of the people over 65 work part-time although they have at least one chronic disease.
- Eighty percent of the elderly have more than one chronic disease that requires medical attention.

Although about 5 percent of the elderly live in nursing homes, the rest live in the community. About 15 percent live in some type of assisted-living arrangement where they receive some help with cooking, housekeeping, or medical care. It is expected that as medicine, nutrition, and the general standard of life improve, the number of aged will increase. As this happens, more and more people who remain at home will need assistance. The home health-care system is changing to meet the needs of these people. Many of your clients who are aged will require assistance so they can remain in their own homes and have some measure of independence and self-respect. Some of your clients will need minimal assistance; others will need maximal assistance. It is important that clients receive the type of help most appropriate for their individual needs.

There are many different types of living arrangements for the elderly. Some live in their own homes; some live in supervised homes with several other clients; and some live in communities with various levels of assistance, such as meals, medical supervision, and/or homemaker services provided by professional caregivers.

The world has changed so much in the past 50 years that the aged are often unfamiliar with what now exists. It is not that they cannot learn about new machines or new systems, but rather that few people take the time to teach them. They often find themselves in a strange world. Adjustment to change is often difficult for clients and their families. Although many clients have a well-tested and strong system of coping that enables them to adjust to changes and new roles, many elderly are unable to cope with all the changes.

geriatrics
knowledge and care of
persons over 65

aging
to become older

The term *geriatrics* refers to the knowledge and care of the elderly. You will use this specialized knowledge as you care for your elderly clients.

AGING

Aging is universal and starts the moment we are born. The way in which society views the aging citizen varies. In some cultures, the aged are of no value and are often neglected because they are unable to contribute to the society. In other cultures and some professions, the aged are well respected and cared for and are given a place of honor. American society often appears to value youth for its beauty and to not value the contributions of its elderly citizens. But it seems that society is also gaining a greater understanding of the aged. There are many signs that our American society is coming to see all ages as valuable. More advertisements for products of interest to the elderly are appearing. Community programs designed for the elderly are gaining popularity. We are also seeing laws passed that meet the concerns of our older citizens and that protect them. American society is coming to the conclusion that, although youth has its value, age has its also (Figure 4.1 ■).

These facts are important for you to remember as you care for older people:

- They want to remain independent.
- They enjoy sexual relationships.
- They can maintain good health.
- Senility is not the same as old age.
- They want to be contributing members of society.
- They can learn, although they often take longer than younger people to do so.

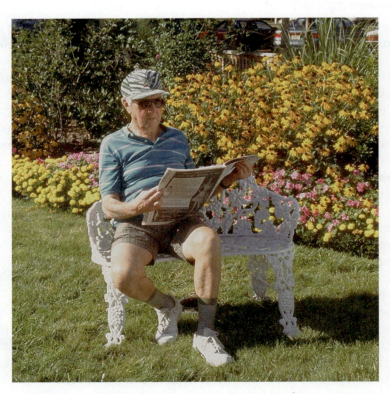

FIGURE 4.1 ■ Elderly people meet their needs differently from when they were younger.

HOW YOU FEEL ABOUT THE AGED

Everyone has feelings about the aged. Some people are afraid of them, or feel sorry for them, and others avoid them because they are a reminder of what may happen when they age. Think about the following statements about the aged. Get to know what your feelings are. Which of these statements are true? Are they true about all older people?

1. Old people are untidy and messy.
2. Old people tend to worry about financial matters.
3. It is normal for the elderly to withdraw from society.
4. Old people prefer to be with people their own age.
5. Old people have no friends.
6. Old people live in the past, and that is boring.
7. Old people only talk about death and are afraid of dying.
8. Old age is a problem for poor people, but not for rich people.
9. Old people prefer to be waited on hand and foot.
10. Old people remind us of what is in store for us when we age.

The **aging process** has many phases (Figure 4.2 ■). The exact combinations of physical, mental, and social changes vary from person to person. Changes may be obvious, or not. Some changes are more easily acceptable than others. There are several theories about how we age, but the results of aging are the same.

As people age, they have the same needs as they did when they were younger. The main difference is that the needs of an older person are often met in a different way than are the needs of a younger person.

aging process
changes in the body caused by growing older

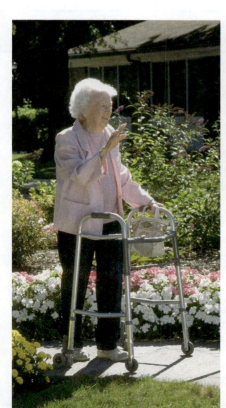
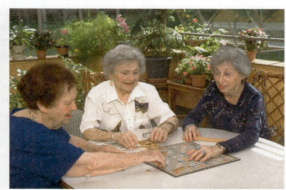
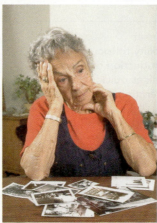

FIGURE 4.2 ■ Putting the many phases of the aging process into perspective is the best way to ensure a well-balanced life.

PHYSICAL CHANGES

As we age, visible changes occur in our body and the way it functions (Table 4.1 ■). It takes longer to walk, longer to make decisions, and longer to execute a task. The physical changes of aging are the most obvious and, for some, the most difficult to accept. These changes occur at different rates and at different ages. Every individual has his own unique schedule. Physical changes that occur in everyone are:

- Reflexes slow.
- Circulation becomes less efficient.
- Hair turns gray and may change in texture.
- All bodily processes slow.
- Skin loses elasticity and underlying fat and becomes thin and more fragile.
- Senses become less acute and aids, such as glasses or hearing aids, are needed.
- Posture becomes more stooped, and walking becomes more difficult.
- Muscles lose strength, and familiar tasks become more difficult.
- Sensing of temperature of water and air becomes less accurate.
- Healing takes longer.
- Short-term memory often decreases so directions have to be repeated often.

Table 4.1: Physical Changes of Aging

Body System or Organ	"Normal" Aging Change	Possible Problems Consequence
Skin	Decreased response to pain sensation, temperature changes, and vibration Loss of fat under skin (subcutaneous fat) and fatty padding over bony prominences (i.e., hips); change in number of blood vessels Decrease in number of sweat glands Decrease in oil production Formation of pigment cell clusters	Accidents; inability to feel hot and/or cold objects, weather changes, injury and/or pain Veins appear more prominent; wrinkles, especially facial, and folds in skin appear; occurrence of pressure sores (bedsores); slower healing; loss of hair; fluid balance of skin is difficult to maintain Difficulty in regulating body temperature Dry skin, itching, easily injured Moles and "old-age spots" (liver spots), graying of hair
Eyes	Clouding of lenses Decrease in ability to focus Decrease in production of tears Inability to blink as quickly Muscle degeneration in 50 percent of people over 70 Less light reaching retina Eyelids tend to evert or invert	Development of cataracts Difficulty seeing at night or in fluorescent lighting Dry eyes Easier to get a foreign body in the eye Central vision loss Need for adequate lighting Irritation
Ear	Decrease in ability to hear high-frequency sounds (presbycusis) Stiffness and inflexibility of ear structure	Hearing loss Distortion of sound and pain if volume is too high
Sense of taste	Decrease in number of taste buds Salty taste decreases the most, sweet next	Food may become tasteless Use of salt and sugar

Table 4.1: Physical Changes of Aging (*continued*)

Body System or Organ	"Normal" Aging Change	Possible Problems Consequence
Sense of smell	Generally declines	Difficulty smelling smoke, gas, etc., or enjoying pleasant odors
Mouth and teeth	Loss of gum and bone structure around teeth	Periodontal disease, loss of teeth
Brain	Change in reaction time and in verbal and vocabulary skills Memory loss may occur after age 50 Decrease in deep sleep Decrease in need for sleep	Slowed reactions and reflexes; inability to learn quickly Recall, recognition may slow slightly (i.e., "Where are my keys?") Periods of wakefulness during sleep hours Hours of sleep may change
Lungs and chest	Stiffness of respiratory muscles Decrease in elasticity of rib cage Decrease in area for oxygen and carbon dioxide exchange Diminished activity of cilia (help to clean lung) and diminished cough reflex	Expansion of the lungs Mild barrel chest due to structural changes Less oxygen available during physical exercise and activity Difficulty coughing and eliminating foreign particles from lung; incidence of bronchitis and pneumonia
Heart and circulatory system	Decrease in cardiac muscle strength Narrowing of arteries and veins	Cardiac output is decreased Blood pressure is increased
Musculoskeletal system	Decrease in absorption of calcium Decrease in bone replacement Loss of muscle mass and tone	Osteoporosis (thinning of bone) Incidence of fractures increases Fatigue and weakness
Balance	Less-efficient balancing mechanisms and reactions	Incidence of falls increases; standing position tends to be with flexed hip and knees
Gastrointestinal system	Decrease in esophageal muscle action Decrease in large bowel mobility, nervous stimulation Decreased sensitivity to thirst	Indigestion is more frequent, slower Constipation, diminished frequency of BMs, incomplete emptying of the bowel Dehydration
Renal system	Decrease in size of urinary bladder Decrease in kidney size Slowing of filtration, blood flow to kidney	Increased frequency of urination Increased sensitivity to medications Decreased ability to eliminate toxic wastes
Genitalia	Men Enlarged prostate gland Increased time needed to urinate Penis may be less hard Women Decreased vaginal and cervical secretions, thinning of vaginal walls Changes in estrogen after menopause	 Urinary system obstruction Increased urinary retention, frequency, and infections Decreased ability to delay ejaculation Uncomfortable intercourse, longer time to experience orgasm Changes in secondary sexual characteristics
Hormones	Decreased insulin response	Blood sugar elevation

MENTAL CHANGES

It was once thought that all older people became senile. This is a myth. Not all older people become confused, forgetful, and dependent. Those who do must be treated carefully just as you would treat any other impaired client, not as an object of pity or as a child.

Decreased circulation to the brain can cause mental changes. Medications can cause mental changes. Some changes are temporary, and some are permanent. Obvious changes in brain function are forgetfulness, disorientation, and irritability. A physical change may cause mental changes. Other mental changes are brought about as a reaction to social changes.

dementia
• loss of mental powers

Dementia is the gradual decrease in a person's ability to make judgments. This is not a normal part of the aging process. The presence of dementia and the type of dementia can be diagnosed only by a physician. Dementia used to be called senility.

Two main types of dementia are reversible dementias and those that are not. Reversible dementia is often caused by a physical, social, or chemical stimulus. When that stimulus is removed, the person reverts to his pre-dementia status. Irreversible dementia can be caused by small portions of the brain losing function due to small strokes. This condition leads to confusion, decreased mental acuity, decreased physical abilities, and decreased ability to make judgments. The client may not have the same problems all the time; he may have "good days" and "bad days." Irreversible dementia can also be caused by Alzheimer's disease (see Chapter 19, Section 8).

It is important for you to discuss with your supervisor the reason for your client's behavior. Knowing why people act in a certain way will help you in caring for them. Aged clients who are confused and forgetful require special precautions. It may be necessary to remind them where they are, who they are, and who you are. Safety is the key to the care of these clients because they are unable to make judgments on their own.

Caring for these clients takes time, understanding, and patience. It can be tiring for you to be continually with a mentally impaired client. When you feel no longer able to handle your feelings, talk with your supervisor. It may be time for a change of assignment. After all, to care for a client at the expense of a homemaker/home health aide is not good home health care.

Families of elderly clients are often stressed. Caring for an elderly relative brings with it several responsibilities. Caring for a mentally disabled elderly client is an additional set of responsibilities. Encourage your client's family to discuss their feelings with professionals. It would not be helpful for the caregivers to suffer family problems.

SOCIAL CHANGES

Many social changes affect the elderly. Some are brought about as a result of physical changes, some are brought about by society, and some just happen. Changes include:

■ Retirement
■ Change in income
■ Change in level of activity
■ Fear of illness
■ Isolation from friends and family
■ Death of a spouse

- Change in housing
- Increased dependence on others

One or two of these changes may not cause any change in your client's behavior. However, several of these changes can cause a person to change his usual behavior patterns because he will no longer be able to cope with the situation. Your client's reaction to change will depend on his usual coping ability and the result of the changes. He may become anxious, depressed, or withdrawn, or he may increase his activity. His eating habits, sleeping habits, or memory may change. He may no longer show interest in those things he used to enjoy. He may suddenly develop an interest in activities he always disliked. If you notice any of these changes in your client's behavior, report them to your supervisor immediately.

REALITY ORIENTATION

Reality orientation is a technique using the remaining brain cells to reduce the confusion often seen in clients with dementia. This program must be carefully individualized by your supervisor and requires the continued backup of the client's family and caretakers. Usually, the reality orientation board, visible to the client, contains simple, useful information so that he can function at home (Figure 4.3 ■).

The homemaker/home health aide must continually reinforce the use of this program. Your supervisor will want to know how the program is progressing, so report the following:

- Does the client understand the subjects on the board?
- Does the client remember the information? For how long?
- Is the family supportive of the reality orientation program?
- Any other observations you may make.

reality orientation
a technique to orient people to their surroundings

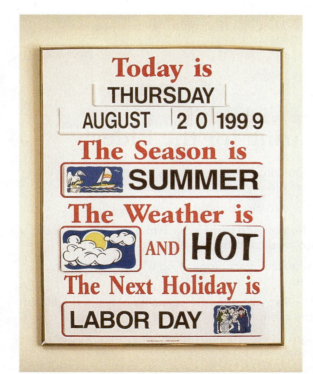

FIGURE 4.3 ■
Orienting a client to his surroundings assists him in feeling secure.

Your Role as a Homemaker/Home Health Aide

The needs of the aged are the same as the needs of all other people. It will be your responsibility to help meet these needs. By giving necessary assistance in a safe, warm, understanding manner, you help the client remain at home in familiar surroundings and be an independent person.

- Assist with all phases of personal care. A complete bath may not be necessary every day. Remember that many clients have dry, flaky, fragile skin. Lubricate the skin with lotion or oil as the client wishes. Expensive lotions are not necessary, but lubrication is.
- Observe the client for irritation, redness, bruises, and areas on the body that do not heal.
- Teach the client how to maintain his own personal hygiene when you are not in the home. A squeeze bottle filled with warm soapy water can be used after urination and bowel movements while the client is seated on the toilet. Remind him to rinse the area thoroughly.
- Provide an environment for safe, simple exercise, such as walking up stairs or moving from room to room.
- Plan your care around the client's usual household schedule and ethnic customs.
- Provide for warmth and ventilation in the home. Aged clients often react to temperature differently from younger people. They often wear sweaters in the summer. Dress and groom them in what makes them comfortable and is appropriate for their age.
- Protect them from extreme heat or cold.
- Do not disturb personal belongings, letters, pictures, and so on. You may suggest moving them, however, to another obvious place where the client can still enjoy them so that you can give better care.
- Do not use baby talk with the client.
- Do not speak about the client to others as though he were not there.
- Have patience!

SECTION 2

Special Considerations in Caring for the Elderly

OBJECTIVES

What You Will Learn to Do

1. List the important safety measures to remember while caring for an elderly client.
2. Discuss how exercise benefits the elderly client.
3. List considerations to remember while assisting elderly clients with medications.
4. Discuss your role in accompanying a client to the physician's office.
5. Become familiar with the role sexuality plays in the life of your elderly client.
6. List the signs of elderly abuse and your responsibility for reporting this.

Introduction: Areas of Special Concern as You Care for the Elderly

Although caring for an elderly client is much the same as caring for a younger client, you must be aware that the elderly often need special attention in certain aspects of their care. You will have to be extra alert in the areas of safety and exercise and in assisting them with medication. In addition, because an elderly person often is unable to report abuse or to find someone to talk to outside of his home, you will have to be his voice. This is an important role.

Because you may be the only person who sees the client regularly, you will develop a special relationship with him and will be able to notice changes in mood and activity. Report to your supervisor every change, no matter how slight, so that your client's status can be assessed and monitored. Remember, your overall goal as you care for your client is to preserve his independence, self-worth, and safety.

SAFETY

Safety for the elderly is always a prime concern. As their activity level changes, so do those things that are considered safe (Figure 4.4 ■). A situation that at one time was considered safe may, as a person ages, become a hazard. Poor eyesight, decreased reflexes, and poor hearing all contribute to accidents. In addition, many elderly attempt tasks they cannot execute and, thus, cause themselves harm. In an effort to be independent, a client may take unnecessary risks.

As people age, their ability to sense and then react to hot water is decreased. Many elderly are severely burned each year because they cannot feel that water is too hot. Teach your client to test his washing and bathing water *before* he uses it. If hot water has been run through a faucet, the faucet itself may be hot enough to cause burns should someone touch it. Briefly running cold water through the faucet after the hot water will cool the metal and prevent such burns.

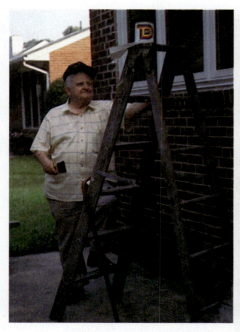 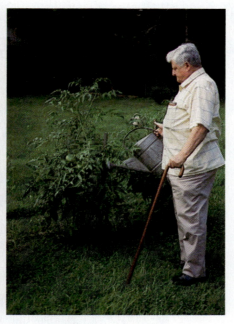

FIGURE 4.4 ■ Assist your client in accepting his limitations and making the right choice for safety's sake.

It is easier to prevent accidents than it is to heal. People who fall and break bones take months to heal and then may never regain full use of the limbs. The elderly heal slower than younger clients, so fall prevention is even more important for your elderly clients than for younger patients. Safety remains one of your primary responsibilities as a homemaker/home health aide. Help your clients maintain a safe environment in the following ways:

- Encourage your clients to discuss their capabilities realistically.
- Help provide good lighting with switches that are easy to operate.
- Encourage the use of banisters and properly installed grab bars.
- Encourage safe practices in the kitchen. Never let clients wear long, flowing sleeves while cooking.
- Set the thermostat on the water heater at a safe temperature.
- Plan emergency exits.
- Help provide for smoke detectors.
- Encourage clients to discuss their driving capabilities with their physicians.

It is important to discuss your activities with your supervisor. If you find yourself in an unsafe situation, both you and your supervisor may have to confront the client. Although we can never forget that the client has the right to act in any way he wants in his own house, it is not part of your job to remain anywhere unsafe. It is also important to determine if the client is acting in such a way as to cause harm to others. For example, does he smoke in bed? In this case, your supervisor will have to report the situation to the appropriate source. Should your client want and need structural changes in the house, your supervisor will be able to arrange for a reputable person to perform this work. Often community groups do such work for minimal pay.

EXERCISE

Health professionals now believe that planned exercise is important for everyone (Figure 4.5 ■). The benefits are many:

- A feeling of well-being
- Increased strength of bones

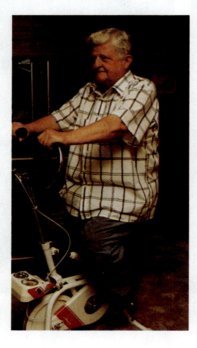

FIGURE 4.5 ■
Advise your client to always consult his physician before starting an exercise regime.

- Increased cardiac and respiratory capacity
- Increased strength and tone of muscles
- Decreased weight
- Decreased blood pressure
- Decreased anxiety
- Better sleep habits

All clients should consult their physicians before they start an exercise regime. There are many considerations before the proper regime is chosen, and only a physician can make the most informed decision. Be sure to report any change in a client's level of exercise or if you notice him having difficulty.

SLEEP CHANGES

Many elderly clients experience changes in their sleep patterns. Among the changes may be the total hours of sleep, the time of sleep, and the effect of medications. Before you suggest changes to your client's routine, try to determine what the routine was before his illness. In that way, you can compare his former activity with his present activity. Consider the following suggestions as you discuss the sleep regime best for your client.

- Limit caffeinated drinks.
- Create a relaxing, pleasant atmosphere before going to sleep.
- Develop a regular sleep schedule.
- Limit naps and time spent without activity.
- Create a regular exercise routine.
- Review medications.

Sleep is necessary to the body for optimum function. A rested client is better able to take an active part in his care and interact with others in an alert and calm manner. If your client is unable to create a regular healthful sleep routine, discuss this with your supervisor.

MEDICATIONS

Elderly clients react to medications differently from younger clients. Often elderly clients have several diseases and disabilities and take several medications for each one. The interaction of these medications often results in unexpected side effects (Figure 4.6 ■). The following can also be problems:

- The older body retains medications at a rate different from a younger body.
- Clients may stop taking medications for financial reasons, through forgetfulness, or because they read or hear news about the drug.
- The kidneys and liver of an older client remove waste products more slowly than do those of a younger client.
- Older clients often forget they have taken medications and repeat them.
- Clients may save medications that become outdated and then start taking them again.
- Older clients may have several physicians, each of whom may not be aware of all the medications that have been prescribed by other physicians.
- Clients may not discuss their reactions to medications with the physician because they believe the physician will be disappointed in their inability to take the drug.

Your role as a homemaker/home health aide is to assist your client with a safe medication schedule. Help your client maintain a foolproof, organized method of taking his medications. This method should be established by your supervisor

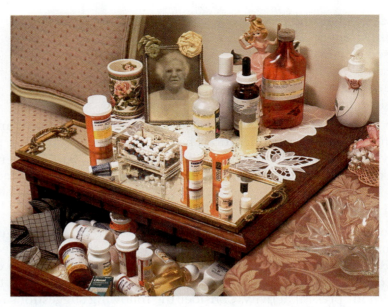

FIGURE 4.6 ■ Keeping medication in a cluttered manner fosters medication errors.

with input from you and the client. Be sure all your client's medications are prescribed for him. Borrowing medications can be dangerous! Report all side effects, no matter how slight, to your supervisor.

Be sure your client knows why he is taking his medication and the possible side effects. Talk to your supervisor if you think your client is unaware or confused about this.

When your client visits a physician, encourage him to take all his medications with him. In that way, the physician will have a clear picture of the medications your client is taking and can prescribe new ones accordingly.

Encourage your client to throw out old, outdated medications and to return medications that are not his.

Many medications are now packaged in childproof bottles. These bottles are difficult for the older client to open. Help your client order his medications packaged in containers easy for him to open and close. Clients often fail to take their medication because they cannot open the bottle.

ACCOMPANYING A CLIENT TO THE DOCTOR

You may be asked to accompany a client to a physician's office. Do not go with the client unless you have been specifically asked to do so by your agency. If the family or client asks you, check with your supervisor before you undertake this task.

It is important that you discuss your role with your supervisor. Be sure you are comfortable in the role and that you understand exactly what is expected of you. It is also important that the client and the family understand your role.

- Are you going to ensure the client's safety?
- Are you expected to discuss the client's status and care?
- Are you expected to relate to the family and to your supervisor changes in the client's medication, exercise level, or medical regime?
- What should you bring with you?

It is unwise to drive the client in your car. You should however, be sure that you know how you and the client will travel to and from the doctor's office or clinic. Be sure plans are safe and you are comfortable with them.

At the doctor's office, it is important that the client feels in control. Give the client and the physician privacy. Allow the client to speak directly to the physician whenever possible. If the information is not correct, find a respectful way to communicate this to the physician. If the physician gives you instructions or changes medication, be sure you have these changes in writing.

When you return from the doctor's visit, document the entire experience, including the time you left the house and the time you returned. Include:

- Mode of transportation
- The client's reaction to the whole experience
- Information or instructions you received from the physician's and what you did with them
- Status of the client when you left

SEXUALITY

The need for intimacy does not disappear with age, although sexual response gradually slows and frequency of activity decreases. Sex and the need for closeness, companionship, and touching are not the same. Sexual performance may decrease, but the need for human companionship does not. Sexual desire, response, and activity also are often affected by medications. Therefore, any change in sexual activity or any concern expressed by your client should be referred to your supervisor immediately.

Some medications can affect sexual desire and performance. When that is the case, clients may stop the medications rather than discuss the problem with their physicians. Often, the medications can be changed and desire and performance return. Some diseases affect sexual performance and desire. This situation should be discussed with the client so that he is aware of this possibility. If you are uncomfortable discussing this or do not have the answers to his questions, refer them to your supervisor. Do not forget about them. The fact that the client has discussed this with you indicates this is of great concern to him and his family (Figure 4.7 ■).

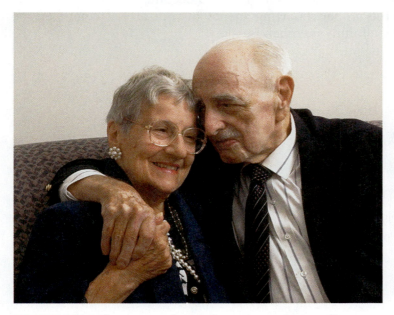

FIGURE 4.7 ■ Closeness and sexuality are necessary at all ages.

You may have preconceived notions and feelings about sexual activity between older people. It is important for you to prevent these ideas from interfering with your relationship with your client. Clients may have sexual practices unfamiliar to you. If you have concerns or questions, talk to your supervisor.

Your role as a homemaker/home health aide is to encourage your client to continue his sexual activities. If you are caring for a couple, respect their privacy and confidentiality. If your clients or their families have questions or concerns, report them to your supervisor so that counseling can be arranged.

ABUSE

abuse
any act that causes
another harm; using a
substance to excess

Abuse is any act that causes another person harm. Abuse of anybody is a disturbing situation. Abuse of the elderly is especially disturbing because the abused are often helpless to fight back and unable to call for help. Today, health professionals are seeing more and more cases of the elderly being physically and emotionally abused and neglected. There may be many reasons for abuse, but the result is always the same—an elderly person is hurt or in danger.

As you work in your client's home, you will be privileged to see and hear activities that no one else sees or hears. Be alert for signs of abuse or neglect. Common signs are:

- Bruises on a client that are hard to explain
- Fear of one particular person
- A request from a client not to be left alone with a particular person
- Conflicting stories from family members
- A "feeling" that things are not right
- Lack of nourishment and care for the client
- Lack of family concern for the safety of the client
- Exchange of abusive words between family members
- Unexpected deterioration of the client's health

The accusation that a person is abusing an elderly client is serious. Do not make it lightly. But do report immediately all activities you see that indicate the possibility of abuse. Most states require that any case of suspected elder abuse be reported. It is your responsibility to become familiar with the laws of your state and the proper reporting agency in your area. Remember, most abuse is inflicted by a family member. Be alert!

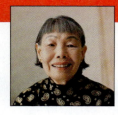

Case Study

Review the case study that appears on the first page of the chapter. Answer two sets of questions about the case study contained in the Explore and Apply sections below.

EXPLORE

1. You visit Mrs. Lee three times a week. You have been assigned to help her with her personal care, accompany her on a walk around her neighborhood, and do light housekeeping. Mrs. Lee often does not let you help her with a bath or shower. She refuses to take off her clothes to change them. Most days she does not want to go outside. You are, however, able to dust and vacuum the apartment as long as you do not go into Mrs. Lee's bedroom. Why do you think Mrs. Lee refuses your help? How do you feel about this?

2. You discuss with your supervisor your experience in this home. It is decided that you will not return to the home but be assigned to another client. The supervisor says she will call the daughter to tell her of the decision. How do you feel about this decision? Could you have done anything differently?

APPLY

1. Although Mrs. Lee seldom goes out and appears to be in good health and able to walk around, you are alert for signs of abuse. Why? What signs might you see?

2. Many Asian people live in your area, and you are sure you will be assigned to care for one of them in the future. How would you obtain more information about their culture? About the role of the aged ? About the role of the younger generation?

Certification Exam Review Questions

Choose the best answer for each question or statement.

1. **Most elderly people in the United States**
   a. *live in nursing homes.*
   b. *live with their relatives.*
   c. *have at least one chronic disease but live independently.*
   d. *have good income because of Social Security.*

2. **Most elderly people in the United States**
   a. *want to remain independent as long as they are able.*
   b. *want to be taken care of because they deserve it.*
   c. *have family who would willingly take them into their homes.*
   d. *live alone because they cannot enjoy sexual relationships any more.*

3. **Physical changes as people age**
   a. *are predictable and happen to everyone at the same age.*
   b. *often can be incorporated into a person's daily life with only a small amount of change.*
   c. *always result in the client becoming unsafe to be alone.*
   d. *can all be counteracted with medication if noticed soon enough.*

4. **Elder abuse**
   a. *is always written about but happens only in poor and rural families.*
   b. *should always be pointed out to family members when it is noted by the homemaker/home health aide.*
   c. *may be missed by one home care professional but noticed by another.*
   d. *is the private business of the family.*

5. **When going to the doctor with a client,**
   a. *it is always best to drive your car because you are familiar with your car.*
   b. *it is best to drive the client's car because then the client pays for the gas.*
   c. *it is best to take transportation that leaves you free to care for the client.*
   d. *if the client is well enough to go to the doctor, you are there only as a friend.*

CHAPTER 5

Working with Children

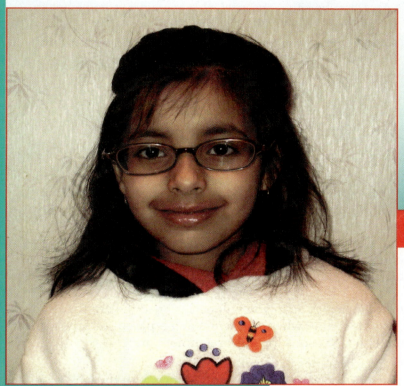

CASE STUDY

Sybil is the youngest of five children. Although she is 7 years old, she still sleeps in a crib in the same room as her 11-year-old brother. She is quiet and does not talk unless the speaker is directly in front of her and speaks slowly and loudly. Her grandmother, hoping to encourage Sybil to play with her toys, thought she needed glasses, so she bought them in a store. Sybil wears them, but because her siblings tease her she wears them only when she is alone. All the children in the house go to school; Sybil attends, but not regularly. When asked about this, her grandmother says, "She is not ready." Sybil's father works nights and sleeps most of the day. He seldom sees his other children, but when he reads the newspaper or watches television, Sybil curls up next to him.

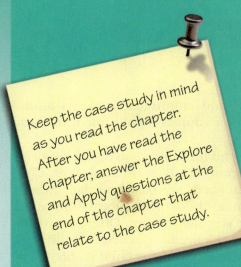

Keep the case study in mind as you read the chapter. After you have read the chapter, answer the Explore and Apply questions at the end of the chapter that relate to the case study.

Basic Needs of Children

OBJECTIVES

What You Will Learn to Do

1. List the basic physical and emotional needs of children.
2. List common ways in which children react to the stress of illness.
3. Know the difference between discipline and punishment.
4. Describe situations in which a homemaker/home health aide would care for a child as a client.
5. Describe ways in which a homemaker/home health aide would relate to a child who is not a client.

Introduction: Caring for a Child

You will relate to children when they are in the homes of your assigned adult clients. They may live there or just be visiting. This interaction calls for a different relationship than when the child is your assigned client. It is important for you to know what your relationship is with the child and his parents or guardian. When meeting a child, bend down so you are at eye level. If the child is your client, spend a few minutes alone with the child. This will signal the child's importance and allow both of you to get to know each other. You will also be able to learn about any special concerns or questions the child may have.

As a homemaker/home health aide, you will be assigned to care for children. In addition, there may be a time when you will teach a parent or family member how to care for a child. Reasons for this assignment are:

- The primary caregiver becomes ill or suffers a disability.
- The primary caregiver needs a rest from or assistance with the care of a child with an illness or disability.
- The primary caregiver must be taught, by your example, how to care for the child.
- The primary caregiver must leave the house to work.
- Child abuse or neglect has been reported or suspected.

BASIC NEEDS OF CHILDREN

Children have many of the same physical and emotional needs as adults (Figure 5.1 ■). However, they often depend on adults for fulfillment of these needs.

Just as adult needs change in importance and fulfillment, so do the needs of children. The age of the child may make certain needs more important. Children are not little adults. Their reactions and needs are based on their experiences as children. Researchers believe that a child must successfully meet specific needs at a certain age before he or she can mature. Often, when the child is ill or a family member is ill, meeting the needs completely is difficult. That is your most important role—to meet the needs of the child (Table 5.1 ■, page 76).

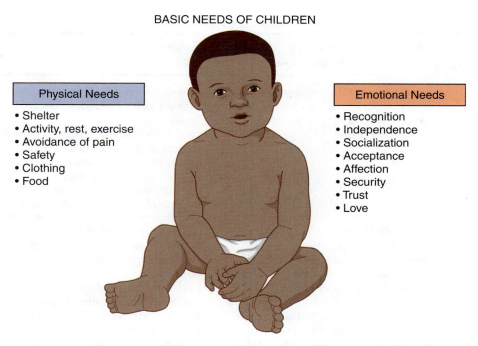

BASIC NEEDS OF CHILDREN

Physical Needs
• Shelter
• Activity, rest, exercise
• Avoidance of pain
• Safety
• Clothing
• Food

Emotional Needs
• Recognition
• Independence
• Socialization
• Acceptance
• Affection
• Security
• Trust
• Love

FIGURE 5.1 ■ Children often cannot meet their own needs and may be unable to ask to have them fulfilled. Be alert to signals that your help is needed.

CONGENITAL ANOMALIES—BIRTH DEFECTS

A **congenital anomaly** is "any abnormal organ or part of an organ present at birth, even though it may not be noted at that time." Such conditions may result from a genetic disorder or from external factors, such as exposure to toxic substances, drug use, or alcohol abuse during pregnancy. Congenital anomalies may be visible, such as a child born with a shorter arm or one born with no fingers or invisible, such as a child with a malformation of his heart.

When you work in a home with a child who has a congenital anomaly, you will assist family members as they learn to cope with the situation and the way it will affect the whole family. It is not unusual for the family to experience anger, guilt, denial, and emotional difficulties as they learn to care for this child. You must show an accepting behavior and encourage the family to seek help and support.

Discuss your feelings with your supervisor so that your actions will complement the plan of care for the whole family. Do not be disturbed if you need support during this assignment. This situation may cause you to have feelings that you will need help to understand. As you work in this house, however, be alert to separate your feelings from those of the family.

CHILDREN UNDER STRESS

Everyone reacts to stress and change differently. Children are especially sensitive to threats to their security and familiar routines. This is true both of children who are ill and those who are in homes where there is illness. You may notice a child behave in a manner that is unusual, offensive, and difficult to explain. You may notice:

■ Refusal to follow familiar household routines
■ Shyness, fear, withdrawal

congenital anomaly
a deviation from the normal, present at birth

Table 5.1: **Stages of Childhood from Birth to Adolescence**

Stage of Development	Age	Key Characteristics or Tasks of the Age	Guidelines for Activities
Infancy	Birth–1 yr.	Rapid growth; totally dependent on adults; experiences first relationship; starts to distinguish the world through his senses	Provide calm routine, taking into account infant's schedule; encourage family to participate in care; stimulation includes brightly colored objects held high or tied to crib, music, different shapes and textures, swings, carriages, rockers; toys he can put into larger containers, smooth objects that do not injure
Training period	1–3 yrs.	Attachment to mother and regular caregivers is strong; begins independence and exploration; learns to say "no"; puts everything in mouth; shows food likes and dislikes; frightened of loud noises and absence of primary caregiver; can understand simple honest explanation; may or may not share; usually starts to toilet train by age 3	Tell familiar stories again and again; do not lie, as the child does not know fact from fiction; help child become familiar with objects that are part of his care; help toilet train as the family wishes without punishment but with positive reinforcement; provide pull toys, balls, stackable objects, mirrors, threads, large beads, windup toys
Love triangle	3–5 yrs.	Girls mature more quickly; discovers sharing of friends and parents; affection and jealousy apparent; imitation; attempts to please; assumes some of his own personal care; assists with simple household chores; vivid imagination leads to stories; likes to use familiar objects over and over; approval of family important; older children like to take active part in care	Activities with hands and crayons, simple puzzles; simple ball games, and tag; always give simple reasons for activities
Middle childhood	6–12 yrs.	Peer acceptance important; easily embarrassed; asserts independence and makes his friendships; secretive; argues with adults; growth spurts; 10–12 yrs: sexual curiosity	Reasons for actions important; explain; give timeframe for schedule; provide scientific play, jigsaw puzzles, table games, board games, electronic and video games, music, puppets, sewing and crafts, model building
Adolescence	13–18 yrs.	Rapid change physically and emotionally; sexual development; mood changes; relationship sensitive; need for privacy; peer relationships important; independence important; enjoys reading, use of telephone, music; may reject familiar objects or foods; exerts his opinions, may reject suggestions from parents or caregivers but accept them from strangers; idol worship is common; concern for appearance and virility	Respect need for privacy, sexual concerns; explain all actions logically, honestly; encourage child to express his desires and interests

- Aggressive behavior
- Jealousy
- Nightmares and fears
- Denial of the condition
- Overdependence
- Bed-wetting
- Regression

When illness is present in a home, many things affect the child indirectly:

- Noise restrictions
- Attention restrictions
- Financial conditions
- Family fears
- Activity restrictions

DISCIPLINE AND PUNISHMENT

You may be faced with the subject of discipline or punishment. There is a difference. Remember, you are not the parent or guardian but the home-maker/home health aide in a work setting. **Discipline** is a set of rules that govern conduct and actions, resulting in orderly behavior. Discipline can be strict or loose. The rules can be well known or not well known. Discipline can be accepted or just followed for fear of punishment. **Punishment** is a harsh act given as a result of an offense or wrongdoing, as when a rule or discipline is broken.

The goal of directing children is to teach them behavior that is accepted by society and will foster self-reliance and independence. Children must feel good about themselves and their actions. They should not act because it will prevent punishment. Self-esteem is developed early in a child's life and is directly related to the way in which behavior is taught and reinforced.

Your role is usually to maintain the discipline already in the home. If you are going to set up new rules in the house, your supervisor will plan this carefully with you. Remember, you will be leaving this house but the other people will stay. You must set up rules they can live with when you are gone. Should you be unable to follow the discipline already in the household, report this to your supervisor. If discipline seems unusually harsh or punishment seems severe, report this with objective data. Punishment is not within your role as a homemaker/home health aide. If you believe that a child deserves punishment, discuss this with your supervisor. As you work with children, remember:

- Treat each child as an individual.
- Discuss with the child the expectations related to his behavior or a particular task. "I expect ____. Do you understand?"
- Encourage and praise children whenever possible.
- Use positive suggestions—avoid saying "Don't." Rather, say, "Please make your bed," or "Please lower the television because it is disturbing your grandfather and he cannot sleep now. Thank you."
- Explain the limits set upon the behavior before the child makes a mistake. "You may play outside until it is dark. Then you are to come in. Do you understand?"
- Make mealtime a pleasure.
- Prepare food the child enjoys.
- Encourage parents to take an active part in making decisions.
- Do not take sides in arguments.

discipline
a system of rules

punishment
action performed as the result of wrongdoing

- Suggest that people separate during an argument before harsh words are said or physical punishment takes place.
- Do not be judgmental.
- Report changes in family members.
- Report changes in family activities.
- Report feelings or suggestions and the objective happenings that lead you to your suspicions.
- Report child abuse or neglect.

Your Role as a Homemaker/Home Health Aide

Your role in each family will be different. Be sure you discuss your role with your supervisor so you understand exactly what is expected of you. Usually, you will be expected to assume one or more of the following roles:

- Teacher
- Primary caregiver
- Observer
- Stabilizer
- Assistant caregiver

Try to maintain the routine familiar to the family. The fewer the changes, the better. Familiarity maintains a feeling of security. If a child has always been involved in household tasks, it would be best to continue this. However, if the child has never taken an active part in the house or its care, this time of illness might not be the best time to start. On the other hand, it might. Use your judgment. Discuss your opinions and plans with your supervisor. It is most important that your plan reflects the best possible plan for that house and that child.

Report all your observations of behavior changes of the child and the adults in the house. You may notice many changes or few. When caring for children, remember that they are part of a unit and depend on that unit. Therefore, the behavior of other family members is important.

Be alert for observations concerning behavior in the home when you are not there! What does the child say? Do your observations agree with the child's report or the adult's report? Your personal opinions as to the responsibilities children should or should not have are not important at this time. The most important point is what works in this house!

SECTION 2

Child Abuse

OBJECTIVES

What You Will Learn to Do

1. Define and recognize various kinds of abuse.

2. Become familiar with reasons for child abuse and why children do not report it.

3. Discuss your role as a homemaker/home health aide when working in a home where child abuse has taken place.

Introduction: Child Abuse

Abuse is any act considered improper and that usually causes harm or pain to another person. No one knows exactly how many children are harmed, and no one knows why some people abuse children. Many possible reasons for abuse have been explored. Abuse may be linked to increased stress in a house and may only happen once in a while. Even if it occurs only occasionally or even once, it must be reported to protect the child and help the family as a whole.

No matter what the reasons for abuse of children, all of them result in children being either physically or emotionally traumatized. Sometimes the children report these events; but most often, they do not (Figure 5.2 ■).

abuse
any act that causes another harm; using a substance to excess

SOME REASONS FOR ABUSE

- The abuser was also abused and learned this type of behavior.
- The abuser cannot cope with the stress of having children.
- The abuser is not the parent, but the parent is unable to stop the event.

REASONS CHILDREN DO NOT REPORT ABUSE

- They are ashamed.
- They do not know whom to tell.
- They do not know any other type of behavior.
- They are afraid the abuse will increase.
- They believe they deserve it.

KINDS OF ABUSE

There are three main kinds of child abuse:

1. ***Physical:*** This form of abuse is seen when a child is beaten, tied up, and/or burned. Evidence of this abuse is usually visible, except in the case of broken bones when the evidence must be verified by X-ray.

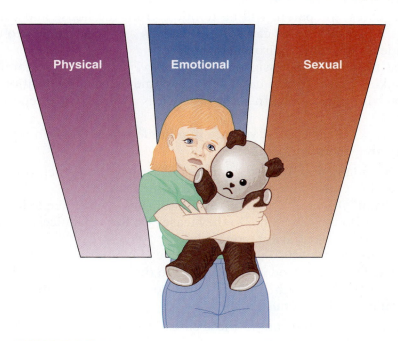

FIGURE 5.2 ■ Abuse comes in many forms. Be alert and report any concerns you have regarding abuse or neglect.

2. *Emotional:* This form of abuse is seen when a child is scared, neglected, screamed at, not permitted to feel safe, or is confined.
3. *Sexual:* This form of abuse exists when a child is forced to submit to sexual acts because of fear of either physical or emotional harm or because the child cannot prevent it.

YOUR FEELINGS ABOUT CHILD ABUSE

Many people have strong feelings about child abuse and the punishments they feel are appropriate for abusers. Some people think children should be removed from the house where they were abused. Some people feel the abusers should be put in jail. It is important to think about your feelings on this subject. It is also important to be able to work in a home where there has been abuse without judging the people. Your responsibility will be to care for the child in the family without punishing the parent or family member who is the abuser. If at any time you feel unable to work in a home where abuse has occurred, report your feelings to your supervisor.

YOUR ROLE AS A HOMEMAKER/HOME HEALTH AIDE

It is possible that you will have different roles in different cases. You must understand what is expected of you in each house. Keep in close contact with your supervisor so she can reinforce your actions and alter the plan of care as is necessary.

Your role will be determined by the situation. Sometimes, the courts will insist that a homemaker/home health aide be in the home. In this case, the parents may feel you are acting as "the police." Your main role is to provide a safe environment for the child and to support the parent in learning to cope with the problem. Learning new behavior is difficult, and your support is crucial in this situation. You will be calm and nonjudgmental and will demonstrate the proper way to interact with the child.

In some cases, the parent will be removed from the house and you will be placed there instead. In this case, you will act in a supportive way to the child and provide a safe, calm environment.

It is possible you will be assigned a client who is a member of a family where abuse is taking place. In this case, you will come by this information by accident. Report it immediately! In some states, it is a crime *not* to report such information.

No matter what the case, if you are in a home where child abuse has taken place, here are general guidelines:

- Do not be judgmental. Do not compare one case with another. Do not compare their life with yours. Be supportive to the parents.
- Be observant! Observe the family dynamics. How do the people in the family interact? Do they scream? Do they tease? Do they talk nicely to one member and in a hostile tone to another?
- Are there any signs of further abuse? Do the children have marks on them? Are they fed? Is there food in the house? Do they have a place to sleep? Are they clean? Do they laugh? Do they play? Do they seem afraid?
- Have you noticed any unusual behavior?

Your feelings are important in these cases. If you suspect something wrong in the family dynamics, report your feelings and objective observations to your supervisor immediately. Do not wait! Children cannot always protect themselves. They need adults to do it for them. The following are important to notice:

- Do the parents have activities that can be considered "adult"? Do they have friends? Do they go out?
- Is the family keeping its counseling appointments?
- Listen to what the children say. If you do not understand what they are saying, report the entire conversation to your supervisor word for word.

SECTION 3

Developmental Disabilities

OBJECTIVES

What You Will Learn to Do

1. Discuss the concept of developmental disabilities.
2. Discuss the role of a homemaker/home health aide when caring for a child with developmental disabilities.

Introduction: What is a Developmental Disability?

A **developmental disability** is any condition that interferes with the proper development of a person. There was a time when developmentally disabled people were put into institutions and not taught to be part of society. The most familiar developmental disabilities are mental retardation and cerebral palsy. These conditions interfere with the way in which a person speaks, learns, and performs activities of daily living. Although these conditions are permanent, with proper care and teaching these people can live productive and happy lives.

The exact reason people are born with developmental disabilities is not known. However, we do know that these conditions are not contagious. Four reasons people have developmental disabilities are:

1. Deficiency in the development of the fetus
2. Infection or injury during birth
3. Accident during developmental stages of a child
4. Heredity

Your Role as a Homemaker/Home Health Aide

As you care for children who have developmental disabilities, remember that they have the same needs as other children. As they become adults, they are expected to meet more and more needs themselves. If your client cannot meet all his needs, you or another adult will have to continue to help him meet his needs throughout his life.

Your feelings as you care for your client are important. Do you feel as though you are doing a worthwhile activity? Do you feel as though you are contributing to the family life of your client? Do you feel that your activities are a waste of time? Discuss your feelings with your supervisor so that the two of you can put your activities into perspective.

developmental disability any condition that interferes with the normal development of a person

Clinical ALERT

Observations About Children

Whether a child is your client or not, if you witness, hear about, or find out about something hurtful, cruel, or dangerous to a child you must report this immediately to your supervisor. Different cultures treat children in different manners, but ALL children in the United States are entitled to be safe and free from harm regardless of the culture in which they live. This is one time when cultural differences are not acceptable and should be reported.

As you work with your client, the plan of care will be determined by what your client can do when you receive the assignment and by what is expected of him in the future. You will be instructed in ways to specially feed, carry, and ambulate your client. It is important that each step be carefully planned so that the client does not get discouraged or attempt an activity that is dangerous for him. In addition, it is necessary to establish a plan the family can follow when you are not in the home and they must assume the care of the client.

Stimulation of the client is an important activity of the caregiver. You may be asked to "play" with the client. Do not neglect this activity, as it is necessary for proper development of the senses. However, different activities are appropriate for different ages and stages of development, so do not assume an activity is correct until you discuss it with your supervisor. All of your activities will fall into one of these categories:

- Supporting the family in the form of demonstration, respite, or discussion
- Encouraging independence up to the ability of the client
- Providing physical and emotional care
- Providing a safe general environment, in particular with feeding and ambulation

As you work in the home, observe the family dynamics. How do the members of the family interact with each other? With the client? Do they consider him a part of the family or merely an imposition? Are family members following the care plan when you are not in the home? The care of a developmentally disabled child can be a draining experience on all family members. Each one is affected in a different way. It is your role to observe and report family interactions that may affect the care and safety of your client. With prompt reporting, your supervisor can intervene and provide support, counseling, or other aid to the family.

SECTION 4

Newborn and Infant Care

OBJECTIVES

What You Will Learn to Do

1. Assist the mother in breast-feeding the baby.
2. Prepare infant formula.
3. Sterilize water, bottles, nipples, and caps.
4. Carry, feed, and burp a baby.
5. Provide care for an infant's umbilical cord.
6. Provide care for a male after circumcision.
7. Give a baby a bath. *pg 85*

Introduction: Care of the Infant in the Home

You may be assigned to care directly for the child or you may be caring for the mother and other family members may care for the child. Or you may be assigned to care for both mother and child.

Reasons you may care for an infant include:

- The mother is recovering from surgery.
- The mother is unable emotionally to assume the care of the child alone.

- There are many other children in the house.
- The child is ill.
- The child has been abused.

The most important part of your role in this house is to teach by example. You will not be in this house forever, and it is important that someone can take over when you leave. One of the tasks you will teach is how to hold the baby comfortably and safely.

Most infants are fed six times a day or about every 3 to 4 hours. Nursing babies, however, may be fed as often as every 2 hours. It is important to remember that some will eat more often and some less. Stick to the schedule already in place in the house. If the mother is breast-feeding her baby, it may be your responsibility to bring the baby to her when it is time for feeding. If the baby is being bottle-fed, you may need to prepare the formula. You will be given detailed instructions by your supervisor about your responsibilities. If you have a question, ask.

CARRYING AN INFANT

Carrying an infant is a big responsibility. It is important to pay close attention to many details and safety factors.

- Always support the child's head (Figure 5.3 ■).
- Hold the infant close to you.
- Do not carry other objects while you are carrying a baby.
- Do not hold an infant while you are talking on the phone or cooking at the stove.

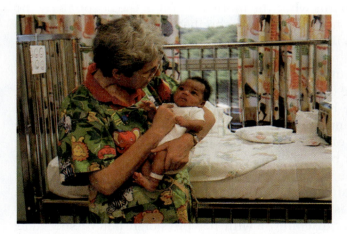

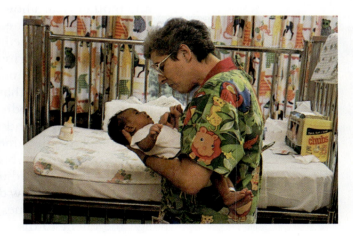

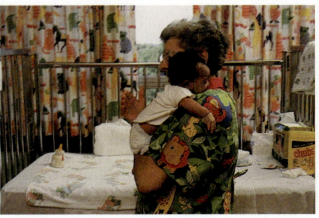

FIGURE 5.3 ■
Support the baby in a comfortable, safe, and secure manner so that you can see where you are going and can quickly reach the baby if needed.

- Do not carry a baby into a dark room. Turn on the light before you enter.
- Be alert to basic household hazards such as liquid spills, shoes, clothing on the floor, and loose rugs.
- Be alert while carrying a baby up and down stairs.
- Wear good supporting shoes with nonskid soles while you are carrying a baby.

DIET

Children's diets vary. Different pediatricians add cereal to diets at different ages. Some pediatricians insist on breast-feeding; some do not. It is important to support the family members as they learn to follow the diet their physician has prescribed. Although you may have definite feelings about the manner in which the child's diet has been ordered, do not change it. Do not change a diet or routine without discussing it with your supervisor.

Observe the pediatric client for his acceptance of the diet. If you notice the child has a great deal of gas following a meal, cries a great deal, has diarrhea or is constipated, or refuses food on a regular basis, report this to your supervisor immediately. Remember, the child is unable to ask for help himself. He needs you to report his distress.

ASSISTING WITH FEEDING INFANTS

Breast-Feeding

You will be asked to assist in the feeding of infants. In some homes, the mother will breast-feed the baby. Breast-feeding is a natural act. Most babies and mothers learn how to do this while the mother is still in the hospital. By the time they come home, the mother will probably have had an opportunity to learn basic breast-feeding skills. She will have pamphlets with pictures. If they are not enough information, ask your supervisor for additional literature.

The body makes milk about 2 to 4 days after the birth. The clear yellow fluid in the breast before that time is called colostrum. This is a nourishing substance and contains antibodies the baby needs. When breasts start to fill with milk, they become hard and full and may be uncomfortable. As the baby nurses, the body regulates the amount of milk needed to satisfy the baby, the discomfort disappears, and the breasts become soft. As the baby grows and needs more milk, the body will adjust the supply.

During the first few days after birth, nursing may stimulate the client's uterus to contract. Sometimes this is uncomfortable, and sometimes it is not. Encourage the client to discuss any discomfort with her physician before she takes medication to relieve the pain.

Most experts recommend feeding the baby from both breasts at each feeding—usually 6 to 8 minutes at each breast. The mother's nutrition greatly influences the quality of milk the body produces. The mother should eat a balanced diet, take vitamins if the physician recommends them, and increase calorie intake slightly. Some medication, alcohol, and caffeine will pass through the blood stream to the milk and to the baby. It is generally advised to avoid these substances while nursing. The client should drink 6 to 8 glasses of fluid each day. If the baby sleeps well and nurses 7 to 10 times a day during the first months of life, the milk is sufficient and the baby is nursing well.

Some families feel comfortable with having a mother feed her baby while other family members are present. Some women prefer privacy. Support the mother and the family in their decision.

■ **GUIDELINES**

Assisting with Breast-Feeding

■ Remind the mother to wash her hands before each feeding. Hands should be washed with a mild soap. Nipples are usually washed with soapy water and rinsed thoroughly during daily bathing. Washing the nipples before each feeding is not usually necessary. The mother should use circular motions, from the nipple outward, when she washes.

■ Assist the mother with nursing aids such as breast shields or pumps.

■ The decision to stop nursing is a personal one and will affect both mother and child. Suggest the mother discuss this with her physician before any decision is made.

■ If the baby does not take the breast, have the mother stroke the cheek closest to the breast with her nipple. This will cause the child to turn toward the breast (Figure 5.4 ■).

■ Support the mother as she learns the skill of breast-feeding. Provide quiet time between feedings so the mother can rest.

■ While the nipple is in the baby's mouth, remind the mother to keep the breast tissue away from the baby's nose with one or two fingers (Figure 5.5 ■).

■ If milk drips from the breast not being sucked, clean the breast. This is normal.

■ To remove the nipple from the baby's mouth, the mother should break the suction by either inserting her little finger in the corner of the baby's mouth or pushing on her breast tissue near the baby's mouth (Figure 5.6 ■).

■ The feeding routine and length of nursing will vary and should be decided by the mother and baby.

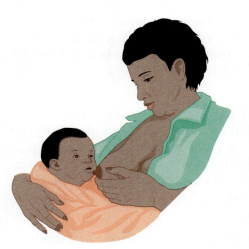

FIGURE 5.4 ■ Stimulate the baby to turn toward the breast.

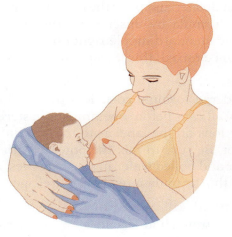

FIGURE 5.5 ■ Keep breast tissue away from the baby's nose so he can breathe more easily.

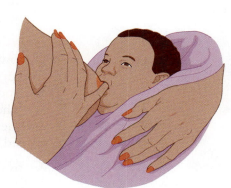

FIGURE 5.6 ■ Break the suction before removing the nipple from the baby's mouth.

You may be asked to help the mother ready herself to breast-feed. This may involve assisting the mother in getting comfortable, removing distractions, or bringing the baby, after you have changed the diaper, to the mother. Some women nurse sitting up and others lying on their side.

The mother may have questions about the timing of the feeding, ways in which to interest the baby in feeding, her diet, or care of her breasts. Assist the mother in reading the material given to her by her physician and the hospital. This material will include advice on whether to feed from both breasts in one feeding, how long to nurse, and how to supplement feedings if necessary. If this material does not answer her questions or if you have questions, call your supervisor.

Bottle-Feeding

The decision to bottle-feed an infant, or to supplement breast-feedings with formula, is made by the mother and her physician. Choosing the type of formula is also made with medical advice. Your role is to support the mother and the family with their decision. In some cases, the mother will use a special pump to remove her breast milk and put it in a bottle for use later.

STERILIZING BOTTLES AND NIPPLES

Bottles and nipples are sterilized to destroy bacteria that might cause illness. There are many opinions as to the age when sterilizing bottles is no longer necessary. Some physicians do not require sterilizing bottles for newborns. You will be asked to follow the instructions of your supervisor. If you do not agree or have questions, ask for an explanation. Do not alter the procedure without being given permission to do so.

Some people sterilize bottles and bottle nipples in the dishwasher. Others use microwave ovens. The most common method of sterilizing bottles and nipples, however, is at the stove.

THREE TYPES OF FORMULA

Ready-to-Feed Formula (Prepared Formula)

The can or bottle of formula does not need to be refrigerated before it is opened. Wash all cans and bottles before opening. This type of formula needs no preparation. Remember to shake it before opening. Open the can with a sterilized can opener and pour the contents into sterile bottles. Open bottles of ready-to-feed formula by unscrewing the cap. All you need to do now is screw a sterilized standard nipple right on the bottle the formula came in and feed the baby. Once mixed, this formula must be kept refrigerated.

Powdered Formula

Powdered formula costs less per serving than ready-to-feed formula. Wash and dry all cans before opening. Use a sterilized can opener. Carefully follow the instructions on the label as to the amounts of powder and sterile water to mix together. Be sure to mix the powder with water that you have boiled. Mix the powder and boiled water in sterile bottles, a sterile pitcher, or a sterile pot. Once mixed, this formula must be kept refrigerated.

Concentrated Liquid Formula

Concentrated liquid is the least expensive type of formula. Shake and wash all cans before opening. Use a sterilized can opener. Be sure to mix the formula according to the directions on the container. *Dilute exactly as the directions state.* Once mixed, this formula must be kept refrigerated.

PROCEDURE 2

Sterilizing Bottles

RATIONALE: Removing bacteria from baby bottles is a major factor in decreasing the possibility of infection and disease in an infant.

1. Assemble your equipment:
   Bottles
   Nipples, caps, and jar
   Bottle brush
   Dish detergent
   Hot water from the tap
   Large pot with cover or a special sterilizing pot for baby bottles
   Small towel
   Tap water
   Stove or heat source for cooking
   Timer, watch, or clock
   Tongs

2. Wash your hands.

3. Scrub bottles, nipples, and caps with hot soapy water. Use the bottle brush to clean inside the bottles. Always squirt hot soapy water through the holes in the nipples to clean out any dried-on formula.

4. Rinse thoroughly with hot water.

5. Fold the small towel to fit in the bottom of the pot and lay it there. This will prevent the bottles from breaking. (This is done when you do not have a bottle rack.)

6. Stand the washed bottles on the towel in a circle around the inside of the pot.

7. Place the caps and nipples into the clean, empty jar. Place into the pot at the center of the bottles.

8. Pour water into and around the bottles and into the jar with the nipples until two-thirds of each bottle is under water (Figure 5.7 ■).

9. Cover the pot.

10. Place the pot on the stove burner and turn on the burner to the high or full setting.

11. When the water comes to a full boil, begin timing. Allow the water to remain at a full boil for 25 minutes.

12. Remove the jar with the nipples and caps 10 to 15 minutes after the full boil begins. With the nipples still inside the jar, stand the jar on the table to cool.

13. Turn off the burner.

14. Take the cover off the pot and allow it to cool.

15. Remove the sterile bottles from the pot with sterile tongs.

16. Empty the water out of the pot. The pot is now sterilized, so you can use it for mixing the formula.

17. Wash your hands.

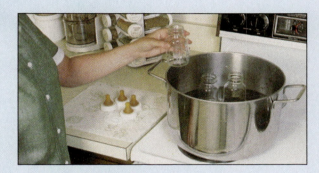

FIGURE 5.7 ■

SAMPLE CHARTING:	11/5/05 12:30 P.M. Mrs. Dow sterilized 8 bottles as per procedure and filled them with formula. Left in refrigerator. Sally Bowles H/HHA

BURPING THE INFANT

Most infants, especially those who are bottle-fed, swallow some air while drinking. Air in the gastrointestinal tract can cause vomiting and abdominal pain. You can prevent a buildup of air by feeding the infant slowly and stopping after every 2 ounces to **burp** the baby. Burping helps the baby get rid of this excess air.

There are two methods for burping a baby.

Method A: Cover your shoulder with a clean cloth. This could be a small towel or a cloth diaper. Hold the baby in a vertical position so his head is

burp
the release of air from the stomach through the mouth

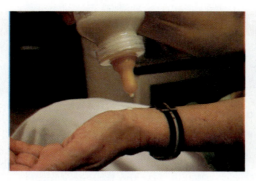

FIGURE 5.8 ■ Always check the temperature of the liquid in the bottle before
giving it to the baby.

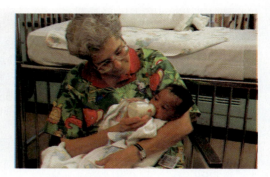

FIGURE 5.9 ■ Infants should be held
during bottle-feeding.

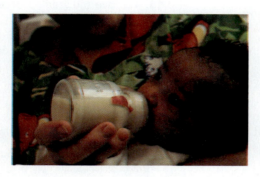

FIGURE 5.10 ■
The nipple should be full of liquid
to prevent the baby from sucking
and swallowing air.

GUIDELINES

Assisting with Bottle-Feeding Using Formula

■ Make sure that the formula is fresh and the bottles have been properly stored.

■ Follow the mother's wishes as to the temperature of the bottles when the baby is fed. If you do not agree with her wishes, discuss this with your supervisor. Check the temperature of the formula before you feed the baby (Figure 5.8 ■).

■ Babies should be held while they are given bottles. Do not prop bottles. Do not leave babies unattended while they are drinking bottles (Figure 5.9 ■).

■ Hold the bottle so that the nipple is full of formula and the baby does not suck air (Figure 5.10 ■).

resting on your shoulder. Gently rub and/or pat the infant's back until you hear the burp (Figure 5.11 ■).

Method B: Sit the infant on your leg so his feet are dangling on your side. Put one of your hands on the infant's chest, and lean the baby over so your hand supports him. Gently rub and pat the baby's back with your other hand until you hear the burp (Figure 5.12 ■).

▪ GUIDELINES

Storing Formula

■ Any opened container of formula can be refrigerated for 2 days without spoiling. After 2 days, it must be thrown away. If you do not know how long formula has been in the refrigerator, discard it. Mark the new can with the date when you open it.

■ Prepared formula will begin to spoil within 2 hours when left at room temperature. Keep the bottle refrigerated until 10 minutes before the feeding.

■ If refrigeration is not available, discuss this with your supervisor immediately, and she will arrange a way to keep the formula safe.

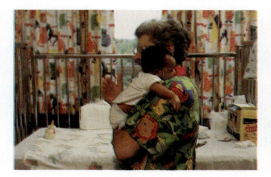

FIGURE 5.11 ■ Support the baby against your shoulder as you gently pat his back.

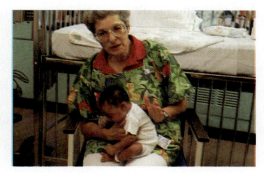

FIGURE 5.12 ■ Support the baby as you gently pat his back. Be sure his head is well supported.

OBSERVING THE INFANT'S STOOL

You will need to observe the infant's **stool** or bowel movement at each diaper change to detect **constipation** or **diarrhea**. A baby is constipated when the stool is hard and well formed. A baby has diarrhea when he has frequent watery bowel movements. When you observe a change from what has been normal for your client, report your observations to your supervisor and to the mother.

The bottle-fed infant will have stools that are yellowish or mustard-colored. They will be lumpy, but soft. One to three bowel movements each day is normal for an infant who is bottle-fed every 3 to 4 hours. It is not unusual for the stools of bottle-fed babies to look as if there are tiny seeds in them.

The breast-fed infant will have stools that are yellowish or mustard-colored, but the color may change slightly and may appear to have a greenish tint, depending on the mother's diet. The stools of infants who are breast-fed will be looser and smoother than those of bottle-fed infants. A bowel movement after every feeding or only once or twice a day is usual for an infant who is breast-fed every 3 to 4 hours.

Diarrhea in infants can be a serious problem and requires immediate attention. An infant with diarrhea can become dehydrated within 2 days. You will see a change in the infant's elimination pattern and in the color and consistency of the stools when an infant has diarrhea. The stools may appear green and watery, running right out of the diaper. There may be a foul odor, and stool frequency will increase as compared to the infant's normal habit. Report to your supervisor at the first sign of diarrhea, and encourage the mother to call the physician.

stool
solid waste material discharged from the body through the rectum and anus. Other names include feces, excreta, excrement, bowel movement, and fecal matter

constipation
having hard, difficult-to-expel bowel movements

diarrhea
abnormally frequent discharge of liquid fecal matter

Diarrhea has many causes in infants. It may be caused by equipment not sterilized properly, by carelessly prepared or spoiled formula, or by allergies. Much diarrhea is caused by passing bacteria to the infant from the hands of those who handle him. This is the reason proper handwashing is essential when caring for an infant. Encourage everyone who handles the infant to wash their hands frequently and certainly before handling the baby or equipment used in his care. Be sure to explain why you are asking them to do this to avoid offending anyone.

DIAPERS

Diapers are used to catch the urine and stool babies expel. By using diapers, you help keep the babies and their environment clean and free of waste material. The methods used to diaper a baby and the types of diaper used vary from house to house. It is important for you to try and follow the wishes of the family as you care for the baby. Remember, they will continue to care for the child after you have left the home.

CARE OF THE UMBILICAL CORD

Before birth, the **umbilical cord** serves as a lifeline, connecting the **fetus** with the mother's **placenta**. All nourishment is passed from mother to fetus through the umbilical cord. At the time of delivery, the cord is clamped and cut and the healing process of the umbilicus begins. Within 5 to 10 days, the cord will become dry, turn black, and eventually fall off, forming the **umbilicus**. This does not hurt the baby.

CIRCUMCISION

Circumcision is the surgical removal of the loose piece of skin, the **prepuce** (foreskin), from the end of the penis (Figure 5.13 ■). It may be done to increase the cleanliness of the penis. Circumcision can be done in the operating room before the baby comes home. It is always a voluntary procedure. That means that

umbilical cord
long, flexible, round organ that carries nourishment from the mother to the baby. It connects the umbilicus of the unborn baby in the mother's uterus to the placenta

fetus
developing infant in the uterus, after the first 2 months

placenta
oval, spongy structure in the uterus from which the unborn baby receives its nourishment. Sometimes called afterbirth, the placenta is discharged from the mother's body soon after childbirth

umbilicus
small depression on the abdomen that marks the place where the umbilical cord was originally attached to the fetus; belly button

circumcision
removal of the foreskin of the penis by a surgical procedure

prepuce
foreskin of the penis, often removed in a procedure called a circumcision

▪ GUIDELINES

Changing Diapers

- Change the diapers often to decrease odor and irritation of the baby's skin.
- Clean the baby's genital area each time you change the diaper. Apply lotion or cream as you have been instructed.
- If you use cloth diapers, rinse the stool from them in the toilet before you put them into a diaper pail.
- If you use rubber pants on top of cloth diapers, be sure the elastic is loose enough to allow air to circulate in the pants.
- Do not use rubber pants over disposable diapers, as they already have moisture-proof protection.
- Do not flush disposable diapers down a toilet. Dispose of them as the family wishes and as you know to be aseptically correct.
- Observe the baby's skin each time you change the diaper for color, texture, and discharge. Report any changes to your supervisor.

◦ GUIDELINES

Care of the Umbilical Cord

■ Keep the diaper folded down away from the cord. A wet diaper on top of the cord could cause an infection.

■ Ask your supervisor if you may use alcohol. Follow her instructions.

■ At every diaper change, wash the cord with plain rubbing alcohol on a cotton ball. The alcohol will help speed up the drying process and will keep the cord clean.

■ Never pull on the cord. Let it fall off by itself. Laying the infant on his abdomen will not hurt the cord. Binders or belly bands are not advised.

■ Never give the infant a tub bath until the cord has fallen off.

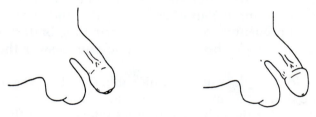

FIGURE 5.13 ■ The choice of whether or not to circumcise a son is a personal one. Support the family with their decision.

the mother of the baby must give her permission to have it done. In the Jewish faith, there is a ritual circumcision on the seventh day after birth. This is done either in the hospital or at home.

The physician will give the mother special instructions as to the care of the penis. Be sure and follow these instructions carefully to prevent complications.

BATHING THE INFANT

Sponge Baths

While the umbilical cord is still attached to the baby, a sponge bath with warm water or baby lotion can be given daily. More frequent bathing is usually unnecessary. A tub bath is not permitted until the cord has fallen off.

◦ GUIDELINES

After Circumcision

■ Keep the penis protected from rubbing on a diaper. The pediatrician will leave instructions.

■ Ask about bathing the child. If the physician does not leave instructions about bathing the baby, ask your supervisor.

■ Keep the penis clean and free of fecal matter.

■ Observe for bleeding or drainage. Report these to your supervisor.

Sponge bathing an infant means gently washing each part of the baby's body with mild soap and warm water, but not submerging the infant in water. Safety of the infant is most important. Whenever in doubt about anything, call your supervisor. A safe table or counter is a convenient place to give a sponge bath. Clear off the counter and wash it well. Spread a towel on the counter to make a soft warm place on which to place the baby. Prepare warm water, mild soap, washcloth, blankets, and towels before bringing the baby to the counter. Only one part of the body is washed at a time. Wash, rinse, and dry each body part or area well. Then cover the body part right away with a towel or blanket.

Tub Baths

After the cord has fallen off, the infant can be given a tub bath. You can use a large sink or a baby bathtub. If you are using a sink, be sure to clean the sink and counter. Scrub the sink with a cleanser and rinse it thoroughly. Assemble your equipment before you begin so you will not need to leave the room for something you may have forgotten. Lock the front door so no one can come in and distract you or the infant's mother. Taking the phone off the hook, if the mother agrees, will prevent it from ringing during the bath. You cannot leave the infant in the tub or on the counter while you answer the phone or the doorbell.

Bath time should be a pleasant and enjoyable time for the mother and baby. Try to involve the mother as much as she is able, and take the opportunity to teach her how to care for the baby. The infant's safety is your first responsibility. Keep your hands and eyes on the baby throughout the bath.

INFANT SAFETY

When you care for an infant, you must take special precautions to protect the baby from preventable accidents. Even if an infant has not yet learned to roll over, he can wiggle and kick until he falls off beds, chairs, tables, or counters. Never leave an infant unattended on any of these surfaces. If you are far from the infant's crib and you must leave him unattended for a few seconds, put him on the floor. The safest place for an infant is in his crib with the side rails up. Some people keep babies in a carriage or a drawer because they do not have a crib. Here are other ways you can prevent accidents when caring for an infant:

- Wash your hands before handling the infant or his supplies.
- Place the infant on his side or belly after feeding to prevent aspiration.
- Keep the crib rails in the up position when the infant is sleeping or playing.
- Use only 1 to 2 inches of bath water, and never leave the infant alone in the water.
- Never place an infant in an infant seat on tables, chairs, beds, or counters.
- Keep all medications and cleaning solutions out of the reach of all children.

ASSISTING WITH MEDICATION

A child you are caring for may require medication. In that case, the family will take responsibility for giving the medication. Although you may assist, you may not be the person who assumes the responsibility of giving the medication. (See Chapter 18.)

Your role is to observe the child after he has received the medication. If you notice any change in his behavior, call your supervisor immediately.

PROCEDURE 3

Giving an Infant a Tub Bath

RATIONALE: Bathing an infant removes bacteria, increases circulation, and allows close interaction between infant and caregiver.

1. Assemble your equipment:
   Infant tub or sink
   Two bath towels (soft)
   Cotton balls
   Washcloth
   Warm water (warm to the touch of the elbow)
   Baby soap
   Baby shampoo (optional)
   Baby powder, lotion, or cream
   Diaper
   Clean clothes

2. Wash your hands.

3. Wash the sink or tub with a disinfectant cleanser and rinse thoroughly.

4. Line the sink or tub with a bath towel.

5. Place a towel on the counter next to the sink or tub, as you may want to lay the infant down to dry him.

6. Fill the tub or sink with 1 to 2 inches of warm water (warm to the touch of the elbow).

7. Undress the infant, wrap him in a towel or blanket, and bring him to the tub or sink (Figure 5.14 ■).

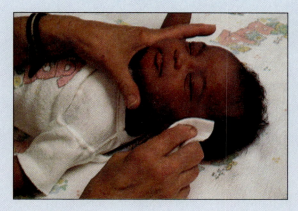

FIGURE 5.15 ■

9. To wash the hair, hold the infant in the football hold, with the baby's head over the sink or tub. This will free your other arm to wet the hair, apply a small amount of shampoo, and rinse the hair.

10. Dry the infant's head with a towel.

11. Unwrap the infant, and gently place him on the towel in the sink or tub. One of your hands should always be holding the baby. Never let go, not even for a second.

12. Wash the infant's body with the soap and the washcloth, being careful to wash between the folds (creases) of the skin (Figure 5.16 ■).

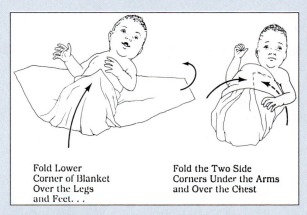

Fold Lower Corner of Blanket Over the Legs and Feet. . .

Fold the Two Side Corners Under the Arms and Over the Chest

FIGURE 5.14 ■

8. Using a cotton ball moistened with warm water and squeezed out, gently wipe the infant's eyes from the nose toward the ears. Use a clean cotton ball for each eye (Figure 5.15 ■).

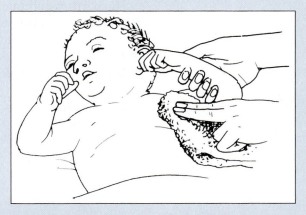

FIGURE 5.16 ■

13. If the infant is female, always wash the perineal area from front to back (Figure 5.17 ■).

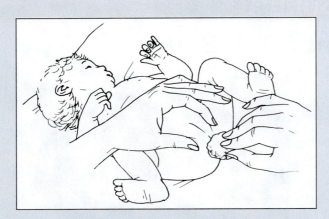

FIGURE 5.17 ■

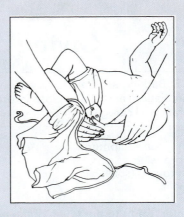

FIGURE 5.18 ■

14. If the infant is male, clean the foreskin by gently retracting it. If the child has been circumcised, this is not necessary.

15. Rinse the infant thoroughly with warm water.

16. Lift the infant out of the water and onto the towel you laid out on the counter.

17. Dry the infant well, being careful to dry between folds of skin.

18. Now you can apply powder, lotion, or cream to the infant, whichever the mother prefers or as instructed by your supervisor.

19. Diaper and dress the infant (Figure 5.18 ■).

20. Place the infant in his crib, or allow the mother to hold him. Show the mother how to hold the infant in either the upright or cradle position.

21. Clean and return equipment and supplies to their proper place.

22. Clean the area where the bath was given.

23. Wash your hands.

SAMPLE CHARTING:	1/15/04 12:00 P.M. Bath given. No red area noted on skin. Baby seemed to enjoy the experience. Queenie Jones H/HHA

Common changes that should be reported are:

■ Rash or any change in the skin color or texture
■ Irritability, confusion, or unusual "fussiness"
■ Change in sleep pattern
■ Pain that persists and is not removed by the medication
■ Vomiting, diarrhea, or constipation
■ Change in breathing pattern
■ Confusion
■ Seizures

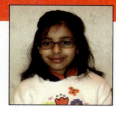

CHAPTER REVIEW

Case Study

Review the case study that appears on the first page of the chapter. Answer the questions contained in the Explore and Apply sections below.

EXPLORE

1. You were asked to visit the home each morning and assist the grandmother with sending the children off to school, setting up the day's routine, and giving the grandmother some time off. You have suggested that she leave the house and visit friends or do something for herself. She refuses and stays home. The case referral from the school nurse indicates concern as to why Sybil does not attend school regularly. It was suggested that another person in the home would assist the grandmother and provide useful information to the authorities. How to you feel about being in a house to gather information? You make several suggestions about simplifying the morning routine, including asking the children to take part in clearing the table and making their beds. This is met with anger by the children and silence by the grandmother. What do you do?

2. How do you deal with the fact that the father of the house is unavailable to the children other than Sybil? What information would you gather about the relationship between the father and his children? What would you do with this information? What information would you gather about the relationship between the father and the grandmother? What would you do with this information?

APPLY

1. Sybil has started following you around the house. Since her grandmother seems interested in broadening Sybil's experience, what help can you offer her as you work around the house?

2. You notice that Sybil sees better with her glasses and seems to want to learn new things. Do you discuss this with your supervisor? Do you discuss this with the grandmother? Do you call the school and talk to the school nurse? Do you suggest that the child must go to school or the grandmother will be violating the law?

Certification Exam Review Questions

Choose the best answer for each question or statement.

1. **The basic needs of children are**

   a. *the same as adults.*

   b. *not the same as adults.*

   c. *your responsibility to meet.*

   d. *the responsibility of an adult to meet until the child is able to meet them.*

2. **Children usually develop according to predictable pattern.**

   a. *Comparing one child to another tells you what to expect.*

   b. *Children within a family usually follow the same developmental schedule.*

   c. *Developmental charts are only guidelines; each child is different.*

   d. *It is not necessary to consider culture when reviewing the developmental stages of a child.*

3. **In your role as a homemaker/home health aide, you will often be in the house with children who may or may not be your clients. Your responsibility pertaining to child abuse is to**

   a. *observe and report to your supervisor what you see.*

   b. *tell the abuser you will call the police if the abuse doesn't stop.*

   c. *take the child out of the house immediately.*

   d. *call your supervisor and objectively report exactly what you observe immediately.*

4. **Assisting someone learning to care for an infant often is difficult because**

   a. *people usually know how to do it and resent being helped.*

   b. *it may not be within their cultural role.*

   c. *they should be able to read books in their native language.*

   d. *homemaker/home health aides are only in the house for a few hours and therefore have nothing to offer.*

5. **When caring for an infant, you should**

   a. *teach the caregiver that what you have experienced is helpful because you know what will work.*

   b. *find out what the caregiver already knows. How the caregiver feels about the baby will provide useful information on which you can build.*

   c. *give the caregiver a book to read, which will always reassure them.*

   d. *observe everyone in the house caring for the baby and then decide which person would be the best primary caregiver.*

CHAPTER 6

Care of the Dying in the Home

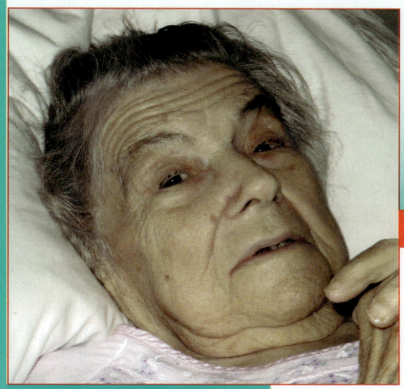

CASE STUDY

Mrs. Bell is 86 years old and lives with her husband of 60 years. She has just been told she has advanced breast cancer. Mr. and Mrs. Bell have decided that she will be cared for at home without any treatment or heroic measures to prolong her life, and they will face this as they have faced everything . . . together. Mr. Bell has learned how to manage the pain medication and, working with the nurses and volunteers, he cares for his beloved wife. He will accept help only once in awhile from you. Mrs. Bell eats small amounts of pureed food and drinks little. The three children and ten grandchildren visit and help with the shopping, laundry, cooking, and cleaning. They update their grandparents on their activities, and the little children draw them pictures, which hang around the bedroom. The children confide in you that they do not know how their father will manage when their mother dies. When they try to talk to their father, he says, "Don't worry, it will work out."

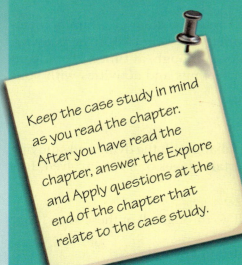

Keep the case study in mind as you read the chapter. After you have read the chapter, answer the Explore and Apply questions at the end of the chapter that relate to the case study.

Dying

OBJECTIVES

What You Will Learn to Do

1. Understand the steps that occur when a person is dying.
2. Understand the client's and family's special emotional needs.
3. Be a good listener to the client and family.
4. Examine your first experience with death and understand how it has affected you.
5. Become familiar with the hospice concept and use part of it when working with the client.
6. Understand the client's choice of a do not resuscitate order.

Introduction: Working with the Client Who is Dying

Many of us feel uncomfortable when we are around a person who is dying. We may not know how to act or what to say to him. We may feel sad or helpless or angry. These feelings may be strong indeed if the person is the same age we are or a member of our family. Sometimes, we deal with our feelings by avoiding working with the person who is dying, or we rush through our tasks as quickly as possible so that we can leave the room. This often leaves the dying person feeling isolated, lonely, or deserted.

To avoid this happening, as a homemaker/home health aide, it will be your responsibility to help meet the special needs of the dying person and his family. Do not be frightened by the thought of helping the client who is dying. Using the same caring, consideration, and understanding you use with clients who will recover will help you work with clients who are dying. After all, we all will die one day, and we must remind ourselves to treat these people as we would like to be treated if we were dying.

Many clients are told they are dying. This must be done by a family member or physician. If a family decides not to let your client know he is dying, you are obligated to carry out their wishes even though, at times, keeping up this charade is most difficult. Discuss your feelings and activities with your supervisor.

STEPS IN THE DYING PROCESS

Dr. Elisabeth Kübler-Ross spent many years talking with the dying and studying how people die (Figure 6.1 ■). She found certain stages or steps involved. It is most important to remember the following:

- All clients are different.
- The family of the person who is dying will go through all of these steps.
- Everyone will not experience every step.
- Clients and families will go from step to step at any time.
- Clients do not go through these steps in any given order.

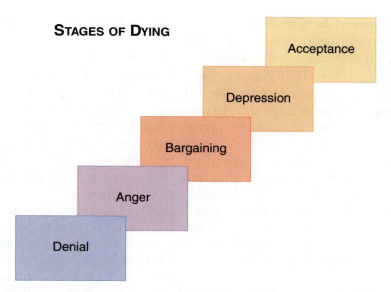

STAGES OF DYING

Acceptance

Depression

Bargaining

Anger

Denial

FIGURE 6.1 ■ Everyone passes through these stages at different rates and sometimes in a different order.

STEP 1: *Denial*—"Not me!"

STEP 2: *Anger*—"Why me?"

STEP 3: *Bargaining*—"Me, but . . ."

STEP 4: *Depression*—"Ah, me."

STEP 5: *Acceptance*—"Yes, me."

SPECIAL EMOTIONAL NEEDS OF THE DYING

Clients who are dying are still living people and have the same needs as you, including:

■ *The need to be normal:* to know that their thoughts and feelings are like those of others in their situation.

■ *The need for meaningful relations:* a chance to talk to friends and family members on a meaningful level.

■ *The need for love:* to feel that they are the object of someone's love (Couples may have sexual exchanges).

■ *The need for recreation:* ways to pass the time. These may include knitting, playing cards, watching TV, reading books, or talking to loved ones.

■ *The need for safety and security:* to know that they will be cared for carefully up until the moment of death.

BE A GOOD LISTENER

When a client suspects that he is going to die, he may react in various ways:

■ He may ask everyone about his chances for recovery.

■ He may be afraid to be alone and want a lot of attention from you.

■ He may ask a lot of questions.

■ He may seem to complain constantly.

■ He may make requests that seem unreasonable.

Usually, when a client asks questions of his caregivers, he is sending a signal that he wants information. Many times, you may not have all the information needed to answer the questions. Assure the client that you will either find the information or provide someone who will.

Here are guidelines you may wish to use when talking with a client who is dying:

1. *Honesty.* If you don't know, be honest and say so. The client probably does not expect you to know everything about his condition anyway.
2. *Do not offer false hope or reassurance.* By telling a dying person that he will be better soon, the homemaker/home health aide is proving she cannot be trusted. Offer realistic short-term goals or say nothing.
3. *Do not say too much.* A caring look, an unhurried manner, a nod, or word at the right time tells the client that you care. Example: "I understand how you feel. I think I would feel the same way."
4. *Let the client take the lead.* Often, a question represents a fear or concern of the client. He may feel relieved if you allow him to express the concern. Example: "I don't know when you'll die. Why do you ask?"
5. *Do not destroy hope.* If the client really believes that he will recover, even if you know he won't, do not destroy this hope. Hope is an important part of life. The client who has hope usually lives longer than the client who does not. Example: "I'm happy to hear of your plans to go on a trip next year."

✔ **hospice**
program of care that allows a client who is expected to die within 6 months to remain at home and die at home while receiving professionally supervised care

palliative care
✔ a multidisciplinary approach to managing care of people who are dying that includes curative medical intervention

Many areas of the country have **hospice** programs. These are organized systems of professional care that help families care for clients who are expected to die within 6 months at home up to and including the time of death. The hospice concept is not appropriate for everyone because not everyone is able to die at home without any heroic methods. You can apply many principles of hospice care to your work with clients without actually having a hospice program.

Most hospice clients do not wish any treatment except to remain comfortable and pain-free. This is often difficult for families to accept. These programs support and help the dying client and his family without the use of curative methods. **Palliative care** is a multidisciplinary approach to managing pain and caring for a client and family when the client is seriously ill, suffers from a chronic illness, or is dying. Clients who have palliative care programs may not be expected to die within 6 months and need not forego curative medical treatments.

The primary goal of palliative care is to give the client the best possible life during their illness through pain and symptom management and client and family support. Support and/or physical care may last a short time or an extended time such as months or years.

Hospice and palliative care programs share many elements, including philosophy and caregivers, but the requirements of each program may differ. It is important for the family and client to understand all elements of the program in which they enroll. Refer all questions or concerns to your supervisor or the program director.

While you are in the home, your responsibilities for clients in either program will be much the same and will include:

■ Treating the client/family as a unit of care.
■ Allowing the client/family as much choice as possible in determining care in the home.
■ Making use of team professionals experienced in home health care.
■ Helping the family through the dying process.
■ Helping the family after the death of their loved one.

Both programs use trained volunteers to help with transportation, shopping, and assisting the client with hobbies and other important things that paid

Clinical ALERT

Palliative Care
The principles of palliative care can be applied to all clients. The way in which different cultures and individual clients view pain and medication is important when creating a focus of care. Be aware of your personal views because they influence the client. Always report your observations of the client, his family, and the effects of medication and other therapies in a timely and objective manner so any needed changes can be made.

employees seldom have time to do. Program volunteer training sessions prepare community members to work with the dying and their families.

If you find yourself caring for a client in a family where you consider hospice or palliative type care appropriate talk to your supervisor. She will discuss the client's situation with the physician. Do not take it upon yourself to recommend either program.

You may also have a client who has refused aggressive treatment and has decided to die. This may be hard for you to accept. Remember, this is the client's decision and you must accept it. If you have difficulty working in this house, discuss it with your supervisor.

ADVANCE DIRECTIVES FOR HEALTH CARE

All Americans have the fundamental right to make choices about their health care treatment. They can accept or refuse treatments so long as they are able to understand the consequences of those choices.

However, when a person suffers from a disease or injury that takes away their ability to understand and make decisions about health care, they often suffer through treatments that they may not have wanted. Family members often consent to treatments for their loved one because they do not know what the patient would have wanted and they are afraid to withhold any treatments. Such treatments may include ventilators, feeding tubes, dialysis, and other aggressive life-prolonging interventions.

Laws have been created in all states to allow competent adults to create a document that makes choices about life-sustaining and life-prolonging treatments before an illness or injury strikes and before they may lose the capacity to make decisions for themselves. These documents are called "**advance directives for health care**," commonly called "**living wills**." The document is created by someone who has decision-making capacity and can describe their wishes with regard to future health care treatment choices. The document may also name a "**health-care proxy**" whom they designate to make treatment choices for them in the event they become unable to do so. Each state has specific requirements for the advance directive to be valid. Therefore, the document should be tailored to the state in which the client lives.

It is important to know if your client has an advance directive and that the doctor and your supervisor are aware of it. A copy should also be on the medical chart. Some clients keep living wills in a drawer or file, and no one knows where it is or even to look for it. Unless everyone is aware of it, the advance directive cannot be followed in the event the patient loses his or her ability to make decisions. *Remember:* As long as a client can understand and make choices, the advance directive is *not* effective. It is implemented only if the client loses the capacity to make health care decisions. In addition, an advance directive becomes effective only after these three steps:

1. A physician determines that the patient has lost decision-making capacity
2. A physician determines the patient's diagnosis and prognosis
3. A physician has evaluated the wishes as expressed in the document to determine what the patient may want or not want.

This means that advance directives do not become "operative" in a medical emergency setting. If a call for emergency medical services (EMS) is placed, the EMS providers will not take time to read the advance directive and do not have the expertise to determine the patient's prognosis. Advance directives are often confused with do not resuscitate (DNR) orders, but they are **_not_** the same.

advanced directive for health care/living wills
Legal documents that describe the wishes of a person regarding health care to be used when they can no longer make choices for themselves

health-care proxy
a person designated to make health-care-related decisions when a person can no longer do so

Patients who have advance directives do not necessarily have DNR orders; and patients with DNR orders do not necessarily have advance directives. A discussion of DNR orders follows.

Do Not Resuscitate Orders

do not resuscitate (DNR)
A legal document that states a person's wishes for no attempt to reverse his death when his heart stops beating

In most states, a client at home may elect a **do not resuscitate (DNR) order**. This means that if his heart stops beating or if he stops breathing, no attempts will be made to reverse his death. No CPR should be initiated for patients who have DNR orders. This DNR order may be indicated by a special bracelet or a special DNR document located in a prominent place. DNR orders must always be written by the patient's physician (or in some states by an advanced practice nurse). A decision to write a DNR order for a setting other than a hospital is always discussed with the patient and/or the patient's surrogate decision maker (family or guardian) prior to writing the DNR. A DNR order may be rescinded by the patient or by the patient's surrogate/guardian. In all other cases, it should be respected and honored by all health-care providers and EMS professionals.

Different states have different DNR practices for outside of the hospital and it is important that you are familiar with the practice and the forms used in your state. It is also important to know if the EMS organization in your area will honor these DNR orders when they are called to a client's home.

CPR and resuscitation attempts at the end of life for patients in whom death is expected are not appropriate interventions. DNR orders are meant to allow death to occur naturally and with respect for the patient's dignity.

Understanding Your Feelings about Death

A person's first exposure to death (usually as a child) affects how the person will react to death for the rest of his life. The time, place, and manner of death we experience may be different, but the feelings are the same. To help you deal with your feelings, it is often helpful to think about death and your feelings. You may want to think about the different feelings you experience when you discuss the death of a baby, a young person, an older person, or a terminally ill person. Some people feel differently about the death of a person when it occurs suddenly. You may want to share these feelings with a close friend, member of the clergy, or someone you trust.

There is no right or wrong way to feel about death or to react to death. It is an individual experience.

Some families treat death as a solemn religious experience; some do not. You will be asked to support the family as they deal with this experience within their culture, their coping mechanisms, and their family dynamics.

SECTION 2

Physical Care of the Dying

OBJECTIVES
What You Will Learn to Do

1. Make a dying client as comfortable as possible.
2. Help meet the physical needs of the client and family.

Introduction: Physical Needs

The client who is dying usually needs careful attention to physical needs. You will have to attend to many needs that the person used to attend to himself. Allow the client to do as much as possible for himself. This permits him to be independent for as long as he is able. Discuss with your supervisor your activities and what the family will do. Here are guidelines for care:

- *Skin care.* Bathe daily, with partial bathing as necessary. The skin may be fragile, so wash gently with mild soap. Apply lotion to bony prominences.
- *Positioning.* Do not allow tight clothing, stockings, garters, or tight bed linens. Use pillows and rolled blankets for careful positioning. Change the client's position often, at least every 1-1/2 to 2 hours. Change soiled linens and protective pads. Change nonsterile dressings when soiled. Reinforce sterile dressings.
- *Mouth care.* Cleanse teeth and mouth at least twice daily. Remove dentures, or brush teeth. Cleanse mucous membranes with glycerine swabs, as needed.
- *Bowel care.* Keep a careful record of bowel movements, and notify the nurse if the client has not had a bowel movement in several days.
- *Circulation.* The circulation slows as death approaches, and the arms and legs may feel cold and look ashen. Elevate the limbs as needed to aid blood return and do not allow the limbs to be in a "dependent position."
- *Food/water.* Assist the client to a comfortable position and cleanse the mouth. Wash his hands, refresh the linen. Air the room of any odors. Do not try to mask odors with perfume or spray, but remove the source of the odors. Ask the client and his family about food choices and seek as much variety as possible. Offer small portions of food and frequent sips of water so as not to tire the client with long meals. Arrange portions in a neat, appetizing manner.
- *Breathing.* Remove secretions from the mouth as necessary. Urge the client to cough up mucous for as long as possible. Elevate the head of the bed or prop the client on pillows if this makes breathing easier.

THE MOMENT OF DEATH

Many clients now choose to die at home rather than return to the hospital. Usually, the nurse has prepared the family for the moment of death and related events.

Many clients die as they have lived. The fearful die in fear, the angry die in anger, and the peaceful die in peace. Some simply slip into a coma for days before the death, and others cling constantly to a loved one's hand.

Dying is a spiritual process for some people. Many clients and families ask to see a priest, minister, rabbi, or person who shares the same concept of spirituality. As the time of death nears, services or prayer rituals may be held at the bedside, and privacy will be requested.

Breathing may become irregular and stop for periods of up to 30 seconds or more. This breathing is called **Cheyne-Stokes** breathing, and although it may be upsetting to the family, it is a usual occurrence. As death approaches, the gurgling breathing called the death rattle may begin. At this time, the client is usually unconscious, so it does not bother him, but it may be distressing to the family. Notify the supervisor when it begins.

Cheyne-Stokes
a type of noisy breathing alternating with periods of no breathing; usually precedes death

Talk openly and in a concerned way to the client, even when he is seemingly unconscious. Hearing is the last sense to be lost, and loving words from a family member, up until the moment of death, are comforting. Plan with your supervisor exactly what you will be expected to do when the death occurs. Whom should you call? What should you do?

Your reaction to the actual death depends on your experience with death, your culture, your religion, and how open you are in expressing and voicing your feelings. Usually, homemakers/home health aides feel sadness and loss when a client dies. This is normal. The agency you work for may hold special "support sessions" for those aides and nurses who have had a client die so that they can discuss their feelings and help each other. Check with your agency regarding the availability of support services.

SECTION 3

Postmortem Care

OBJECTIVES   **1.** Describe postmortem care.
What You Will Learn to Do

Introduction: Postmortem Care in the Home

postmortem
after death

Care of the body after death is called **postmortem** care. Most of the time when death occurs at home, the family has been prepared for what to do by the doctor and nurse who care for the client. Usually, the client's doctor, the nurse from the home health agency, and the funeral director are notified. If the client's doctor is not available to make a home visit, an ambulance may have to be called to take the client to the emergency room so a physician can pronounce him dead. Check with your agency for the policies and procedures to be followed at the time of death.

The body must be prepared for removal in any case. After death occurs, the family may sit at the bedside and say their final goodbyes. Families handle grief in many ways, and they should have time and privacy as they need it. Be sure to inquire as to specific religious practices that should be observed at this time.

When appropriate, prepare the body in the following manner:

- Remove all pillows except one under the head.
- Bathe the body, removing secretions and reinforce dressings.
- Place dentures in the mouth if possible.
- Close the eyes, but do not press on the eyeballs.
- Keep the body flat on its back, straightening the arms and legs.
- Move the body gently to avoid bruising.
- Check with the family regarding any jewelry the client may be wearing.
- Fold the arms over the abdomen.
- Check your agency's policy about the removal of catheters. Usually, you will not be asked to remove a tube after death if you did not care for it when the client was alive.

After the body is removed from the home, strip the bed and air the room. Remove any equipment. Check with the family regarding the proper disposal of these items. Place personal items carefully at the bedside so family members can remove them at the appropriate time.

In addition, the aide may help the family by answering phone calls from friends and neighbors, making coffee, or sitting with grieving family members. Ask the family how you can help, and try to do whatever is necessary to help them through this difficult time.

Some caregivers wish to attend the funeral of the client. It gives them a formal chance to say goodbye and shows the family how much they cared for the client. You must examine your own feelings on the subject and do as you feel best.

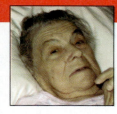

CHAPTER REVIEW

Case Study

Review the case study that appears on the first page of the chapter. Answer two sets of questions about the case study contained in the Explore and Apply sections below.

EXPLORE

1. How do you feel about working with a patient who is dying?
2. While speaking with Mrs. Bell, you discover she has a living will in her dresser drawer. When she indicates that she has not shared it with her husband or her children, you are surprised. What do you do?

APPLY

1. What procedures that you learned in this chapter would you use to help Mrs. Bell with her activities of daily living?
2. What would you be looking for when you take Mrs. Bell's vital signs?

Certification Exam Review Questions

Choose the best answer for each question or statement.

1. **Many clients elect to die at home because**
   a. *they do not know what will happen to them in a hospital.*
   b. *the doctor says when they should.*
   c. *it is a personal choice and often cannot be explained.*
   d. *Medicare wants it that way because it is cheaper.*

2. **Dying is**
   a. *a process, and everyone goes through it at the same rate and the same way.*
   b. *a process, and everyone must go through it at their own speed in their own way.*
   c. *easier when you share with the client ways in which others have reacted to death.*
   d. *not easier when the client talks about dying.*

3. **Your role in caring for a dying client and his family is**
   a. *to be a good listener and support the client in his decisions.*
   b. *to tell the family what they can expect based on your experience.*
   c. *not to bother reporting changes in the client's condition as he is dying.*
   d. *to write down everything the client says so you can tell the family.*

4. **Physical care of the dying client includes**
   a. *skin care and basic mouth care.*
   b. *all the needs of any other client.*
   c. *only care that is not painful.*
   d. *only care a client requests.*

5. **You have been caring for a client for several months. When the client dies you**
   a. *expect to feel sad, but are sure you will go on to care for another client easily.*
   b. *are not sure how you will feel.*
   c. *do not ask your supervisor for permission to attend the funeral.*
   d. *will plan on being absent if you think the client is expected to die.*

CHAPTER 7

Anatomy and Physiology

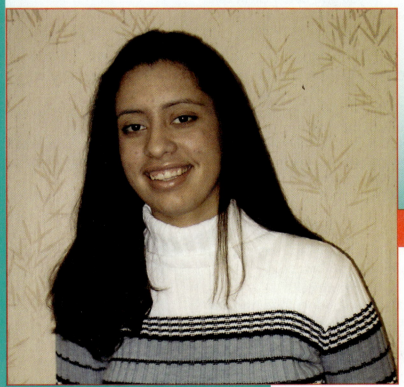

CASE STUDY

Ms. Colin is the niece of your client. She is the main caretaker of her uncle, a 78-year-old man confined to a wheelchair due to his recent leg amputation. When at home, Ms. Colin goes to the health club at least twice a week and enjoys an active social life consisting of various outdoor sports and activities. She works during the day as a 3rd-grade teacher. Ms. Colin lives some distance away and, for the time being, has moved in with her uncle and sleeps on the couch. She plans to go home after he is more self-sufficient and other caretakers can be arranged. Your client used to garden and be proud of the fact that he could walk the mile and a half to the local store for his morning paper, where he met his friends and spent time discussing politics. Now, however, he just sits in his wheelchair and looks outside.

Keep the case study in mind as you read the chapter. After you have read the chapter, answer the Explore and Apply questions at the end of the chapter that relate to the case study.

An Introduction to Anatomy and Physiology

OBJECTIVES
What You Will Learn to Do

1. Describe the structures and functions of cells, tissues, organs, and systems.
2. Explain how body systems work together.
3. Discuss ways your knowledge of body systems will help you give better client care.

Introduction: An Introduction to Anatomy and Physiology

anatomy
study of the structure of the body

physiology
study of the functions of body tissues and organs

cell
basic unit of living matter

Anatomy is the study of the structure of the body. **Physiology** is the study of how the body functions. Knowledge of how the human body is constructed and how it works will help you give better care to your clients. The vocabulary will help you understand and communicate with other health-care workers.

THE CELL

The **cell** is the fundamental building block of all living matter. The human body is made up of millions of cells. Each has a special task within the body, but they all have certain things in common:

■ They come from preexisting cells.
■ They use oxygen to break down food into energy.
■ They need water to live.
■ They grow and repair themselves.
■ They reproduce.
■ They die.

tissue
group of cells of the same type

organ
several types of tissues grouped together to perform a certain function

system
group of organs acting together to carry out one or more body functions

skin
the largest organ in the body. Functions include protection from infection, temperature regulation, and removal of waste products

TISSUES

Groups of cells of the same type that do a particular kind of work are organized into **tissues**.

Tissues to Systems

Tissues, each having a special function are grouped together to form **organs**, such as the heart and lungs. Each organ has a specific function that cannot be carried out without its various tissues. Organs that work together to perform one or more body functions make up **systems**: for example, the digestive system, respiratory system, and circulatory system. A system cannot work by itself. What happens to one system affects all the others (Figure 7.1 ■).

THE SKIN

The **skin**, our largest system, has many functions. It covers and protects internal organs from injury, bacteria, and environmental changes. The skin also contains nerve endings from the nervous system that aid the body in awareness of its environment. The skin helps regulate the body temperature by controlling the loss of heat from the body. To increase heat loss, the blood vessels

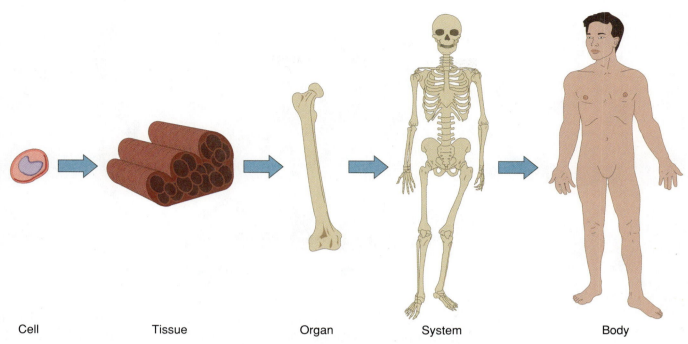

| Cell | Tissue | Organ | System | Body |

FIGURE 7.1 ■ Cells combine to form tissues, tissues combine to form organs, and organs combine to form systems.

near the skin **dilate** or enlarge and the increased blood flow brings more heat to the skin. Then the skin temperature rises, and more heat is lost from the hot skin to the cooler environment. **Evaporation** of fluid **perspiration** from the sweat glands through **ducts** or **pores** to the outside skin also helps cool the body.

When the body is conserving heat, perspiration stops and blood vessels constrict (contract). This prevents the blood from carrying heat to the skin. The skin temperature falls, decreasing heat loss. We know this sensation as goose

dilate
expand; become bigger

evaporation
to pass off as vapor, as water evaporating into the air

perspiration
body moisture given off during physical activity

duct
passage for fluids

pore
opening to the outside of the skin

Table 7.1: Primary Kinds of Tissues

Type of Tissue	Function	Location in the Body
Epithelial	Protect, secrete, absorb, receive sensations	Lining of mouth and nose, skin, lining of stomach
Connective tissue	Connect, support, cover	Tendons, bones, layer of fatty tissue under skin
Muscle tissue 　a. striated 　b. smooth 　c. cardiac	Movement—stretch, contract	Muscle groups in arms, legs, abdomen, back, and internal organs
Nerve tissue	Transmit impulses to and from the central nervous system and to the body systems	Throughout the body
Blood and lymph tissue	Circulate nutrients, oxygen, and antibodies throughout the body; remove waste products	Circulatory system

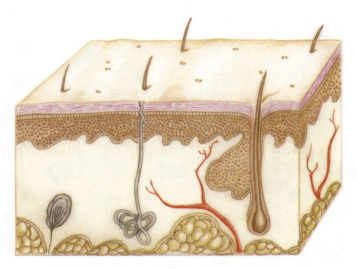

FIGURE 7.2 ■ Magnified cross-section of skin.

bumps. When illness is present and the body cannot release heat as quickly as it is produced, a person is said to have a fever. The body also rids itself of certain waste products through perspiration.

Skin secretes an oily substance through ducts that lead from oil glands to the pores. This protects the skin and keeps it lubricated, soft, and flexible. In elderly persons, these oil glands sometimes fail to function properly and the skin becomes quite dry, scaly, and delicate. In addition, as we age, our skin loses its elasticity and fatty padding, and the skin becomes thin, wrinkly, and saggy.

Other parts of the skin include the hair and the nails. Each hair has a root under the skin into which the oil glands of the skin open. Fingernails and toenails grow from the nailbed at the base underneath the skin. If the nailbed is destroyed, the nail stops growing.

The outer layer of the skin that you see is called the **epidermis** (Figure 7.2 ■). Cells are constantly flaking off or being rubbed off this layer of the skin as they naturally die. Beneath the epidermis is the **dermis**. These cells replace the cells that are lost from the epidermis. **Pigment**, which is responsible for the color of the skin, is found in the epidermis.

Keeping the skin clean removes waste products, those naturally secreted through the skin and those from the environment. Waste products that remain on the skin can cause irritation, disease, and odor.

Watch for changes in your client's skin such as changes in color; temperature; bruises; breaks in skin, such as scratches or cuts; dryness or oiliness; and thinness or thickness of skin. Be particularly aware of whether or not both limbs are the same temperature and color. If you should notice any changes or areas on the client's body that you question, report to your supervisor.

THE SKELETAL SYSTEM

The **skeletal system** is made up of more than 206 bones. The bones act as a framework for the body, giving it structure and support. Bones also protect several internal organs. The bones of the skull, joined together during the first year of life, totally surround the brain. The **vertebral column**, or spinal column, protects the spinal cord. The rib cage guards the heart, lungs, and major

epidermis
outermost layer of skin

dermis
the skin in general; specifically, the second layer of skin

pigment
substance that gives the skin color

skeletal system
bones of the body that give the body shape and protection

vertebral column
backbone

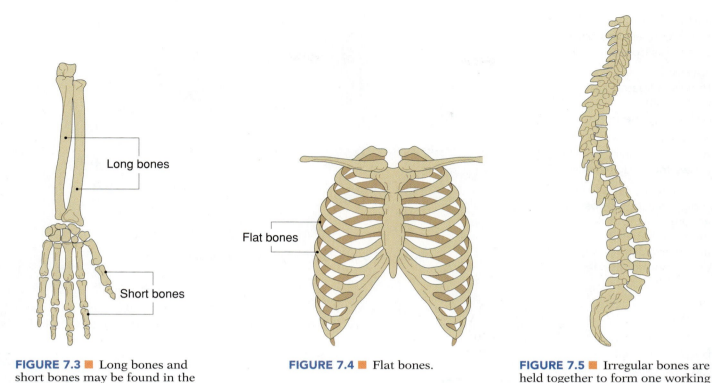

FIGURE 7.3 ■ Long bones and short bones may be found in the same limb.

FIGURE 7.4 ■ Flat bones.

FIGURE 7.5 ■ Irregular bones are held together to form one working structure.

blood vessels. Bones do not move by themselves. They must be moved by muscles, which shorten or contract. This is an example of how systems work together. Bones also store minerals necessary for many other body activities and involved in the constant reproduction of blood cells. There are four types of bones:

1. *Long bones,* like the bones in your arm, provide support (Figure 7.3 ■).
2. *Short bones,* like the bones in your fingers, provide flexibility.
3. *Flat bones,* like the bones of the rib cage, provide protection (Figure 7.4 ■).
4. *Irregular bones* include the vertebrae that make up the spinal column (Figure 7.5 ■).

Broken, or **fractured**, bones usually mend solidly, but the process is slow and gradual. Bone cells grow and reproduce slowly compared to other types of cells. The hardening of the new bone is a gradual process of depositing calcium. As we age, our bones become more brittle. The blood supply is often decreased, calcium is not as readily stored, and the body's powers of general resistance to infection and healing are decreased. For this reason, an elderly person who breaks a bone will require a longer time to heal than a younger person. In addition, an elderly person who falls is more subject to fractures than a younger person is because his bones are so brittle.

Joints are areas in which one bone connects with one or more other bones. The tough white fibrous cord that connects a bone to a bone is called a **ligament**. The fibrous material that connects muscle to bone is called a **tendon**. Shoulder, hip, and knee joints are each enclosed in a strong capsule lined by a membrane that secretes a lubricating fluid. This is called a **bursa**. Movable joints are constructed so that two ends of the bones do not rub against each

fracture
break

joint
part of the body where two bones come together and there is movement

ligament
a tough band of tissue connecting bone to bone

tendon
tough cord of connective tissue that binds muscles to bony parts

bursa
sac of fluid within a joint capsule that provides lubrication for joint movement

cartilage
tough connective tissue that holds bones together

sprain
to twist a ligament or muscle without dislocating the bones

muscular system
group of organs that allows the body to move

antagonistic groups
groups having opposing actions; for example, muscles that flex the upper arm act in opposition to muscles that extend it

flex
to bend

contract
become smaller

extend
straighten an arm or leg

flexion
bending of a joint

abduction
to move an arm or leg away from the center of the body

adduction
to move an arm or leg toward the center of the body

voluntary
muscles moved consciously

involuntary
action taken without conscious input

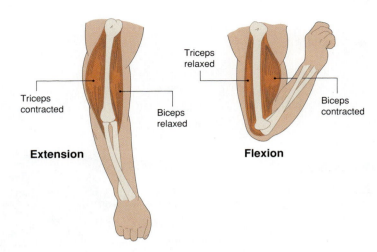

FIGURE 7.6 ■ Adduction moves a limb toward the body.

other. A pad of **cartilage** at the end of the bone absorbs jolts and cushions bone ends. Injury to joints may strain a ligament or tendon in what is called a **sprain**.

THE MUSCULAR SYSTEM

The **muscular system** makes all motion possible. Groups of muscles work together to perform a body motion (Figure 7.6 ■). Two groups of muscles that work together are called **antagonistic groups**. For example, **flex** your forearm, bending it toward your shoulder. Your biceps **contract**, or shorten, and the triceps relax. **Extend** your forearm. The biceps muscle relaxes while the triceps contracts. *Flexion* and *extension* are two terms you should know (Figure 7.7 ■). Two others are *abduction* (Figure 7.8 ■), which means moving a part away from the body, and *adduction* (Figure 7.9 ■), which means moving it toward the body.

Muscles can also be classified as **voluntary** (those muscles we move consciously, such as an arm), **involuntary** (those that move without conscious

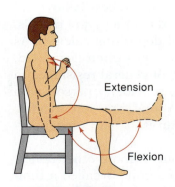

FIGURE 7.7 ■ Abduction moves a limb away from the body.

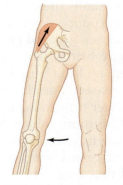

FIGURE 7.8 ■ Muscles work in coordination with each other to move bones and provide movement.

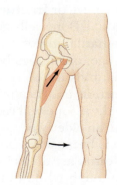

FIGURE 7.9 ■ Every muscle has two activities: flexion—bending the limb, and extension—straightening out the limb.

control, such as the heart), or **smooth** or **striated** (depending on what they look like under a microscope).

Muscles not only move the body but also help keep the body warm, especially during activity. If a muscle is kept inactive for too long, it tends to shrink and waste away. This is called atrophy. **Contracture** is a permanent muscle shortening or loss of function and a permanent flexed position of the limb. Range-of-motion exercises are often given to inactive clients to prevent these problems.

THE CENTRAL NERVOUS SYSTEM

The central **nervous system** controls and organizes all body activity, both voluntary and involuntary (autonomic nervous system). The nervous system is made up of the **brain**, the **spinal cord**, and the **nerves**. The nerves are spread throughout all areas of the body. Nerve tissue is made up of specialized cells called **neurons**. All body organs receive messages from the brain by way of the nervous system (Figure 7.10 ■). Any strong enough change in our external or internal environment will set up a nervous impulse in these receptor organs. This impulse is carried through the spinal cord to the brain. The impulse is then interpreted by the brain, which sends other impulses to a body part that must respond to the first impulse.

When part of the brain is damaged, as in a stroke or accident, either the path along which impulses travel or the brain itself is damaged. Nerve cells do not grow back once they die. If possible, another part of the brain or impulse pathway can be trained to take over the function of the damaged part. You will work with rehabilitation therapists helping clients learn to do things again after such damage has occurred.

The right half of the brain controls most activity on the left side of the body, and the left half of the brain controls activity on the right side of the body. Specific parts of the brain are responsible for movement, emotions, thoughts, learning, and memory.

smooth muscle
appears smooth under a microscope; usually associated with involuntary actions

striated muscle
appears to be lined under a microscope; usually associated with voluntary action

contracture
a permanent muscle shortening that often result in loss of function

nervous system
system that controls all body functions

brain
main organ of the central nervous system, found in the skull

spinal cord
one of the main organs of the nervous system; carries messages from the brain to other parts of the body and from parts of the body back to the brain; is inside the spine (backbone)

nerve
bundle of neurons held together with connective tissue; nerves go to all parts of the body from the central nervous system, that is, from the brain and spinal cord

neuron
cell that is part of all nerves

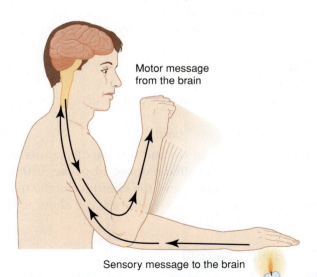

Motor message from the brain

Sensory message to the brain

FIGURE 7.10 ■
All messages travel to the brain, which directs appropriate activity in response to the messages.

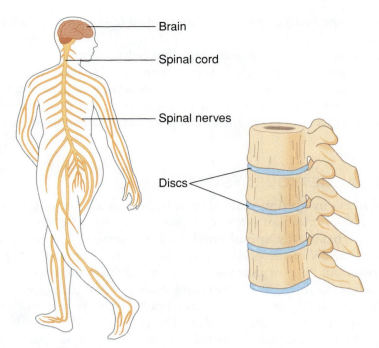

FIGURE 7.11 ■ The nervous system provides pathways for messages to and from the brain.

vertebrae
bones of the spinal column

disc
round piece of cartilage between the vertebrae

autonomic nervous system
part of the nervous system that carries messages without conscious thought

sense organs
groups of tissue that make us aware of the outside world through sight, hearing, smell, taste, and touch

stimuli
activity that causes the body to respond

nerve impulse
regular wave of negative electrical impulses that transmit information along a neuron from one part of the body to another

hormones
protein substance secreted by an endocrine gland directly into the blood

endocrine glands
ductless glands in the body that secrete hormones into the blood

feedback mechanism
process whereby system output is fed back into the system (input) to change the way the system works or what it produces (output)

The nerves that serve your entire body as pathways to and from your brain branch off the spinal cord housed inside the spinal column (Figure 7.11 ■). The small cushion of cartilage that separates the **vertebrae** or back bones is called a **disc**. It prevents the two bones from rubbing each other and squeezing the nerve. When the disc is damaged and pressure on the nerve increases, pain is often the result.

Much of the body's organ activity is involuntary. In other words, we cannot regulate it. The part of the nervous system that controls such activity is called the **autonomic nervous system**.

Sense organs contain specialized endings of the sensory neurons. These are activated by sudden changes in the outside environment called **stimuli**.

■ Eyes respond to visual stimuli.
■ Ears respond mainly to sound stimuli.
■ Membranes of the nose respond to odors.
■ Taste buds, located mostly on the tongue, respond to sweet, sour, and other sensations.
■ Skin responds to touch, pressure, heat, cold, and pain.

Sense organs must send their messages to the brain and receive directions as to how to respond to the stimuli. This message is called a **nerve impulse**. If this pathway is broken, the sense organ cannot function and the client loses the use of it. For example, if the nerve pathways to the eye are damaged, the client will be unable to see.

HORMONES AND THE ENDOCRINE SYSTEM

The endocrine glands secrete liquids called **hormones** into the bloodstream (Figure 7.12 ■). These chemicals are secreted in one place, but work in another. The organs that manufacture the chemicals are called **endocrine glands** (Table 7.2 ■). The endocrine gland works by a "**feedback mechanism**." When

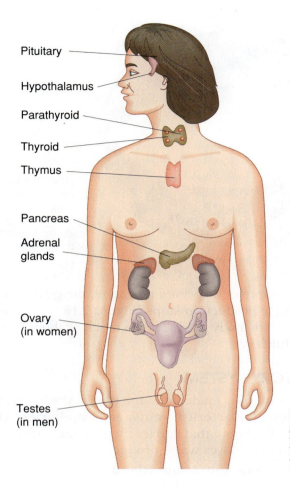

Pituitary

Hypothalamus

Parathyroid

Thyroid

Thymus

Pancreas

Adrenal
glands

Ovary
(in women)

Testes
(in men)

FIGURE 7.12 ■ Endocrine glands secrete hormones that travel throughout the body to regulate proper body function.

Table 7.2: Endocrine Glands and Their Functions

Gland	Function

Pituitary
   Direct (hormones into bloodstream)
   Indirect (acts on other glands)
	Regulates growth and sexual development; salt and water in body; milk production in women after birth; metabolism of food; body reaction to stress; sexual development; circulation; respiration; and urinary output

Thyroid	Regulates growth and general metabolism; stores iodine
Parathyroid	Works with thyroid to regulate levels of calcium and phosphorus; affects muscle and nerve function
Pancreas	Produces insulin
Adrenal	Produces adrenalin; helps regulate body fluid and electrolyte balance; influences metabolism; influences sexual organs; helps body cope with stress
Ovaries (female)	Produce estrogen and progesterone, which regulate menstruation and female characteristics
Testes (male)	Produce testosterone, which causes sperm production and is necessary for male characteristics

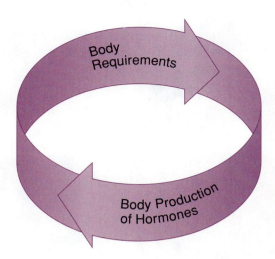

FIGURE 7.13 ■
Hormones are produced as the body needs them. Any imbalance in this system leads to illness, disease, or body changes.

circulatory system
organs of the body concerned with circulation

blood
fluid that circulates through the heart, arteries, veins and capillaries; carries nourishment and oxygen to the tissues and takes away waste matter and carbon dioxide

heart
four-chambered, hollow, muscular organ in the chest cavity, pointing slightly to the left, that pumps blood throughout the body

lymph
clear, colorless fluid carried by an independent system of vessels that returns the fluid to the heart

blood vessels
tubes that carry blood throughout the body

arteries
blood vessels that carry blood away from the heart

veins
blood vessels that carry blood to the heart

capillaries
minute blood vessels that connect arteries to veins

nutrients
food substances required by the body to repair, maintain, and grow new cells

the body requires more of a specific hormone, the gland supplies it. When the level is high enough, production stops (Figure 7.13 ■). If this feedback mechanism is not perfect, the body produces too much or too little of a hormone. This causes body misfunctions.

THE CIRCULATORY SYSTEM

The **circulatory system** is made up of the **blood**, the **heart**, the **lymph** system, and the **blood vessels—arteries**, **veins**, and **capillaries**. The heart acts as a pump for the blood, a liquid that carries the **nutrients** (food) and oxygen to the cells of the body and removes waste products.

Important Facts to Know About Blood
- Blood carries oxygen from the lungs to the cells.
- Carbon dioxide is a waste product carried by the blood from the cells to the lungs.
- Nutrients are absorbed by the blood from the duodenum (small intestine) and brought to the cells.
- Hormones from the endocrine glands are transported by the blood.
- Dilation and contraction of the blood vessels help regulate body temperature.
- Blood helps maintain the fluid balance of the body.
- White cells of the blood help defend the body against disease.
- Blood is continually recirculated through a closed system in our bodies.
- Red blood cells exchange oxygen, iron, and other nutrients for waste products from all body tissues.

The blood vessels leading away from the heart are called arteries. Usually, these vessels carry blood rich in oxygen. (This is true of all arteries except the pulmonary artery.) Arteries have thick, elastic walls that can absorb the pressure of the heart's constant pumping of blood (Figure 7.14 ■).

Arteries branch into a vast network throughout the body and become smaller and smaller until they are so small that they become capillaries. The walls of the capillaries are only one cell-layer thick. Through these walls, gases, nutrients, waste products, and other substances are exchanged between the red blood cells in the capillaries, the tissue fluid, and the tissue cells.

After the blood has given up its oxygen, which is carried on the surface of the red blood cells, it returns to the heart through the veins. The veins, which carry blood to the heart, have valves in them that function as trapdoors, so that the

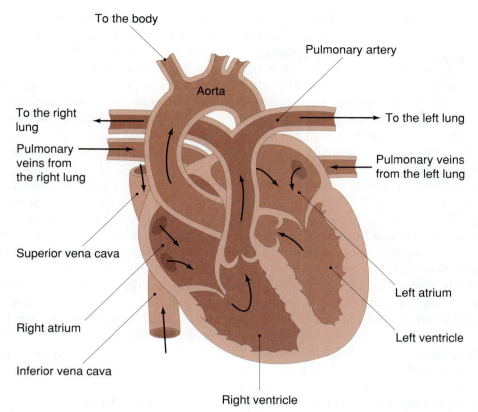

FIGURE 7.14 ■ The heart acts as the pump that moves the blood and nutrients through the circulatory system.

blood flowing against gravity will not fall backward. When these valves do not work well and blood pools in veins, they stretch. This condition is known as **varicose veins**. People who have too few red blood cells have anemia; people with too many red blood cells have too much iron and oxygen in their circulatory system.

The heart is made up of four chambers—the two **atria** and the two larger and more powerful **ventricles**. The right atrium receives blood from the body that is high in carbon dioxide and other waste products. This blood flows into the right ventricle. Then it is pumped through the **pulmonary** artery to the lungs. Here, in the lungs, the blood exchanges the carbon dioxide for oxygen and returns to the heart through the pulmonary veins. It reenters the heart in the left atrium, flows to the left ventricle, and is pumped out to the body through the aorta. The **aorta** is the largest blood vessel in our body. This cycle then repeats.

It is necessary that the heart muscle be supplied with blood carrying oxygen. The **coronary** arteries, which surround the heart, carry the needed oxygen and nutrients to the cardiac muscle tissue. When one of the branches of the coronary artery is blocked, as by a blood clot, the client suffers a heart attack. This can result in death of heart tissue. This event is called a **myocardial infarction (MI)**.

The liquid portion of the blood, called **plasma**, transports both the red blood cells (carrying oxygen and iron) and white blood cells (that fight infection). When a person has an **inflammation** or injury, white blood cells rush to the infected area to help fight the foreign material. The waste product of this battle is **pus**.

varicose vein
abnormal swelling of a vein

atria
the two upper chambers of the heart

ventricles
lower two chambers of the heart

pulmonary
refers to the lungs

aorta
major artery that carries blood away from the heart

coronary
pertaining to the heart

myocardial infarction (MI)
death of part of the heart due to blockage in a blood vessel

plasma
liquid portion of blood

inflammation
reaction of the tissues to disease or injury; usually includes pain, heat, redness, and swelling of the body part

pus
a waste product of inflammation

liver
body's largest organ located in the upper right quadrant of the abdominal cavity, which helps process waste products

toxin
toxic substance

stabilizes
returns to normal

lymph nodes
organs of lymph tissue

spleen
abdominal organ

thymus
ductless gland, part of the lymphatic system, located in the chest cavity just above the heart

involuntary
without conscious control

pharynx
area behind the nasal cavities, mouth, and larynx that opens into them and the esophagus

trachea
organ of the respiratory system located in the throat area, commonly called the windpipe

larynx
area of the throat containing the vocal cords

diaphragm
muscular partition between the chest cavity and the abdominal cavity

bronchi
two main branches of the bronchial tree that lead to the lungs

lungs
primary organs of breathing

epiglottis
a flap of tissue located in the back of the throat that covers the larynx while swallowing

The **liver** is where **toxins**, or poisonous substances, are removed from the blood. Damage to the liver can be caused by drinking alcoholic substances or taking drugs harmful to its tissue. The liver is also responsible for the production and storage of elements necessary for proper circulation of the blood and for blood clotting. Blood clots are not always bad. When a blood vessel has been injured, a clot may form that holds the blood within the closed vessel until healing occurs. Sometimes, however, a blood clot can be dangerous because it may prevent new blood from passing through the vessel. This means that part of the body will not receive its nutrients or rid itself of waste.

A person's circulation tends to slow down when in bed. Therefore, when you have orders to help a client out of bed, remember that his circulation is not at its peak. Make sure that he moves carefully and slowly. Allow him to sit at the edge of the bed until his circulation **stabilizes**, that is, returns to normal. Then assist him to a standing position. If the client becomes dizzy or feels faint, have him sit down again.

The lymphatic system is considered part of the circulatory system. This system assists the circulatory system in draining fluid from the body tissues. Lymph channels are located in the body near veins. The channels become bigger as they near the heart. Two large lymph vessels empty into the venous blood system in the neck area. Lymph fluid is always moving toward the heart. Lymph contains fluid plasma, white blood cells, carbon dioxide, and other chemicals, depending on what the body must flush out.

Lymph nodes are organs of lymph tissues. They help the body fight infection. While doing this, they often enlarge and become tender. This is called enlarged nodes or swollen glands.

Two glands, the **spleen** and the **thymus**, are also part of the lymphatic system. The spleen produces, stores, and destroys blood cells. We know little about the thymus gland. We do know, however, that the body uses it to fight infection.

THE RESPIRATORY SYSTEM

The respiratory system provides a pathway for oxygen to travel from the air into the lungs and for the blood to exchange carbon dioxide for this oxygen. Breathing is regulated in part of our brain. It is an **involuntary** act.

The organs that make up the respiratory system include the nose, mouth, **pharynx** (throat), **trachea** (windpipe), **larynx** (voice box), **diaphragm**, **bronchi**, and **lungs** (Figure 7.15 ■). Because this exchange must take place all the time, it is necessary that this pathway always be kept open. The structures themselves help do this. The trachea and bronchi are kept open by their anatomical structure. The tiny hairs in the nose trap dust so that it does not reach the lungs. On the top of the trachea, opening from the pharynx, is a structure known as the larynx. It is not only the opening to the trachea; it also contains vocal cords that make it possible for us to have a voice. An important piece of cartilage, the **epiglottis**, covers the opening to the trachea. When food is swallowed, the epiglottis prevents the food from going into the lungs.

A weak client or one having trouble breathing must be watched carefully while eating so that food does not enter the trachea. This is known as **aspiration** of food. An unconscious client who vomits may also be in danger of aspirating that material. Turn the client's head to the side at once.

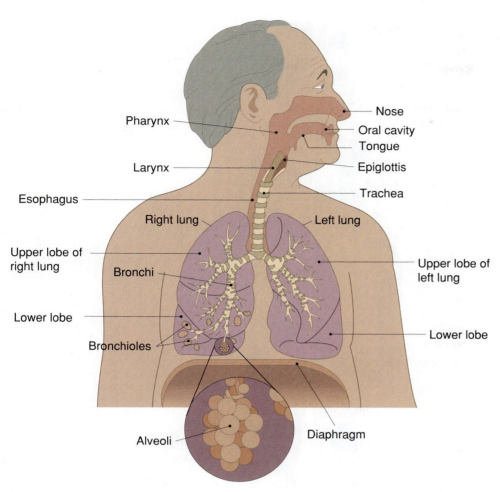

Pharynx

Nose

Oral cavity

Tongue

Larynx

Epiglottis

Esophagus

Trachea

Right lung

Left lung

Upper lobe of
right lung

Upper lobe of
left lung

Bronchi

Lower lobe

Lower lobe

Bronchioles

Alveoli

Diaphragm

FIGURE 7.15 ■ The respiratory system exchanges waste products for oxygen through a filtering system in the lungs.

The exchange of oxygen and carbon dioxide occurs in the small air sacs (**alveoli**), which are the last branches of the bronchi. As you **inhale** and the diaphragm moves toward the abdominal cavity, oxygen fills these sacs and is exchanged for carbon dioxide that the blood brings to the sacs from the heart. As you **exhale**, the diaphragm compresses the lungs and forces the carbon dioxide out of the lungs into the air. The oxygen-rich blood then returns to the heart to be sent around the body. If your client has difficulty breathing, that means he has difficulty exchanging the carbon dioxide in his blood for fresh oxygen in his lungs. As a result, all the cells in his body have less oxygen.

If the weather is humid or pollution is thick, people with heart or lung disease may have difficulty breathing. This may signal to you that a client has a blocked airway. If you are assigned to a client who may have difficulty swallowing or breathing, be sure to discuss with your supervisor any emergency procedures of which you should be aware.

THE DIGESTIVE (GASTROINTESTINAL) SYSTEM

The **digestive system** is responsible for breaking down food into a form usable for body cells. This action is both chemical and mechanical. The digestive tract

aspiration
when food or fluid is taken into the lungs

alveoli
microscopic air sacs in the lungs where oxygen passes into the blood in exchange for waste products

inhale
to breathe in air in respiration

exhale
to breathe out air in respiration

digestive system
the group of organs responsible for converting food into energy for the body

digestion
the act of converting food into energy the body can use

saliva
secretion of the salivary glands into the mouth; moistens food and is necessary for digestion

esophagus
muscular tube for the passage of food. Extends from the back of the throat (pharynx), down through the chest and diaphragm into the stomach

stomach
part of the digestive tract between the esophagus (food pipe) and duodenum

duodenum
first part of the small intestine

small intestine
the digestive tract between the stomach and large intestine

pancreas
an organ producing both digestive juices and hormones

bile
substance used in digestion, secreted by the liver and stored in the gallbladder

gallbladder
a reservoir that holds the bile secreted by the liver

villi
tiny fingerlike projections in the lining of the small intestines into which the end products of digestion are absorbed and distributed through the bloodstream

peristalsis
movement of the intestines that pushes food along to the next part of the digestive system

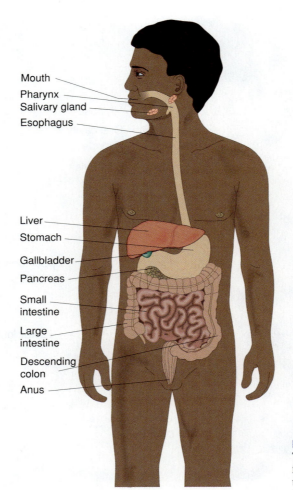

Mouth
Pharynx
Salivary gland
Esophagus

Liver
Stomach
Gallbladder
Pancreas
Small intestine
Large intestine
Descending colon
Anus

FIGURE 7.16 ■
The digestive system changes food into chemical nutrients the body can use or store for future use.

is about 30 feet long. Its entire length is important in reducing food to the form of body needs (Figure 7.16 ■).

    Digestion begins in the mouth, where food is chewed and mixed with **saliva**. During swallowing, the food moves in a moistened ball down the **esophagus** to the **stomach**. The stomach churns and mixes the food as it is broken down chemically. The most important part of digestion and absorption of nutrients occurs in the **duodenum**. This is the first part of the **small intestine**. Here digestive juices from the duodenum and **pancreas** and **bile** from the **gallbladder** finish the job of breaking down food.

    The lining of the duodenum is composed of thousands of tiny fingerlike projections called **villi**. Each villus is capable of absorbing the end products of digestion. The products are then moved into the bloodstream, where they are carried to individual cells.

    A lot of water is necessary to chemically reduce food into its end products. Food is moved along the length of the intestines by the rhythmic contraction of the muscle walls called **peristalsis**. What is left of the food, after some has been absorbed by the small intestines, moves through the **large intestine**, where water is reabsorbed into the body. The material not used by the body is excreted from the rectum through the **anus** as **feces**, or waste.

    The liver is part of the digestive system. Besides manufacturing bile, the liver is a storage area for **glucose**. This form of sugar is released in large amounts when the cells need it for energy.

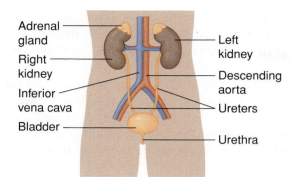

FIGURE 7.17 ■
All blood passes through the kidneys so that chemicals can be filtered out in the form of urine.

On the right side of the **colon**, or large intestine, at the junction between the small intestine and the large intestine is a pouch with a projection called the **appendix**. Because there is little peristalsis in this area, the appendix may trap material and become infected. This is known as appendicitis. Surgery is usually performed to remove the appendix and correct this condition.

The lowest portion of the large intestine curves in an S shape into the **rectum**, with an internal and an external **sphincter** muscle. When the rectum has fecal matter in it, a message is received by the brain. The brain returns a message to the muscles of the rectum, allowing them to relax. This is called a bowel movement. Sometimes blood vessels that supply the rectal area become enlarged and filled with blood clots, resulting in **hemorrhoids**.

THE URINARY SYSTEM

One of the systems that rids the body of waste products is the **urinary system**. This system filters out waste products and toxins from the blood and disposes of them in the liquid called **urine**. The organs that make up the urinary system include the **kidneys**, the **ureters**, the urinary **bladder**, and the **urethra** (Figure 7.17 ■).

As all blood passes through the kidneys, an exchange of substances takes place between the capillaries and the filtering units of the kidney, which are tiny **tubules**. There are hundreds of these tubules in each kidney. As the filtered material flows through these tubules, the blood vessels surrounding them reabsorb those materials still needed by the body, particularly the water. Near the end of the winding tubules, substances from the blood, such as toxins and some drugs, pass into the urine. The material that is left is collected in a larger tube, the ureter. From here it drips steadily through the ureter, helped by a peristaltic motion very similar to that of the gastrointestinal tract, to the urinary bladder. The urinary bladder is capable of expanding and storing about 500 cc of urine. When **stretch receptors** in the muscular bladder wall are stimulated by a full bladder, messages are sent to the brain, causing urinary tract muscles to release the urine from the bladder. This is called **urinating**, or **voiding**.

Because the urethra is open to the outside of the body, it may also provide a passageway for disease-causing microorganisms to enter the bladder. A bladder infection is known as **cystitis**. The infection may also spread through the ureters to the kidneys, causing kidney damage. Cystitis is most commonly found in women because of the shortness of the urethra.

You may have a client who has a urinary **catheter** in the urethra. This is a tube from the bladder to a bag that collects the urine. (This does not have to hamper women's sexual activity. If your client has questions about this, tell your supervisor.)

large intestine
the last section of colon starting at the end of the small intestine and ending at the rectum

anus
opening of the rectum onto the body surface

feces
solid waste material discharged from the body through the rectum and anus

glucose
sugar

colon
large bowel

appendix
slender growth attached to the large intestine

rectum
lower 8 to 10 inches of the colon

sphincter
ring-like muscle that controls opening and closing of a body opening

hemorrhoid
swollen vein near the anus

urinary system
organs that work together to produce urine

urine
liquid waste manufactured in the kidneys and discharged from the urinary bladder

kidney
organ lying in the upper posterior portion of the abdomen that removes wastes from the bloodstream and discharges them in the form of urine

ureters
tubes leading from the kidneys to the urinary bladder

bladder
membranous sac that serves as a container within the body, such as the urinary bladder, which holds urine

urethra
tube-like structure that carries urine from the bladder to the outside of the body

tubules
small tubes

stretch receptors
nerve cells that relay messages to the brain as the organ enlarges

voiding/urinating
passing urine

cystitis
inflammation of the bladder

catheter
a tube used to remove body fluids from a cavity

ovaries
organs in the female that produce mature eggs and the primary female sex hormones, estrogen and progesterone

fallopian tubes
also called the oviducts, through which an egg travels from the ovary to the uterus

uterus
expandable female reproductive organ in which an embryo grows and is nourished until gestation is complete

vagina
the birth canal leading from the cervix to the outside

ovulation
period of time in which the ovum is pushed out from the surface of the ovary and usually picked up by the oviduct

ovum
egg

The urinary system determines the water content of the blood, and the blood content, in turn, determines the content of the tissue fluid. The urinary system also determines the content of other nutrients in the blood, such as salt and potassium.

When ill, a client is sometimes unable to void. This condition must be reported to your supervisor immediately. You will notice the color, odor, and amount of urine your client voids as you care for him. Observe usual color, odor, and amount for your client so you will be alert to changes and report them. Many changes in client kidney functions can be detected from changes in urine.

THE REPRODUCTIVE SYSTEM

Female Reproduction

In the female, the reproductive organs are two **ovaries**, two **fallopian tubes**, the **uterus**, and the **vagina** (Figure 7.18 ■). The main task of the ovary is production of eggs (ova). These are specialized cells that may unite with a sperm cell (released from the male during sexual intercourse) and then grow over a period of 40 weeks into a new human being.

Ovulation is the process whereby an **ovum** (egg) is released from one ovary into the opening of a fallopian tube and moves through this tube to the uterus. This occurs approximately once each month, usually 14 days before the onset of the next menstrual period. During this time, a woman is **fertile** (able to become pregnant). During ovulation, the hormone estrogen is released into the bloodstream. This causes a buildup of the **endometrium** (lining of the uterus), preparing it for a possible pregnancy. If the ovum is fertilized, the mouth of the uterus closes to protect the developing embryo.

The uterus lining now helps to nourish the embryo. If the ovum is not fertilized, the lining of the uterus is not necessary and is shed. This process is called **menstruation**. Menstruation is the periodic loss of blood and a small

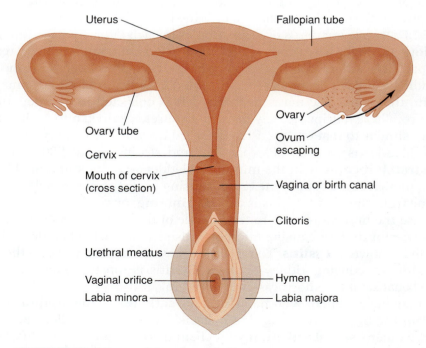

FIGURE 7.18 ■ Internal female genitalia.

part of the lining of the uterus. The discharge flows out of the vagina for 4 to 7 days.

The process of ovulation is controlled by hormones from the pituitary gland and the ovaries. These hormones from the pituitary gland are involved in ovum development and in maintaining pregnancy.

Ovulation and menstruation usually begin between ages 10 and 13. At this time, a girl develops breasts and body hair and starts to look more and more like a woman. Once a female starts to menstruate, she can become pregnant, no matter how young she is. Menstruation usually continues uninterrupted, except for pregnancy, until a woman enters menopause.

When a woman is about 45, her menstrual cycles change. They become farther apart and finally stop. In addition, she may have emotional changes and changes in her skin and hair. This process is called **menopause**, or "the change of life." Some women may feel depressed, have hot flashes, or have sexual difficulty. If a client or family member mentions to you that she finds this time of life difficult, suggest she discuss this with her physician. Of course, you will report this conversation to your supervisor. Many cultures have customs or superstitions connected with menstruation. As a homemaker/home health aide, you will have to show tolerance and understanding for customs that may be different from your own.

The human female reproductive or excretory systems has three openings from the body to the outside area: (1) the external urinary **meatus**, the end of the urethra; (2) the vagina, which is not only the organ for intercourse, but also the birth canal; and (3) the anus, the last portion of the gastrointestinal tract (Figure 7.19 ■). These three systems are not connected and function independently of each other.

You may have a client who has had a **hysterectomy**. At the time of surgery, the physician removes the uterus and ovaries. This procedure is done for many reasons. Women who have had this operation are often concerned about their sex lives. This operation will usually have no effect on your client's sex life. If a client voices concerns to you, communicate them to your supervisor and discuss the most appropriate plan of care.

fertile
the period of the month when a woman is able to conceive

endometrium
lining of the uterus

menstruation
cyclical discharge of blood from the uterus

menopause
period of life in the female usually between the ages of 45 and 50 when menstruation stops; change of life

meatus
opening of the urethra to the outside of the body

hysterectomy
removal of the uterus

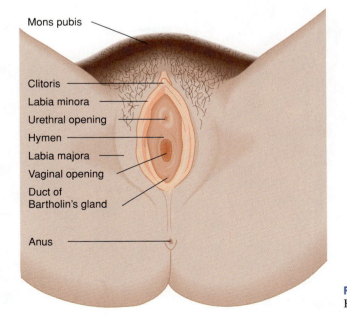

FIGURE 7.19 ■
External female genitalia.

testes
pair of reproductive organs in the male that lie in the scrotum hanging from the perineal area, dorsal to the penis

epididymides
organs attached to the testes

seminal ducts and vesicles
small glands in the male near the prostate and urethra where semen is stored before it is discharged

ejaculatory ducts
part of the male reproductive system

spermatic ducts
tubes containing sperm

Male Reproduction

The male internal reproductive system has two **testes**, two **epididymides**, two **seminal ducts** and **vesicles**, two **ejaculatory ducts**, two **spermatic ducts**, the urethra, and the **prostate gland**. The **penis** and **scrotum** are considered external reproductive organs (Figure 7.20 ■).

Testicles, or testes, are paired glands that lie outside the body in a sac called the scrotum. The testes produce **sperm**, the male cell of reproduction. During intercourse, sperm travel up the **vas deferens**, or sperm ducts, to a point where they enter the urethra. They enter along with secretions from other glands in the male reproductive system. These glands—the seminal vesicle, the prostate gland, and Cowper's glands—contribute water, nutrients, and vitamins, which, added to the sperm, make up the **semen**, a fluid **ejaculated** (expelled) at the same time the male has an orgasm. There is only one duct in the penis. It is used for the flow of urine and for the ejaculation of sperm in its carrying medium, the semen. During intercourse, the internal sphincter of the male's urinary bladder closes tightly, so there is no chance for urine to mix with semen. The penis has three columns of spongy tissue. During sexual excitement, blood rushes in through the penile artery and the veins constrict, trapping the blood so it fills these spaces. Then the penis becomes erect and hard. All of this activity occurs under the influence of **testosterone**, the primary male sex hormone, which also is manufactured in the testes. It is secreted into the blood through the influence of hormones from the pituitary gland.

Sometimes during the aging process the prostate gland, which encircles the urethra like a doughnut, becomes enlarged. When the prostate expands, it

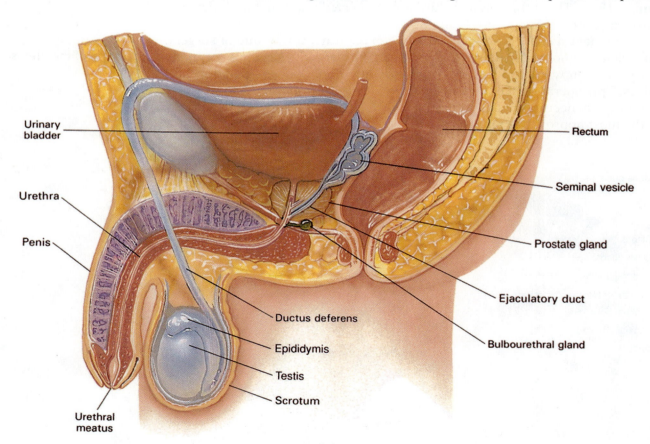

FIGURE 7.20 ■ A cross-section of the male genitalia.

Table 7.3: **The Body Systems**

System	Function	Organs
Skeletal	Supports, protects the body; provides a place for muscles to attach	Bones, joints
Muscular	Gives movement to the body; protects	Muscles, tendons, ligaments
Gastrointestinal (digestive, GI)	Processes nutrients into usable units of absorption for the body; eliminates waste	Mouth, teeth, tongue, esophagus, salivary glands, stomach, intestines, liver, gallbladder, pancreas
Nervous	Controls movements and activities of the body	Brain, spinal cord, nerves
Urinary (excretory)	Removes waste from the blood, produces urine, and eliminates urine	Kidneys, ureters, bladder, urethra
Reproductive	Reproduces the species	Male: testes, scrotum, penis Female: ovaries, uterus, fallopian tubes, vagina
Respiratory	Eliminates carbon dioxide; supplies oxygen	Nose, pharynx, larynx, trachea, bronchi, lungs
Circulatory	Carries nutrients, oxygen, and water to the body cells and removes wastes	Heart, blood, arteries, veins, capillaries, spleen, lymph nodes, lymph vessels
Endocrine	Secretes hormones directly into the blood, regulating body function	Thyroid and parathyroid glands, adrenal glands, testes, ovaries, pancreatic islets of Langerhans, pituitary gland
Skin	Provides first line of defense against infection; maintains body temperature, regulates fluids, and rids body of waste	Skin, hair, nails, sweat and oil glands

squeezes the urethra, causing painful urination. Many men fear surgery on their prostate glands, because they believe it will end their sex life. The amount of semen ejaculated will be less, but otherwise, men who have had prostate surgery are almost always capable of having normal sexual relations.

prostate gland
male gland behind the outlet of the urinary bladder

penis
male sexual organ; urine is also ejected through the penis

scrotum
pouch below the penis, contains the testicles

sperm
male reproductive cell

vas deferens
tubes carrying sperm from the testicles to the glands where they are stored in preparation for ejaculation

semen
the fluid of ejaculation

ejaculate
to discharge fluid suddenly, especially the discharge of semen from the male urethra

testosterone
a male hormone

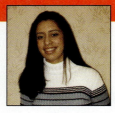

CHAPTER REVIEW

Case Study

Review the case study that appears on the first page of the chapter. Answer two sets of questions about the case study contained in the Explore and Apply sections below.

EXPLORE

1. Can you remember any superstitions you have heard about how the human body functions?

2. You have been asked to help your client increase his daily activity. What might you suggest? How would you explain the benefits of this activity and how would you observe them?

APPLY

1. Ms. Collin tells you that she is not feeling well. She says she thinks it is stress.

   a. What do you tell her?

   b. What suggestions do you make to relieve her stress?

2. Your client can no longer do as much physical activity as before.

   a. How do you explain to him the benefits of at least some physical activity?

   b. What steps would you take to incorporate more physical activity into your client's daily routine?

Certification Exam Review Questions

Choose the best answer for each question or statement.

1. **Understanding the way each body system functions is important because**
   a. each system affects the other.
   b. clients do not know anything about their anatomy.
   c. you will be responsible for reporting how each system is functioning.
   d. you will be responsible for discussing with the family the client's disease.

2. **Some people do not discuss the way the human body functions because**
   a. they are embarrassed, it is not discussed in their culture.
   b. it is your responsibility to know this.
   c. the doctor will be upset if they do.
   d. the client will be upset if family members talk about him.

3. **Understanding the way body systems function**
   a. permits you to know when a system is not functioning correctly.
   b. helps you speak to the doctor about your client's condition.
   c. indicates to the family that you are a member of the health team.
   d. impresses your family.

4. **One of your roles is to discuss the client's status.**
   a. This is usually easy because all people want to know how their bodies work.
   b. This may be difficult because cultural moves may limit subjects you can discuss with members of the family.
   c. Children should always be told how their bodies work.
   d. It is not necessary to chart what you tell the client since this will change each time you visit.

5. **You regularly point out to the client how the body systems he is concerned with function because**
   a. the body has many separate systems, and your client should learn about what affects him.
   b. when one is not functioning well, the others are unaffected.
   c. when one is not functioning well, vitamins will heal it.
   d. this will include him in his care and will provide a basis for him to judge how he is doing.

CHAPTER **8**

Infection Control in the Home

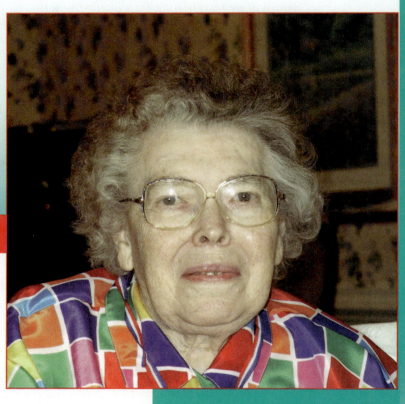

CASE STUDY

Mrs. Day lives alone in her own home. She has not changed anything in the past 25 years, saying that it was fine when her husband was alive so everything will be fine now. Although she has never worked, she is financially secure. She has managed to keep up the house and the garden. She admits to being somewhat forgetful and finding physical work a challenge. This bothers her. She rejects, however, help in the house, memory aids, or other minor assistances with her daily activities. The house is tidy but has not had a thorough cleaning in awhile. It is dark and the windows are seldom opened. She eats three regular meals, which she prepares herself. To save water, Mrs. Day washes her dishes once a day. Her three children are attentive, calling frequently. Only one daughter lives close by, and she is the primary caretaker while the other children only visit or call on special occasions.

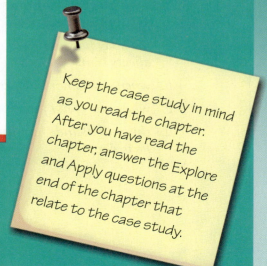

Keep the case study in mind as you read the chapter. After you have read the chapter, answer the Explore and Apply questions at the end of the chapter that relate to the case study.

SECTION 1

Medical Asepsis in the Home

OBJECTIVES

What You Will Learn to Do

1. Explain the relationship between microorganism control and infection control.
2. List the conditions necessary for microorganisms to grow.
3. Explain the chain of infection and your role in interrupting it in the house.
4. List the ways microorganisms are spread.
5. Define medical asepsis.
6. Define clean and dirty.
7. Demonstrate the procedures for sterilization of equipment in the home.

Introduction: The Nature of Microorganisms

People once believed that sickness was caused by evil spirits. About 500 years ago, scientists began to suspect that some diseases were caused by small living things called **microorganisms.** *Micro* means tiny. An **organism** is a living thing. Microorganisms can be seen only under a microscope. Some microorganisms are helpful to people. Microorganisms in the human digestive system break down foods not used by the body and turn them into waste products (feces).

There are some microorganisms, however, that are harmful. They cause disease and infection. Disease-producing microorganisms are called **pathogens.** Pathogens destroy human tissue by using it as food and give off waste products called **toxins.** Toxins are poisonous to the human body. Every living organism has its own natural environment where it can exist without causing disease. When an organism moves out of its normal environment and into a foreign one, it can become a pathogen. For example, the **bacterium** *Escherichia coli* belongs in the colon, where it helps to digest our food. When it enters the bladder or bloodstream, it can cause a urinary infection or a blood infection.

Conditions Necessary for Bacteria Growth

Just as human beings need proper conditions to live, so do microorganisms. Microorganisms need six conditions to grow (Figure 8.1 ■).

Chain of Infection

A pathogen travels from one **host** to another by the **chain of infection** (Figure 8.2 ■). All parts of the chain must be present for a pathogen to successfully move from one host to another and cause a disease. A person can harbor a pathogen without displaying any symptoms of the disease. That person is said to be a **carrier.**

If one of these six elements of the chain of infection is not present, the pathogen cannot cause disease in the second host.

- **Causative agent**—the pathogen (agent) that causes a disease
- **Reservoir of the agent**—the place where the pathogen lives and/or reproduces

---

Clinical ALERT

Chain of Infection
Every time you break the chain of infection, you are preventing pathogens from infecting someone. Hand washing and keeping a clean and orderly environment is both soothing and healthful for the client and his family. Set a good example to the family and tactfully point out ways they too can change behaviors to break the chain of infection and spread of pathogens.

microorganism
living thing so small it can be seen only through a microscope

organism
living thing

pathogen
disease-causing microorganism

toxin
toxic substance

bacteria
microorganisms that may or may not be pathogens

host
the place where an infection develops

chain of infection
the process by which an infection is transmitted to and develops in a host

carrier
a person who has a disease that can be transmitted to others but who does not display any signs or symptoms of the disease

causative agent
the pathogen responsible for a disease

reservoir of the agent
the place where a pathogen can live and reproduce

portal of exit
the place where the pathogen leaves the host

portal of entry
the method by which the pathogen enters the new host

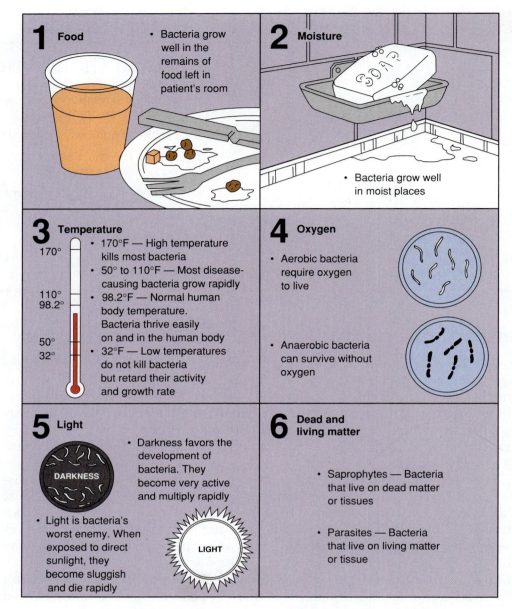

1 Food
• Bacteria grow well in the remains of food left in patient's room

2 Moisture
• Bacteria grow well in moist places

3 Temperature
170°
110°
98.2°
50°
32°
• 170°F — High temperature kills most bacteria
• 50° to 110°F — Most disease-causing bacteria grow rapidly
• 98.2°F — Normal human body temperature. Bacteria thrive easily on and in the human body
• 32°F — Low temperatures do not kill bacteria but retard their activity and growth rate

4 Oxygen
• Aerobic bacteria require oxygen to live
• Anaerobic bacteria can survive without oxygen

5 Light
DARKNESS
LIGHT
• Darkness favors the development of bacteria. They become very active and multiply rapidly
• Light is bacteria's worst enemy. When exposed to direct sunlight, they become sluggish and die rapidly

6 Dead and living matter
• Saprophytes — Bacteria that live on dead matter or tissues
• Parasites — Bacteria that live on living matter or tissue

FIGURE 8.1 ■ Bacteria growth is affected by these six conditions.

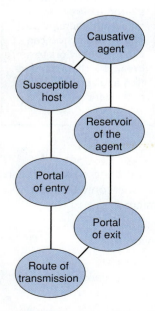

FIGURE 8.2 ■ The chain of infection.

■ **Portal of exit**—the means by which the pathogen leaves the host
■ **The portal of entry**—the means by which the pathogen enters the new host
■ **Route of transmission**—the way in which the pathogen travels from the portal of exit of one host to the portal of entry of another
■ **The susceptible host**—a body that cannot resist the new pathogen and its disease-producing toxins.

Interrupting Bacteria Transmission

One of the most effective ways of decreasing disease is to interrupt transmission of bacteria from one host to another. Transmission occurs in one of six ways.

■ **Direct contact**—direct body-surface-to-body-surface contact
■ **Indirect transmission**—contact with a contaminated object

- **Droplet transmission**—small moisture particles containing pathogens move from one person to another.
- **Airborne transmission**—pathogens in the air are moved by the air from one person to other.
- **Nosocomial transmission**—infections are acquired as a result of being in a health facility

Medical Asepsis

Medical **asepsis** means creating an environment free of disease-causing organisms by preventing conditions that allow pathogens to live, multiply, and spread. As a homemaker/home health aide, you will share responsibility for preventing the spread of disease and infection by using aseptic techniques. Creating an aseptic environment does the following:

- Helps the client overcome a current infection or prevent the spread of that infection.
- Protects the client against a second infection by the same microorganism. This is called **reinfection.**
- Protects the client against infection by a new or different type of microorganism from a visitor or member of the health care team. This is called **cross-infection.**
- Protects the family and health-care team against infection by microorganisms passed from caregiver to client, client to caregiver. Diseases that can be passed from person to person are called **communicable** diseases.
- Protects the client from infection from his own organisms. This is called **self-inoculation.**

Clean and Dirty Areas in the House

One way to control the spread of disease is to have a **clean** area in the house and a **dirty** one. The kitchen is considered clean, and the toilet is considered

GUIDELINES

Aseptic Techniques

- Wash your hands after using the bathroom or blowing your nose, before handling food, after caring for the client, before any procedure, and before meals.
- Practice good personal hygiene.
- Cover your nose and mouth when you sneeze or cough. Turn your face to the side when you cough. Wash your hands after you cough into your hands.
- Clean wastebaskets often.
- Wash, dry, and put away all client-related equipment after each use.
- Dispose of contaminated articles in the proper way.
- If you have an open area on your skin, check with your supervisor before you give client care.
- Wash your hands before you put on gloves and after you take them off.
- Report to your supervisor conditions in the house that contribute to bacteria growth and transmission.

route of transmission
the method by which the pathogen moves from the reservoir to the new host

susceptible host
a host that possesses the optimal conditions in which the pathogen can live

direct contact
body-surface-to-body-surface pathogen transfer

indirect transmission
contact with a contaminated object and pathogen transfer

droplet transmission
pathogen transfer via droplets propelled through the air by coughing, talking, or sneezing

airborne transmission
pathogen transfer via evaporated droplets or dust particles moving through the air

nosocomial transmission
an infection acquired while in a health-care facility

asepsis
the process of creating an environment free of disease-causing organisms

reinfection
to become ill again with the same microorganism

cross-infection
infection by a new or different microorganism from a visitor or health-team member

communicable
spread from one person to another

self-inoculation
infecting oneself with one's own organisms

clean
uncontaminated by harmful microorganisms

dirty
contaminated by harmful microorganisms

MICROORGANISMS ARE IN MANY PLACES	MICROORGANISMS ARE SPREAD IN MANY WAYS
• In the air we breathe • On our bodies • In our bodies • On our clothing • In liquids • In food • On animals • In animals • In human waste • In animal waste	• Touching secretions, urine, feces • Touching objects (dishes, bed linen, clothing, instruments, belongings) • Sneezing, coughing, talking • Contaminated food, drugs, water, blood • Dust particles and moisture in the air

FIGURE 8.3 ■ Microorganisms are in many places and spread in various ways during the day.

dirty; and the area of dishwashing is considered clean, and the area of toileting is considered dirty (Figure 8.3 ■).

Clean: This means uncontaminated. It refers to articles and places from which disease cannot be spread. Clean areas contain food, dishes, and clean equipment. No waste material is ever brought into this area.

Dirty: This refers to areas that have come in contact with disease-causing or -carrying agents. In the home, there are differing degrees of dirty. We make a distinction between items that are dirty with human waste, such as wound drainage or fecal matter, and bedsheets that are only soiled. Articles that are dirty with potentially infectious material are brought into the dirty area for initial cleaning or disposal. This could be linen, bath water, or equipment. Articles that are only soiled are cleaned in the usual way.

SECTION 2

Handwashing

OBJECTIVES

What You Will Learn to Do

1. Discuss the importance of handwashing.
2. Demonstrate the correct method of handwashing in the home.
3. Discuss when you wash your hands.

Introduction: The Importance of Handwashing

In your work, you will use your hands constantly. You will touch clients. You will handle supplies and equipment used in the treatment and care of clients. Microorganisms will get on your hands. They will come from clients or from the things they have touched. Your hands could carry these microorganisms to other persons and places. They could also be moved to your own face and mouth. Washing your hands frequently with lots of soap and friction is the best way to prevent this transfer of microorganisms.

◾ GUIDELINES

Handwashing

- ◾ Wash your hands before and after each task and before and after direct client contact.

- ◾ The water faucet is always considered dirty. This means it may harbor pathogens. Use paper towels to turn the faucet on and off.

- ◾ If your hands accidentally touch the inside of the sink, start over. Do the whole procedure again.

- ◾ Take soap from a dispenser, if possible, rather than using bar soap. Bar soap leaves pools of soapy water in the soap dish, which is then considered contaminated.

- ◾ Wash your hands before you put on gloves for a procedure and again after you remove the gloves.

PROCEDURE 4

Handwashing

> **RATIONALE:** Proper handwashing technique is the most effective way to prevent the spread of disease.

1. Assemble your equipment:
   Soap or detergent
   Paper towels
   Warm running water (if possible)
   Wastepaper basket
   Nail brush

2. Open a paper towel near the sink. This is considered your clean area. Put all your equipment on it. Leave it there until you are ready to leave the house.

3. Turn the faucet on with a paper towel held between your hands and the faucet. Adjust the water to a comfortable temperature.

4. Discard the paper towel in the wastepaper basket.

5. Completely wet your hands and wrists under the running water. Keep your fingertips pointed downward. Hold your hands lower than your elbows while washing. This is to prevent microorganisms from contaminating your arms. Holding your hands down prevents backflow over unwashed skin (Figure 8.4 ◾).

6. Apply soap.

7. Work up a good lather. Spread it over the entire area of your hands and wrists. Get soap under your nails and between your fingers. Add water to the soap while washing. This keeps the soap from becoming too dry.

8. Use the nail brush on your nails.

9. Use a rotating and rubbing (friction) motion for a minimum of 15 seconds.
   a. Rub vigorously.
   b. Rub one hand against the other hand and wrist.
   c. Rub between your fingers by interlacing them.
   d. Rub up and down to reach all skin surfaces on your hands and between your fingers.
   e. Rub the tips of your fingers against your palms to clean with friction around the nailbeds.

10. Wash at least 2 inches above your wrists.

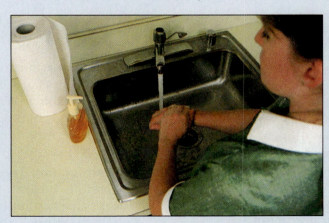

FIGURE 8.4 ◾

continued

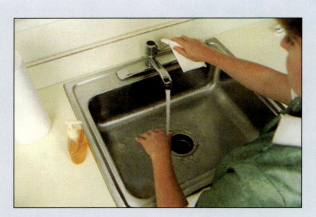

FIGURE 8.5 ■

11. Rinse well one hand at a time. Rinse from 2 inches above your wrists to hands. Hold

your hands and fingertips down under the water.

12. Dry thoroughly with paper towels.

13. Use a paper towel to turn off the faucet. Never touch the faucet with your hands after washing (Figure 8.5 ■).

14. Throw the paper towel into the waste-paper basket. Do not touch the basket.

SAMPLE CHARTING:	5/5/05 11:30 A.M. Hot water not available at the sink. Water heated on the stove for handwashing and bath. Reported this problem to the landlady, who says she will rectify the situation. Valerie Treeman H/HHA

Disinfection and Sterilization

OBJECTIVES

What You Will Learn to Do

1. Discuss differences between disinfection and sterilization.

2. Demonstrate the procedure for wet or dry sterilization in the home.

3. Discuss when wet-heat sterilization would be appropriate and when dry-heat sterilization would be appropriate.

Introduction: Disinfection and Sterilization in the Home

disinfection
process of destroying most disease-causing organisms

sterilization
process of destroying all microorganisms including spores

spore
microorganism that has formed a hard shell around itself for protection. It can only be destroyed by sterilization

While you care for your client, you will always try to prevent the spread of pathogens. Despite the best efforts of health-care personnel, we always have harmful microorganisms around us. They can be made harmless, however, by simple cleanliness procedures. We can keep ourselves clean by bathing and frequent handwashing. We can keep the environment and equipment clean with soap, water, and solutions that assist in keeping down bacterial growth.

Two other important methods for killing microorganisms or keeping them under control are:

1. **Disinfection.** The process of destroying as many harmful organisms as possible. It also means slowing down the growth and activity of organisms that cannot be destroyed.

2. **Sterilization.** The process of killing all microorganisms, including spores, in a certain area.

Spores are bacteria that have formed hard shells around themselves as a defense. These shells are like a protective suit of armor. Spores are difficult to kill. Some can even live in boiling water. Sterilization is necessary if the article comes in direct contact with a wound, as in the case of surgical instruments or solutions used for cleaning a wound. Sterilization is the responsibility of a specialized department within a health-care institution. However, in the home, such specialized equipment does not exist. Depending on the item, it can be sterilized in one of two ways: wet heat or dry heat.

PROCEDURE 5

Wet-Heat Sterilization

RATIONALE: Removing pathogens from instruments decreases one cause of disease.

1. Assemble your equipment:
   Items to be sterilized, cleaned, and dried
   Clean, covered pot large enough to hold items
   Cold water to cover the items in the pot
   Timer or clock
   Sterilized tongs
   Potholder
   Source of heat (stove, Sterno, fire)

2. Wash your hands.

3. Place the equipment in the pot so that water touches all parts of it. If there are glass parts, put a clean piece of cloth in the bottom of the pot to protect them.

4. Cover the contents of the pot with cold water. Be sure to leave headroom in the pot.

5. Put the pot on a source of heat big enough to heat it. Turn handles away from the edge of the stove.

6. Bring water to a boil. Do not open the pot. Note when steam escapes under the cover.

7. Boil the contents undisturbed and covered for twenty minutes.

8. Turn off the heat.

9. Allow the contents to cool undisturbed. Leave the equipment in the pot until you are ready to use it.

10. Use sterilized tongs to remove the contents to a sterilized holder (Figure 8.6 ■).

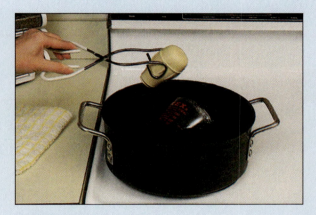

FIGURE 8.6 ■

SAMPLE CHARTING: 1/1/04   12:15 P.M. Instruments for dressing change sterile as per procedure. Left them in the sterile holder for Mr. Rummy's daughter, who will change the dressing on his left hip. Therese Hooper H/HHA

PROCEDURE 6

Dry-Heat Sterilization

RATIONALE: The removal of pathogens from cloth used for dressings is one way to decrease the spread of pathogens.

1. Assemble your equipment:
   Pie tin
   Dressing or cloth to be sterilized
   Oven
   Potholder

2. Wash your hands.

3. Place the clean dressings wrapped in a clean cloth in the pie tin.

4. Place the pie tin in an oven at 350°F. Allow the dressings to bake for one hour. Then allow them to cool (Figure 8.7 ■).   *continued*

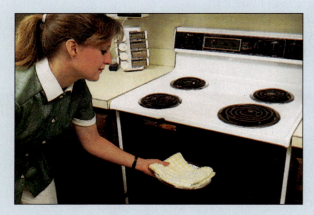

FIGURE 8.7 ■

5. Unwrap carefully. Do not touch the dressings; they are considered sterile.

Note: A hot iron held on dressings for several seconds also sterilizes them; however, the oven method is preferred.

> **SAMPLE CHARTING:**   8/8/04   8:30 P.M.
> Two dressings sterilized as per procedure. Both left in oven to cool. Mrs. Sample's daughter will use one tonight and one in A.M. to change dressing on the decubitus on client's back. Note left for daughter that more clean cloth is needed. Ruth Hawks H/HHA

SECTION 4

Special Infection Control and Isolation Precautions for Transmittable Diseases

OBJECTIVES

What You Will Learn to Do

1. Name two diseases transmitted through exposure to blood and body fluids.

2. Discuss the need for standard precautions.

3. List the standard precautions necessary when caring for clients in their home.

4. Discuss the five areas of concern for basic isolation.

Introduction: Care of Clients with Transmittable Diseases

blood-borne pathogens
disease-causing entities transmitted through contact with blood

The discovery of certain diseases within the past 15 years has alerted healthcare workers to the need to lower the chance of transmission of these diseases from client to caregiver. These diseases are spread through exposure to blood and body fluids and are called **blood-borne pathogens.** Two of these diseases are AIDS and hepatitis B. The human immunodeficiency virus (HIV) causes acquired immunodeficiency syndrome (AIDS). HBV causes hepatitis B. Both diseases are spread through sexual contact, shared intravenous needles, and the exchange of blood and/or body fluids. One problem with caring for clients who have AIDS is that little is known about this disease. The other problem is our personal feelings. This disease may awaken negative feelings because of fear or because some victims may have an unfamiliar lifestyle. The physicians and your agency will determine if isolation precautions should be instituted for a particular client. Remember, not all clients with AIDS and hepatitis B need be on isolation precautions. However, observe standard precautions all the time.

Table 8.1: Different Types of Hepatitis

	Type A	Type B	Type C
Transmission	Oral-fecal; poor sanitation, contaminated water or food; sexual contact	Body fluids; sexual contact; blood-to-blood contact; contaminated needles	Direct blood-to-blood; sexual contact
Complications	Rare	Cirrhosis; cancer	Cirrhosis, cancer
Risk to Health-Care Workers	Poor hand washing	Contact with bodily fluids into open skin; needle sticks	Needle sticks
Vaccine	Available	Available	None available
Prevention	Hand washing; avoid contaminated food and water; cook all food	Standard precautions; safe sex; do not share personal items with people you don't know well	Standard precautions; safe sex; do not share personal items with people you don't know well

The chance of transmitting a disease such as AIDS or hepatitis from any client to a caregiver is small if caregivers follow current regulations from the U.S. Centers for Disease Control (CDC) and the Occupational Safety and Health Administration (OSHA). However, remember that each agency may also have specific policies and procedures to follow when caring for clients.

Hepatitis, an inflammation of the liver caused by a virus, has three types. Although no vaccine is known against type C, a vaccine against type A and B is available to most people. You may elect to receive such a vaccine or you may refuse it. The best way to prevent transmission of this disease remains the use of standard precautions; you may not know who has this disease and who does not (Table 8.1 ■).

MRSA or methicillin-resistant staphylococcus aureus is the staph bacterium strain resistant to usual antibiotics. It can pass from person to person through direct contact or droplet transmission. This infection is often found in hospitals or other health-care facilities. The bacteria is not usually treated unless it infects a person who is already ill or who has a chronic disease. The best way to prevent giving or getting this disease is to practice good hygiene and standard precautions. Washing hands frequently and disposing of used tissues and soiled dressings is important. If you care for a client in whom this has been definitely diagnosed, the physician will institute isolation precautions. You will be instructed in how to work safely in this atmosphere. If you are immunosuppressed or pregnant, discuss this with your supervisor and your doctor.

STANDARD PRECAUTIONS

Medical tests and careful medical history are often not enough to identify clients who have blood-borne pathogens. Therefore, the CDC requires health workers to decrease the risks of being exposed to all body fluids except sweat. These basic activities are called **standard precautions.** An important point to remember is

hepatitis
inflammation of the liver, either chronic or acute

MRSA
methicillin-resistant staphylococcus aureus

standard precautions
those routine activities recommended to protect health care workers from contamination with blood and all body fluids (except sweat)

CDC GUIDELINES

Standard Precautions

- *Disposable Gloves:* Must be worn when contact is possible with blood, all body fluids except sweat (whether or not they contain blood you can see), skin that has breaks in it, and all mucous membranes. This includes activities during direct care and care of equipment.

- *Gowns or Aprons:* Must be worn during procedures or situations when there may be an exposure to blood, body fluids (except sweat) draining wounds, or mucous membranes.

- *Masks, Face-shields, or Goggles:* Must be worn during procedures that are likely to generate droplets of blood or body fluids (except sweat), or when the client is coughing excessively. Discuss with your supervisor the agency policy for reusing masks.

- *Handwashing:* Hands must be washed before gloving and after gloves are removed. Hands and other skin surfaces must be washed immediately and thoroughly if contaminated with blood or body fluids (except sweat) and after all client care activities. Caregivers who have open cuts, sores, or dermatitis on their hands must wear gloves for all client contact or be removed from client contact until the hands are healed.

- *Transportation:* When transporting (moving) any client who may have an infection, ensure that care is taken to use standard precautions to minimize the risk of transmission of microorganisms to others and to limit the contamination of environmental surfaces or equipment.

- Use resuscitation devices as an alternative to mouth-to-mouth resuscitation.

transmission-based precautions
additional isolation precautions that become part of the patient's plan of care if a diagnosis of a specific pathogen is made

protective barriers
equipment to protect you from splashes, spills, droplets, or other sources of contamination

that standard precautions are actions taken on a routine basis for all clients and are designed to protect you against transmission of microorganisms through body fluids. It is the law that standard precautions be incorporated into the routine tasks of all health care workers. In addition to standard precautions, if a definite diagnosis is made, specific types of isolation, called **transmission-based precautions,** will be added to the patient's plan of care.

Each agency has a policy discussing standard precautions and the use of **protective barriers.** Protective barriers are equipment to protect you from splashes, spills, droplets, or other sources of contamination. These include gloves, gowns, aprons, masks, face shields, and goggles. Your agency is required to provide you with this equipment. If you do not have it available, be sure to ask for it. Also, ask for the standard precautions policy and be sure that you understand what it means. The policy will be based on the CDC guidelines for standard precautions.

Using Nonsterile Gloves

Gloves protect you and the client. Use gloves whenever there is a chance you will touch body fluids other than sweat, or nonintact skin, or if you might put your hands in or near a client's mouth.

- Wearing gloves does not mean you do not have to wash your hands.
- Remember to wash your hands before and after you use gloves.
- Never wear gloves outside the client's room.
- Put on a new set of gloves each time you use them.
- Never reuse a pair of gloves!

Note: Once the gloves are on, the outside of the glove is considered "dirty" and the inside is considered "clean." The outside of the gloves should not touch any of your skin surfaces.

Using the Standard Precautions Guidelines

Standard precautions are common-sense guidelines. Wear gloves whenever exposure to body fluids (except sweat) may occur. Clients often feel uncomfortable being cared for by somebody wearing gloves. Explain to them that this is the new standard of care for all clients, and that it is required. If you injure yourself while caring for a client, report it immediately. If you have any cuts or injuries on your hands or body, report to your supervisor before you start to care for your client, and wear gloves while giving care (Figure 8.8 ■).

- *Exposure to body fluids or blood.* Wear gloves if a chance exists for contamination. If splattering is possible, wear a gown or protective apron and mask. Flush waste products down the toilet. Spills should be wiped up with soap and water by a person wearing disposable gloves, then wiped with a solution of 1 part household bleach to 10 parts water. The rag should be thrown out. Change gloves frequently. When removing gloves, do not touch the outside of the gloves.
- *Personal items.* Items such as tampons, peripads, or razors are not considered medical waste and should be disposed of as you would any dressing.
- *Sharp objects, needles, blades.* Handle carefully to prevent cutting yourself. These objects should be placed in a puncture-resistant container and disposed of according to local rules. Do not bend needles or try to recap them.
- *Dressings.* Wrap these items in a plastic bag and dispose of them according to local law. You may have to double-bag them if you are transporting them as medical waste. Check with your supervisor (Figure 8.9 ■).
- *Plates, glasses, dishes.* Use separate utensils—disposable, if possible. Clean reusable utensils in hot water and detergent. Use hot water, friction; dry. Do not let dishes drip dry.

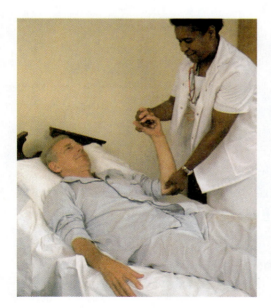

FIGURE 8.8 ■ Gloves are not required when touching a client, provided the skin is not draining. Gloves are not required changing linens, provided the linen is not soiled.

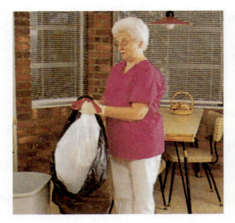
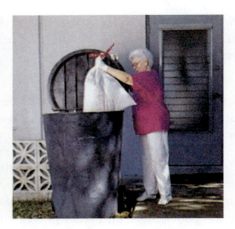

FIGURE 8.9 ■ (a) Double-wrapping dressings protects you, the environment, and the people who handle the bags. Double-bagging may be done as part of isolation technique or as an extra precaution for all heavily soiled trash. (b) Be sure all trash goes into a covered container.

■ *Laundry.* Unsoiled laundry needs no special attention but should be washed or dry-cleaned normally. Soiled linen should be separated and handled with disposable gloves. Keep soiled linen in a double plastic bag lined with a cloth bag or pillowcase. Empty the contents of the plastic bag into the washing machine without touching the items, then throw away the plastic bag. Wash soiled linen each day.

PROCEDURE 7

Putting On Nonsterile Gloves

RATIONALE: Gloves provide a barrier between you and potential contamination.

1. Assemble equipment
   Nonsterile gloves
   Trash can in which to dispose of them
   A place or method of washing your hands

2. Wash your hands

3. Select a clean pair of gloves

4. Inspect the gloves for holes or tears. Discard them if they are not intact.

5. Grasp the gloves just below the cuff and slip your hand into it (Figure 8.10 ■).

6. Straighten out the glove so it does not roll on your wrist.

7. Put the second glove on the same way (Figure 8.11 ■).

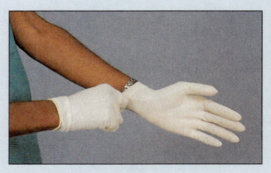

FIGURE 8.11 ■

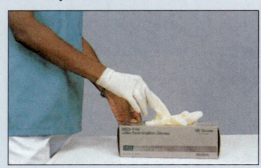

FIGURE 8.10 ■

CHARTING: Not necessary.

PROCEDURE 8

Removing Nonsterile Used Gloves

RATIONALE: Removing gloves correctly will decrease the chance of contamination.

1. Assemble your equipment
   Trash can in which to dispose of gloves
   A place or method of washing your hands
2. Grasp the glove at the palm of your hand with the other gloved hand to loosen it.
3. Pull the glove over your hand while turning the glove inside out (Figure 8.12 ■).
4. Continue holding the removed glove with the gloved hand.
5. Place the index finger and middle finger of the ungloved hand inside the cuff of the glove turning the cuff downward (Figure 8.13 ■).
6. Pull the cuff and glove inside out as you remove your hand from the glove (Figure 8.14 ■).

7. Discard the gloves in the trash (not your pocket).
8. Wash your hands.

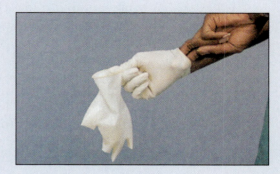

FIGURE 8.13 ■

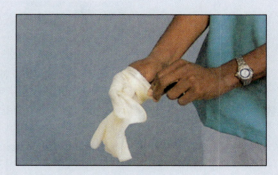

FIGURE 8.14 ■

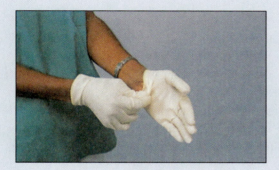

FIGURE 8.12 ■

CHARTING: Not necessary.

Machine washing (colorfast)	1 cup of household bleach in hot water and laundry detergent
Hand washing (colorfast)	2 tablespoons of household bleach in 1 gallon of warm water and laundry detergent; soak for 10 minutes and rinse
Machine washing (noncolorfast)	1 cup of Lysol in warm water and laundry detergent; wash again with water only to remove Lysol
Hand washing (noncolorfast)	2 tablespoons of Lysol in 1 gallon of warm water and laundry detergent; rinse at least 3 times to remove Lysol

ISOLATION TECHNIQUES (TRANSMISSION-BASED PRECAUTIONS)

Beyond standard precautions, additional precautions may be necessary when you care for a client with a highly contagious disease. This helps decrease the chance of spreading the disease to others. Also, when a client is highly susceptible to diseases, caregivers may have to protect the client until his body is able to fight an infection. The physician will determine the type of isolation precaution to use. Transmission-based precautions include contact precautions, droplet precautions, and airborne precautions. Check with your supervisor for instructions on agency policy regarding these procedures.

The use of gown, gloves, and mask should be discussed with your supervisor and individualized. Wearing a gown protects you and the client.

Wearing a mask decreases the spread of airborne pathogens. Mask material filters the air the wearer breathes. Sometimes, a mask is worn to protect the client, too. There are different types of masks, but they all filter the air and should be applied the same way and changed after every patient encounter.

Basic handwashing is necessary even though gloves are worn. Wash your hands before and after every client contact. The client may have additional restrictions

■ GUIDELINES

Basic Isolation—Five Areas of Concern

■ *Dressings:* Always dispose of dressings in plastic bags and according to local regulations. If the dressings are heavily soiled, double-bag them.

■ *Urine/feces:* Flush down the toilet immediately. Clean urinal, bedpan, or commode thoroughly with disinfectant.

■ *Dishes:* Use disposable dishes and cups, if available. Wash dishes separately in hot water and soap. Do not let dishes soak or remain in the sink.

■ *Linen:* Transport to laundry area in separate plastic bags. If heavily soiled, double-bag. Wash separately in hot water. Dry immediately.

■ *Cleaning equipment:* Use a disinfectant. Dispose of cleaning water down the toilet. Dispose of cleaning rags in plastic bags.

■ GUIDELINES

Using a Gown and Mask

■ Gown should be long enough to cover your clothing. The outside is considered contaminated. A wet gown is considered contaminated. Do not touch the outside of the gown when you remove it. Wear a clean gown for each client contact (Figure 8.15a–d ■).

■ Apron should be worn to cover clothing during routine client care.

■ Masks should fit snugly over the nose and mouth. A wet mask is considered contaminated, as is the front of the mask. Do not wear a mask around your neck. A clean mask should be worn for each client contact. There are several different types of masks. Discuss with your supervisor which one is appropriate for your client (Figure 8.16 ■).

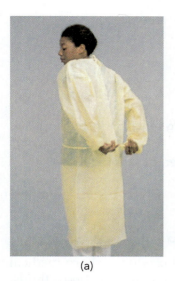
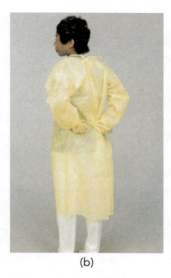
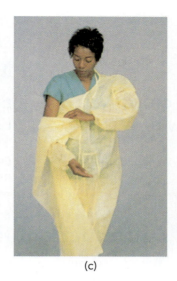
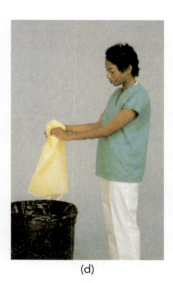

(a) (b) (c) (d)

FIGURE 8.15 ■ Tie the neck piece of the gown and overlap the back flaps. (b) Tie the gown securely. Put on gloves now if you need them. (c) To take off a gown, take off your gloves if you are wearing them. Untie neck and waist. Grasp shoulders. Turn gown inside out as you take it off. (d) Fold up the gown and discard. Do not reuse a gown. Wash your hands.

placed on his activity and the washing of his linen and may need to use disposable dishes. There will be additional laundry. Your help in arranging laundry care will be important in care of the client. Your supervisor will help you and the family incorporate the needed isolation techniques into the plan of care.

Remember, standard precautions require that you protect yourself against contact with blood and body fluids. The use of isolation status may mean additional activities, but basic standard precautions must always be used. **Double-bagging** is a technique of placing contaminated articles in a plastic bag in the isolation room and then placing the closed bag into another plastic bag as it is held outside the doorway. This can be done by either one person or two.

double-bagging
technique of putting contaminated material into two plastic bags for protection

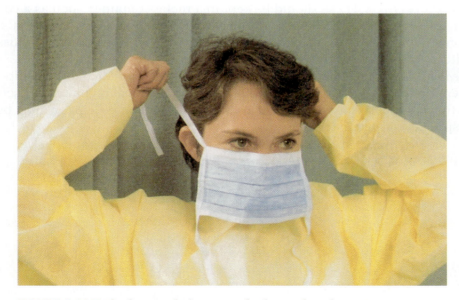

FIGURE 8.16 ■ The face mask that covers both mouth and nose is worn to prevent exposure to blood, body fluids, or when patient is coughing excessively.

Regulated Medical Waste

OBJECTIVES

What You Will Learn to Do

1. Define regulated medical waste.
2. List three reasons for segregating regulated medical waste from ordinary trash.
3. Demonstrate proper disposal methods for regulated medical waste.

Introduction: Regulated Medical Waste

regulated medical waste
waste products
determined by law to be
in need of special
disposal

Regulated medical waste is defined as blood, blood products, sharp medical instruments such as needles, and dressings contaminated with body fluids. Many communities have regulations that specify how the residents may dispose of regulated medical waste. It is important that you know this information so that you can assist the client and his family with proper disposal. In many cases, if the medical waste is not disposed of according to the local regulations, the client can be fined. Some towns make pickups, and some require residents to bring the waste to a central point.

Regulations protect local residents, the people who process the trash and waste, and the environment. If you or the client are not aware of local regulations, your supervisor will be able to obtain the details.

- *Human waste products.* These should be flushed down the toilet immediately and not discarded in the street, backyard, or street sewers.
- *Blood and bloody fluids.* These should be cleaned up immediately. If the liquid can be flushed down the toilet, that is the best disposal method. Contaminated clothes should be washed separately in hot water and dried. Dressings and cleaning rags should be double-bagged in plastic and disposed of according to local regulations.
- *Needles (sharps).* These should be kept in a metal container, such as a coffee tin. Secure the top and dispose of the can according to local regulation. Some items may be kept; some must be disposed of immediately. Discuss with your supervisor the best method of disposal.
- *Medical equipment.* If contaminated, it should be emptied and the equipment double-bagged and disposed of according to local regulation. Discuss with your supervisor whether the used equipment can be kept or must be disposed of immediately.

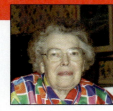

Case Study

Review the case study that appears on the first page of the chapter. Answer two sets of questions about the case study contained in the Explore and Apply sections below.

EXPLORE

1. You have been assigned to visit Mrs. Day three times a week to assist her in changing the dressing on her leg ulcer and help her to maintain a clean environment. What are your main concerns given her home? Safety? Infection control? Cooking, preparing, and keeping food?

2. What concerns do you have about Mrs. Day when you are not in the house? How would you communicate these concerns to her family?

APPLY

1. You notice that Mrs. Day is losing weight. When you question her, she says that the food spoils quickly and she cannot afford to buy food in small quantities. What practices could you establish to help Mrs. Day receive more complete nourishment?

2. As you change Mrs. Day's dressing, she mentions that she does not understand why you wear gloves. How do you explain this practice to her? What would you observe and document? Discuss how you would dispose of the used dressing.

Certificate Exam Review Questions

Choose the best answer for each question or statement.

1. **Bacteria must have all of the following to grow:**

    a. *Food, moisture, temperature*

    b. *Food, moisture, temperature, oxygen, light, living or dead matter*

    c. *Age of the bacteria*

    d. *Sunlight*

2. **The single best way to prevent the spread of bacteria is**

    a. *to wash all clothes in bleach.*

    b. *leave all garbage outside in double plastic bags.*

    c. *feed dogs outside so they don't spill their food.*

    d. *wash hands frequently and dry them with paper towels.*

3. **Gloves should be worn**

    a. *during all client care.*

    b. *when caring for a client who is coughing.*

    c. *when giving a client a bath.*

    d. *whenever there is a possibility of contact with blood or body fluids.*

4. **Standard precautions are necessary**

    a. *because the government might check on your care.*

    b. *because the agency policy says they must be used.*

    c. *because they protect both you and the client.*

    d. *because it makes the client happy.*

5. **Keeping the house clean**

    a. *is the responsibility of the homemaker/home health aide.*

    b. *is the responsibility of the family.*

    c. *is a joint responsibility among all caretakers and the client.*

    d. *must be contracted out to a dedicated person.*

CHAPTER 9

Care of the Client's Environment

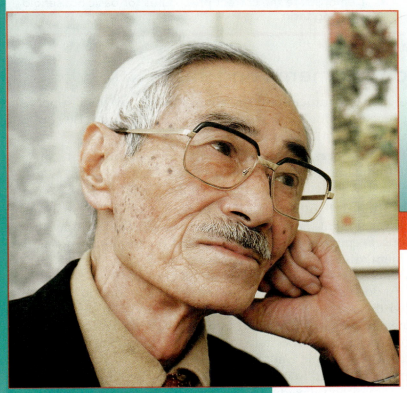

CASE STUDY

Mr. Phom lives with his sister and her two adult children and their families in a small apartment above a bar. The children have all been in this country for 10 years, but only the school-age children speak English. They act as interpreters whenever they are in the house. The family shops in Asian stores, watches Vietnamese television, and reads Vietnamese newspapers. The adults have never attempted to learn English. Mr. Phom is home from the hospital after an abdominal operation. His sister continues to be his primary caretaker, but she has to go to work each day and he is alone. An independent and private man, Mr. Phom does not accept assistance easily, and the language barrier presents a challenge. You assist the client with his meals, which are left by the family, but you are unable to chart what he eats as you are not familiar with the ingredients. You have not been able to develop a way of finding out what Mr. Phom does when you are not in the house. Mr. Phom is in pain and self-medicates with native medication he buys over the counter in the local Asian store. The house is dark and the rugs are worn. You have offered to help with the laundry, but the client's sister has refused this assistance.

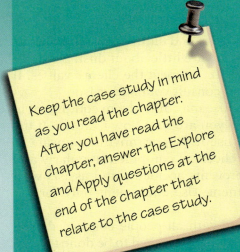

Keep the case study in mind as you read the chapter. After you have read the chapter, answer the Explore and Apply questions at the end of the chapter that relate to the case study.

Homemaking

OBJECTIVES

What You Will Learn to Do

1. Understand your role as a homemaker/home health aide in maintaining a clean environment.

2. Discuss ways of establishing an individual work plan with your client and his family.

3. Demonstrate the correct procedures for basic household cleaning tasks.

Introduction: Homemaking Tasks

When you receive your assignment and the client's care plan, your supervisor will tell you what housekeeping tasks you will be expected to do. Be sure you know the answers to the following questions:

■ Is the task related to the personal and therapeutic care of the client?
■ Can anyone else in the home or family do this task?
■ Who will do this task when you are no longer in the home?

Remember, it is often difficult for families to realize what is important in keeping a house clean and that the homemaker/home health aide is not there to perform all the housekeeping tasks. If the client and his family do not understand your assignment, discuss this with your supervisor.

Clean environments keep harmful bacteria under control. By cleaning bathrooms regularly, you decrease the chances for the spread of communicable diseases. Foods stored in specific places are easy to find and can be used more often with less time and energy being spent to look for them. Accidents are less likely in areas kept orderly. It is especially important to keep clutter away from stairways and areas where people walk frequently.

Clean environments also tend to make us feel better. When things are looking their best, we are more often relaxed and comfortable. It also gives us a feeling of pride when others visit. A client will tend to be healthier and happier in an environment that is clean and comfortable.

CLEANING A CLIENT'S HOME

"Clean" usually refers to an area free of pathogens and clutter. To some people, a dust-free home is the only clean home. Others care little about dust. Such differences in values are important to recognize. Try to meet the client's values. If your values and the client's needs are different, consult your supervisor.

Cleaning equipment available to you in a house may differ from equipment in your house. Do not use any equipment unless you are sure how it works. If the equipment is not in good condition, do not use it. Report anything unsafe to your supervisor. Encourage to the family to check all equipment regularly and maintain it in perfect working order. This prevents accidents and assists with maintaining a clean and healthful environment. Use equipment only for the purpose for which it was intended.

Discuss all housekeeping tasks in the home with all people concerned. You might hold a meeting with the family to decide what jobs need to be done to keep the household functioning. You might want your supervisor at this meeting, or

Table 9.1: **Sample Work Plan**

Day	Task	Who Will Do It
Monday		
Tuesday		
Wednesday		
Thursday		
Friday		
Saturday		
Sunday		

this discussion might be informal. After the group has made a list of jobs, discuss who will do them. Remember, you will not always be in the house. It is important to develop a routine the family can follow when you are gone (Table 9.1 ■).

Encourage all family members to make suggestions and offer help. Remember, the family is in a crisis situation and people who may not usually help in housekeeping may be willing to help at this difficult time. A spirit of cooperation and flexibility should be encouraged. Children are important parts of families. Do not overlook them.

If someone is willing to help but does not know how, a "teacher" (either you or a family member) could be found. In teaching, remember:

- Make the explanation of the job as simple as possible.
- Help the people, but do not do it for them.
- Let them do it their way if it gets the same results.

HOW TO KEEP A HOUSE CLEAN

Make a list of what you need to keep the house clean. Remember to use products already in the home. Do not insist that the client purchase your brand of cleaning products. Your list might look like this:

Necessary Supplies	Nice to Have
Hot water	Dustpan
Soap or detergent	Vacuum cleaner
Broom	Scouring pads
Vinegar	Mop
Scrub pad, scrub brush	Wastebaskets
Baking soda, baking powder	
Bucket	
Trash container	

Table 9.2: **Basic Kinds of Cleaning Products**

Products	Form	Uses	Cautions
Soaps and detergents	Liquid Powder Solid	All types of cleaning; personal cleaning	Read label; protect eyes
All-purpose cleaner	Liquid Powder Solid	All types of cleaning	Read label; protect eyes
Abrasives/bleach	Liquid Powder	Surface soil; kills certain pathogens	Read label; protect eyes and skin
Specialty cleaners	Foam Liquid Powder Spray	Specific jobs: metal, windows, etc.	Read label

Be sure you know how to use the appliances in the house. If you are not sure, ask!

When using any cleaning product (Table 9.2 ■), use the following care:

■ Read the instructions on the label. Follow the directions in the order they are given and use the amount suggested (Table 9.3 ■).
■ Do not mix cleaning products unless you have been instructed to do so. Mixed products may cause a chemical reaction that will hurt you and/or the surface you are cleaning.
■ Do not leave cleaners on a surface for a long time. Use care in how much you scrub a surface.
■ Change the cleaning water when it is only moderately dirty, and rinse if needed to avoid streaking or filming.

Table 9.3: **Using Common Cleaning Products**

Task	Product	Use
Bathtub stains	White vinegar or paste of hydrogen peroxide and baking powder	Rub stain with rag dipped in vinegar; leave paste on stain overnight; rinse
Tile cleaner	Baking soda	Sprinkle on, rub with damp rag or sponge; rinse, as solution makes tile slippery
Windows and painted surfaces	Mix carefully: 5 cups water 1 teaspoon detergent 1 pint rubbing alcohol 1/2 cup sudsy ammonia	Wash area carefully; rinse well; dry
Mattress stain solution	1/2 cup water 1/2 cup white vinegar	Dab solution on stain and let dry; rub area with water and detergent; leave on for 10 minutes; blot dry; rinse; let mattress dry

- Store all cleaning products safely away from children and pets, away from heat sources, and in their original containers. Store cleaning tools and supplies safely as close as possible to where you will use them.
- Line garbage pails with plastic or paper bags. Do not put wet objects directly into paper bags. Wrap them first.

When using equipment, keep in mind the following safety points:

- Keep electrical equipment away from water. Never soak this equipment unless the manufacturer says that you can.
- Use equipment for the use for which it was intended.
- Do not put sharp objects such as hairpins, knives, or screwdrivers into electrical equipment.
- Before repairing an electrical object, unplug it!
- Be sure all equipment is in good condition and does not have frayed cords.

SPECIFIC TASKS

Dusting

Dusting is done to prevent the spread of bacteria. In homes where people are particularly sensitive to dust, you may have to dust often. Dampen the rag with a light spray of water or a commercial spray to keep the dust from spreading. Dust with motions that will gather the dust into the rag and away from you. Dust from top to bottom. Dust pictures on walls, then objects on tables, and finally tables and cabinets. If the rag becomes soiled, change it.

Washing Dishes

Dishes should be washed properly soon after meals. If a dishwasher is used or dishes are to be washed at a later time, scrape the food off the dish (a rubber spatula is a good tool to use for this job). Then rinse or soak the dishes in a basin of water.

- Place dishes on the counter to the left of the soapy dish water in the order in which they are to be washed—least dirty first, (glasses, silverware, plates, cups, and saucers) most dirty last (pots and roasting pans).
- Wash dishes in the hot, soapy water and rinse in clear water in the pan to your right (Figure 9.1 ■).
- Drain dishes on drainboard placed to the right of the rinse water.
- Dry dishes with a clean cloth. If none are available, allow dishes to air dry.

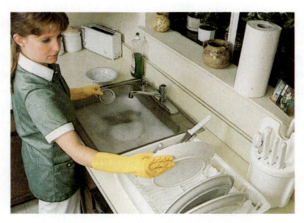

FIGURE 9.1 ■ Carefully place dishes in a clean drainer that has a mat under it to catch the water.

Note: If you are left-handed, reverse the placement of the soapy water pan, clear water pan, and the place where the dishes are stacked and drained.

When water is not plentiful, use water from rinsing dishes for another cleaning task, such as washing the floor. Wash dishes in water hot enough to clean the grease from them and destroy as many microorganisms as possible.

Keeping a kitchen clean is important. Just as food keeps us alive, it also feeds bacteria. Cleaning spills and taking proper care of leftover food is important. Trash should be disposed of regularly (before it falls out of the container). If the trash is wet, put it into a plastic bag first and then into the garbage can. Keep the garbage can clean. Wash it often!

- The stove should be wiped up regularly with soapy water to avoid spills becoming "cooked on."
- The refrigerator (or the place where food is kept cold) should be wiped out on a regular basis. If the refrigerator needs defrosting, discuss this with the family and/or your supervisor. Do not use sharp objects to poke at ice clumps when defrosting the refrigerator. If the refrigerator is self-defrosting, clean up spills promptly. Food tends to dry out faster in these models.
- Small appliances can be wiped down with soap and water or an all-purpose cleaner *after* they have been disconnected.
- Countertops should be free of food spills and grease. Counters are easier to wipe off if they are kept uncluttered. Areas around drawer handles and door pulls should be kept clean by wiping with a cloth (or sponge) and warm soapy water.

Cleaning Bathrooms

Constant moisture in the air keeps bathrooms in need of regular cleaning to keep them free of bacteria and odors. If bathroom floors are ceramic tile, any water spilled on them can make them slippery and dangerous. Keep the floors dry.

Safety in bathrooms should always be on your mind. Before a client uses a bathroom, check it:

- Are there nonskid mats in the tub?
- Are there nonskid rugs on the tile floor?
- Are there grab bars in the shower or tub?
- Is there good lighting?
- Is there ventilation?

Cleaning shower walls and bathtubs can be kept to a minimum if everyone will wipe the area out after each use. People will cooperate more easily if you keep a rag or old towel handy for them to use.

Sinks and other bathroom fixtures should be cleaned regularly with cleanser and a rag. Do not destroy the surface of enamel fixtures by using cleaners that will scratch them.

To clean the toilet bowl, you will need soap or detergent, a toilet bowl brush, and a rag or sponge. *Note:* Do not wipe anything else with this rag or sponge. Wash it after this task (Figure 9.2 ■).

- Lift up the seat and put soap or detergent into the bowl.
- Scrub the inside of the bowl with a toilet bowl brush. Clean under the rim of the bowl.
- Let the suds stay in the bowl while you wash the outside.
- To avoid a possible chemical reaction, do not mix toilet bowl cleaner with any other cleanser.

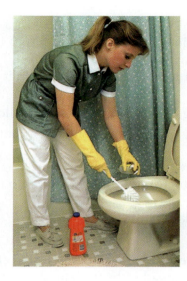

FIGURE 9.2 ■ Store the brush used to clean the toilet in a special container and use it for this purpose only.

■ Use clean hot water to rinse off all parts of the toilet with the sponge or rag.
■ If there are water stains such as rust in the bowl, shake in 1/4 cup of toilet bowl cleaner. Let stand about thirty minutes, then scrub and flush.

Laundry

Clean clothes are important for good health. They also make us look good and feel better about ourselves. Before washing any clothes, repair all tears, loose buttons, and jammed zippers. If you cannot do this, put the clothes aside and either repair them later or tell your client about the need for the repairs. Such precautions will prevent the repair job from becoming a much larger task. Before washing, sort clothes by:

■ *Color.* Dark colors should be washed separately from light colors.
■ *Fabric.* Delicate fabrics cannot take as much scrubbing as can heavy-duty fabrics.
■ *Degree of dirt.* Heavily soiled items should not be washed with lightly soiled ones.

As with any appliances that you use, either ask the client how to operate the washer correctly or read the instructions in the "use and care" booklet from the appliance manufacturer.

After sorting clothes, load the machine, being careful not to overload it. Put in the recommended amount of detergent and select the water temperature and amount of agitation. Add bleach and fabric softener (if needed) after the water has soaked all the clothes.

Clothes dried out of doors conserve energy and have a fresh, clean smell. Take dry clothes immediately from a dryer as they will then need less ironing and you will save energy and time.

Not all homes have a washing machine. After you have found out how the laundry is usually done in the home, discuss with your supervisor what your responsibilities will be. Bending and lifting wet, heavy pieces of linen could cause you to injure your back. If you must do this, use good body mechanics. Protect your back!

Care of Rugs and Carpeting

Ask your client how to care for the carpets and rugs. Frequent vacuuming or sweeping will preserve the rugs and decrease lint and dust.

If the client has a vacuum cleaner, remember:

■ Treat it as you would any electrical appliance.
■ Ask how to change the dirt collection bag inside.
■ Use the vacuum cleaner at a convenient time for the family, when it will not disturb them.

When you find stains on a carpet or rug, you may treat them as follows:

■ Ask the family if the stain is new. If it is an old stain, you will probably not be able to get it out.
■ You may use commercial stain removers.
■ You may mix water and baking soda into a solution and rub it into the stain. After it dries, vacuum.
■ If the spot is sticky, sprinkle baking soda on it, then vacuum.

Care of Floors

Keeping floors clean is important to the general well-being of the client and his family. Clean floors also decrease the spread of bacteria and provide a safe path in which people can walk.

■ Sweep floors frequently, especially before washing them.
■ Ask family members how they usually clean the floors. Wood floors often require special cleaners and are not cleaned with water.
■ Use the detergent or cleanser according to directions. Do not let water remain on the floor.
■ Most households will have a mop for this job. If you do not find one, discuss this with your supervisor.
■ Let the floor dry before walking on it or putting furniture back in place.

Pests and Bugs

Pests and bugs may carry diseases and may annoy you and your client. They may bite, cause skin irritations, or even frighten people. The best way to keep an area free of bugs, rodents, and other pests is to keep it clean and free of clutter.

■ Put food away in closed containers; tin and glass are best.
■ Clean up spills and crumbs.
■ Take out garbage and trash.
■ Keep garbage and trash in covered containers.
■ Roaches and mice can pass through small cracks in walls and near pipes. Talk to your supervisor about having someone caulk up such holes (Figure 9.3 ■).
■ Do not let water stand inside or outside.

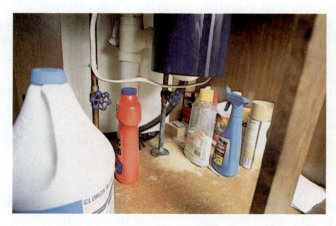

FIGURE 9.3 ■ Wet, damp, dark places left undisturbed attract bugs and pests.

If you or any family member wish to use a commercial product to get rid of bugs or rodents, check with your supervisor to be sure that it is safe.

SECTION 2

Bed Making

OBJECTIVES

What You Will Learn to Do

1. Make a closed bed.
2. Make an open fanfolded bed.
3. Make an occupied bed.
4. List the reasons why a well-made bed is important.

Introduction: Bed Making

You may have a client who spends part of the day in bed. Other clients, though, cannot or must not leave bed at all. As a result, many clients are fed and bathed and use a bedpan in bed.

Homemaker/home health aides should make beds with no wrinkles in the sheets. Wrinkles are not only uncomfortable, they can restrict the client's circulation and cause painful **decubitus ulcers** (bedsores). These open wounds often slow the client's recovery. Decubiti can form quickly and are difficult to heal.

You may care for a client in his own bed. Your client may decide to sleep on a couch or a hospital bed in his home. Your client may have side rails on his bed. Side rails both protect the client and assist him as he moves in the bed by providing him with something to grab for support. If your client needs a side rail to prevent him from falling out of bed, you could put chairs up against the bed with their backs against the mattress. Tie the chairs together and tie them to the bed (Figure 9.4 ■). The same rules and procedures apply for any type of bed.

■ Keep the bed dry and clean—change linen when necessary.
■ Keep the linen wrinkle free.
■ Make the bed to suit your particular client.
■ Keep the bed free of food particles and crumbs.

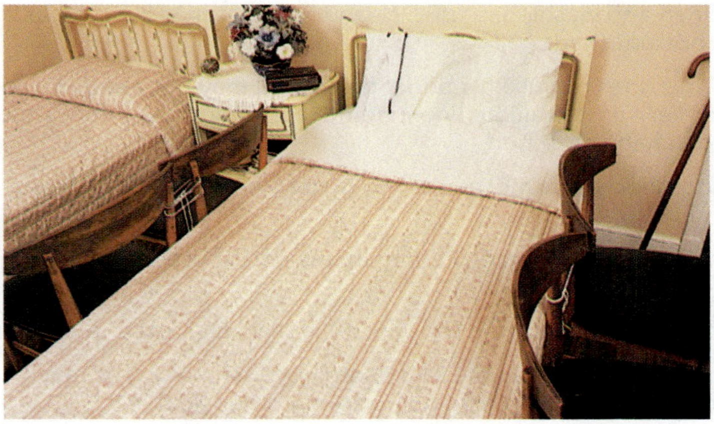

decubitus ulcer
bedsore; open wound that occurs from lack of blood supply to an area usually located on a bony prominence

FIGURE 9.4 ■ This is a good way to remind a client to call for assistance. Permanent side rails have to be provided if the client uses them frequently to change position or to pull himself up in bed.

GUIDELINES

Bed Making

- Use linens the client has available. If you do not have enough, report this to your supervisor.

- Try to make the bed according to the custom of the house. If you must change the custom, explain your reasons to the client and his family.

- Do not use a torn piece of linen. It may tear even more and could be dangerous.

- Never use a pin on any item of linen.

- Do not shake the bed linen. Shaking spreads harmful microorganisms to everything and everyone in the room, including you.

- Never allow any linen to touch your uniform.

- Dirty used linen should never touch the floor.

- Put dirty linen in the place agreed upon by you and the client's family.

- Some clients use fitted bottom sheets. Others use flat sheets with which the homemaker/home health aide makes **mitered corners.** The mitered corners keep the sheets firm and smooth and makes the bed neat and attractive.

- The bottom sheet must be firm, smooth, and wrinkle-free. This is important for the client's comfort.

- By fanfolding the top of the bed, you make it easy for the client to get in and out of his bed.

- The **draw sheet** is about half the size of a regular sheet. When draw sheets are not available, a large sheet can be folded in half widthwise (with small and large hems together) and used. The fold must always be placed toward the head of the bed and the hems toward the foot of the bed. You could also use a tablecloth. If you must protect the bed, a plastic tablecloth makes an excellent protective sheet. Never use plastic from a garment bag or garbage bag.

- The plastic draw sheet and disposable bed protectors protect the mattress. Plastics should never touch a client's skin. When using a plastic draw sheet, be sure to cover it entirely with a cloth draw sheet.

- Some clients do not use a draw sheet. Instead, small disposable bed protectors are placed on the bed under the client as necessary. These are often expensive. Check with your supervisor before you suggest this to the family.

- To save linen and washing, a used clean top sheet may be used as a draw sheet or bottom sheet.

- A client who does not use his bed a great deal may not need the linen changed every day. Evaluate linen, home, client, and the entire situation before you change the bed.

- Always use good body mechanics, no matter what kind of bed your client is using.

- "Bottom of the bed" refers to the mattress pad, if used; the bottom sheet; and the draw sheets.

- "Top of the bed" refers to the top sheet; the blanket, if used; and the bedspread.

- Remember that you save time and energy by first making as much of the bed as possible on one side before going to the other side.

- Side rails prevent the client from falling.

mitered corner
folding the bedding at the corners when making a bed so that the sheet is tightly stretched with no wrinkles

draw sheet
small sheet made of plastic, rubber, or cotton placed across the middle of the bed to cover and protect the bottom sheet and assist in moving the client

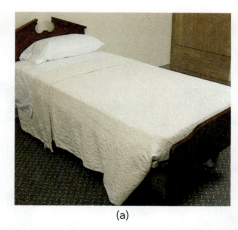

(a)

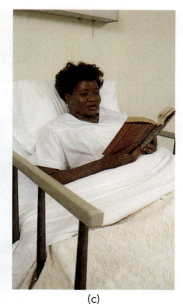

(c)

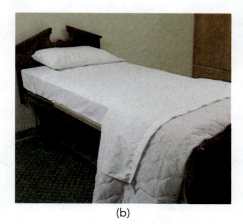

(b)

FIGURE 9.5 ■ (a) Closed bed. The linen is changed only when it is soiled; (b) Open bed. This bed is usually made without a heavy blanket. Have one available if needed; (c) Occupied bed. Change the linen as needed. You may not have to change the entire bed each day.

Three Basic Beds

1. *The closed bed.* This bed is usually made when it will remain empty for a while. You can make it with a bedspread or with only a sheet and blanket (Figure 9.5a ■).
2. *The open bed.* This bed is used when it will be occupied within a short period of time (Figure 9.5b ■).
3. *The occupied bed.* This bed is made with the client in the bed (Figure 9.5c ■).

The Open Bed, Fanfolded Bed, Empty Bed

The procedures for making the open bed, the fanfolded bed, and the empty bed are all the same. You will make an open bed when the client can get out of bed and move around.

The open bed is made exactly like the closed bed except that the top bedding is left open so that the client can easily get back into the bed.

This is done after you finish making the cuff at the head of the bed.

The Occupied Bed

The occupied bed is made when the client cannot or must not leave the bed. The most important part of making an occupied bed is to get the sheet smooth and tight under the client so no wrinkles will rub against the skin. When making the bottom of this bed, your job will be easier if you divide the bed in two parts—the side the client is lying on and the side you are making. By doing this, the weight of the client is never on the side where you are working.

PROCEDURE 9

Making the Closed Bed

RATIONALE: A closed bed keeps linens clean and orderly. Clean linen helps prevent the spread of bacteria.

1. Assemble your equipment:
   Mattress cover, if used
   Bottom sheet
   Cotton and plastic draw sheet (or disposable bed protector)
   Top sheet
   Blanket
   Bedspread
   Pillowcase
   Pillow
   Pillow protector, if used
   Chair

2. Wash your hands.

3. Place a chair near the bed.

4. Put the pillow on the chair.

5. Stack the bed-making items on the chair in the order in which you will use them: first-used items on top, last used on the bottom.

6. If you have a hospital bed, adjust the bed to the highest horizontal position and lock the bed in place. If not, move the bed so you have room to practice good body mechanics.

7. Pull the mattress to the head of the bed until it touches the headboard.

8. Place the mattress pad on the mattress even with the head of the mattress.

9. Fold the bottom sheet lengthwise and place it on the bed:
   a. Place the center fold of the sheet at the center of the mattress from head to foot (Figure 9.6 ■).
   b. Put the small hem at the foot of the bed, even with the edge of the mattress.

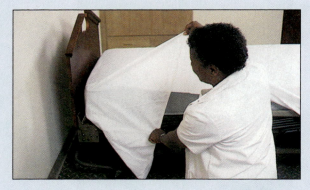

FIGURE 9.7 ■

   c. Place the large hem at the head of the bed with about 18 inches left to tuck in.

Always do this while practicing good body mechanics. Bend your legs, not your back.

10. Open the sheet. It should now hang evenly over each side of the bed.

11. Tuck the sheet in tightly at the head of the bed. Lift the mattress with the hand closest to the foot of the bed and tuck with the other hand. This is good body mechanics.

12. To make a mitered corner:
    a. Pick up the edge of the sheet at the side of the bed 12 inches from the head of the mattress (Figure 9.7 ■).
    b. Place the triangle (the folded corner) on top of the mattress (Figure 9.8 ■).
    c. Tuck the hanging portion of the sheet under the mattress (Figure 9.9 ■).
    d. While you hold the fold at the edge of the mattress, bring the triangle down over the side of the mattress.
    e. Tuck the sheet under the mattress from head to foot (Figure 9.10 ■).

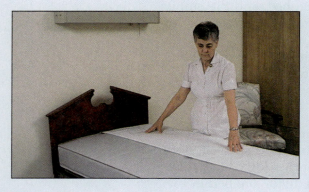

FIGURE 9.6 ■

FIGURE 9.8 ■

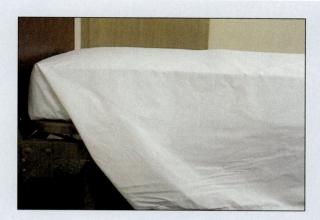

FIGURE 9.9 ■

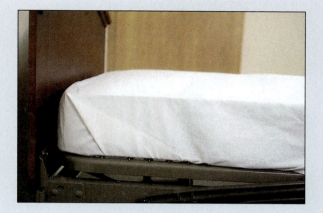

FIGURE 9.10 ■

13. Stand and work entirely on one side of the bed until that side is finished.

14. Place the plastic draw sheet 14 inches (two open handspans) down from the head of the bed. Tuck it in (Figure 9.11 ■).

15. Cover the plastic draw sheet with the cotton draw sheet and tuck it in (Figure 9.12 ■).

16. Fold the top sheet lengthwise and place it on the bed:
   a. Place the center fold on the center of the bed from the head to the foot.
   b. Place the large hem at the head of the bed, even with the top edge of the mattress.
   c. Open the sheet, with the rough edge of the hem up.
   d. Tightly tuck the sheet under the foot of the bed.
   e. Make a mitered corner at the foot of the bed.
   f. Do not tuck the sheet in at the side of the bed.

17. Fold the blanket lengthwise and place on the bed.
   a. Place the center fold of the blanket on the center of the bed from head to foot.

   b. Place the upper hem 6 inches from the top edge of the mattress.
   c. Open the blanket.
   d. Tuck it under the foot tightly.
   e. Make a mitered corner at the foot of the bed.
   f. Do not tuck in at the side of the bed.

18. Fold the bedspread lengthwise and place it on the bed.

19. Now move to the other side of the bed. Start with the bottom sheet.
   a. Straighten the sheet to remove all wrinkles. This should be done three times, first near the head, the middle, and at the foot of the bed.
   b. Miter the top corner.
   c. Pull the sheet tight so it is wrinkle free. Roll the sheet up in your hands so it is near the bed and pull slightly down and tuck in. Do this near the head, the middle, and the foot of the bed.
   d. Pull the plastic draw sheet tight and tuck it in.
   e. Pull the cotton draw sheet tight and tuck it in.

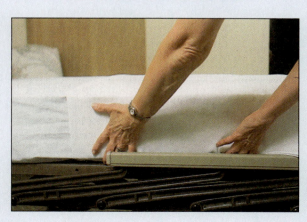

FIGURE 9.11 ■

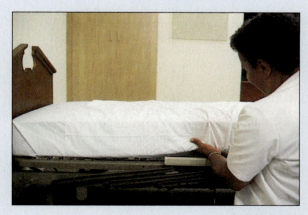

FIGURE 9.12 ■   *continued*

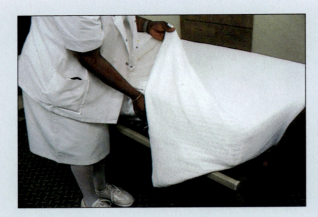

FIGURE 9.13 ■

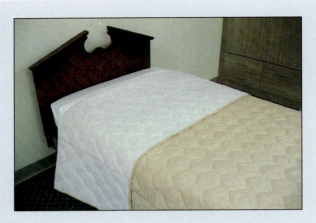

FIGURE 9.14 ■

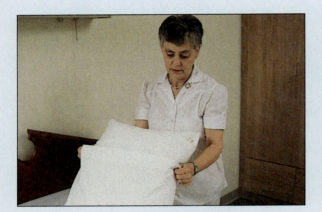

FIGURE 9.15 ■

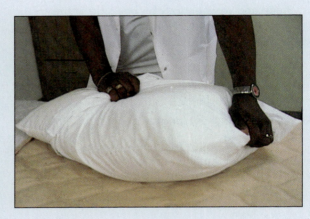

FIGURE 9.16 ■

f. Straighten out the top sheet, making the mitered corner at the foot of the bed.
g. Miter the corner of the blanket.
h. Miter the corner of the bedspread (Figure 9.13 ■).

20. To make the cuff:
   a. Fold the top hem of the spread under the top hem of the blanket.
   b. Fold the top hem of the sheet back over the edge of the spread and the blanket to form a cuff. The hemmed side of the sheet must be on the underside, so that it does not come in contact with the client (Figure 9.14 ■).

21. To put the pillowcase on a pillow:
   a. Hold the pillowcase at the center of the end seam.
   b. With your hand outside the case, turn the case back over your hand.

c. Grasp the pillow through the case at the center of the end of the pillow.
d. Bring the case down over the pillow (Figure 9.15 ■).
e. Fit the corner of the pillow into the seamless corner of the case (Figure 9.16 ■).
f. Fold the extra material from the side seam under the pillow.
g. Place the pillow on the bed with the open end away from the door.

22. Adjust the bed to its lowest horizontal position if you have a hospital bed.

SAMPLE CHARTING:	1/2/04 8:30 A.M.
	Bed made. All linen changed. Bed left closed as client plans to remain out of bed all day. Kathy Brown H/HHA

PROCEDURE 10

Making the Open, Fanfolded, Empty Bed

RATIONALE: An open bed provides easy access for clients returning to bed. Clean linen helps prevent the spread of bacteria.

1. Make a closed bed.
2. Grasp the cuff of the bedding in both hands (Figure 9.17 ■).
3. Pull it to the foot of the bed (Figure 9.18 ■).
4. Fold the bedding back on itself toward the head of the bed. The edge of the cuff must meet the fold.

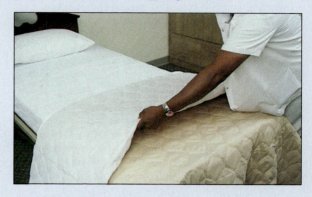

FIGURE 9.18 ■

5. Smooth the sheets on each side neatly into the folds you have made.
6. Wash your hands.

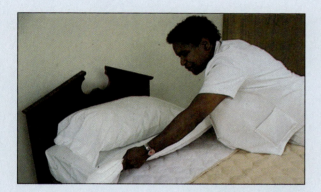

FIGURE 9.17 ■

SAMPLE CHARTING:	1/4/04 8:30 A.M. Bed made. Linen not changed. Bed left open and fanfolded, as client plans to nap after exercises. Kathy Brown H/HHA

PROCEDURE 11

Making the Occupied Bed When Side Rails Are Present

RATIONALE: Clean linen promotes cleanliness, good skin care, and comfort for bed-bound clients. Clean linen also helps prevent the spread of bacteria.

1. Assemble your equipment near the bed, in the order in which you will use them. A chair is useful for this purpose.
   Two large sheets
   One plastic draw sheet, if used
   One cotton draw sheet, if used
   Disposable bed protectors, if used
   One bath blanket, if available
   Pillowcase(s)
   One blanket
   One bedspread
   Container for dirty laundry
2. Wash your hands.
3. Ask any visitors to step out of the room, if appropriate.
4. Tell the client you are going to make his bed.
5. If you are working on a hospital bed, lower the backrest and knee rest until the bed is flat if that is allowed. Raise the bed to its highest horizontal position and lock in place.
6. Loosen all the sheets around the entire bed.
7. Take the bedspread and blanket off the bed, and fold them over the back of the chair.

continued

Leave the client covered only with the top sheet.

8. If using a bath blanket, cover the client with this by placing it over the top sheet. Ask the client to hold the bath blanket. If he is unable to do this, tuck the top edges of the bath blanket under the client's shoulders. Without exposing him, remove the top sheet from under the bath blanket. Fold the top sheet and place over the back of a chair.

9. If the mattress has slipped out of place, move it to its proper position touching the headboard. Remember to use proper body mechanics. If you cannot move the mattress, ask for assistance.

10. Raise the side rail on the opposite side from where you will be working, and lock in place.

11. Ask the client to turn onto his side toward the side rail. Help the client to turn if necessary. If the client cannot turn, have him stay on his back but move as far as possible toward the side rail. Be careful how the client's hands are placed. Adjust the pillow to suit the client's needs. Check it for items such as dentures and eyeglasses.

12. Fold the cotton draw sheet toward the client and tuck it against his back. Protect him from any soiled matter on the bedding (Figure 9.19 ■).

13. Raise the plastic draw sheet (if it is clean) over the bath blanket and client.

14. Roll the bottom sheet toward the client and tuck it against his back. This strips your side of the bed down to the mattress (Figure 9.20 ■).

15. Take the large clean sheet and fold it in half lengthwise. Do not permit the sheet to touch the floor or your uniform.

16. Place it on the bed, still folded, with the fold running along the middle of the mattress. The small hem end of the sheet should be even with the foot edge of the mattress. Fold the top half of the sheet toward the client. (This is for the other side of the bed.) Tuck the folds against his back, below the plastic draw sheet.

17. Tuck the sheet around the head of the mattress by gently raising the mattress with the hand closest to the foot of the bed and tucking with the other hand.

18. Miter the corner at the head of the mattress. Tuck in the clean bottom sheet on your side from head to foot of the mattress.

19. Pull the plastic draw sheet toward you, over the clean bottom sheet, and tuck it in.

20. Place the clean cotton draw sheet over the plastic sheet, folded in half. Keep the fold

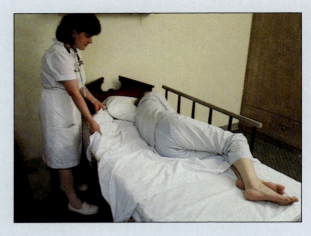

FIGURE 9.19 ■

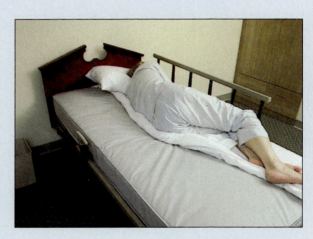

FIGURE 9.20 ■

near the client. Fold the top half toward the client, tucking the folds under his back, as you did with the bottom sheet. Tuck the free edge of the draw sheet under the mattress.

21. Ask the client, or help him, to roll over the "hump" onto the clean sheets toward you.

22. Raise the side rail on your side of the bed, and lock into place.

23. Go to the opposite side of the bed and lower the side rail.

24. Remove the old bottom sheet and cotton draw sheet from the bed. Put them into the container for soiled linen. Pull the fresh bottom sheet toward the edge of the bed. Tuck it under the mattress at the head of the bed and make a mitered corner. Then pull the bottom sheet under the mattress from the head to the foot. Do this by rolling the sheet up in your hand toward the mattress and pull it as you tuck it under.

25. One at a time, pull and tuck each draw sheet under the mattress (Figure 9.21 ■).

26. Have the client turn on his back.

27. Change the pillowcase, and place the pillow under the client's head. If necessary, assist the client to place the pillow under his head.

28. To put the pillowcase on a pillow:
    a. Hold the pillowcase at the center of the end seam.
    b. With your hand outside the case, turn the case back over your hand.
    c. Grasp the pillow through the case at the center of the end of the pillow.
    d. Bring the case down over the pillow.
    e. Fit the corner of the pillow into the seamless corner of the case.
    f. Fold the extra material from the side seam under the pillow.
    g. Place the pillow on the bed with the open end away from the door.

29. Spread the clean top sheet over the bath blanket with the wide hem at the top. The middle of the sheet should run along the middle of the bed. The wide hem should be even with the head edge of the mattress. Ask the client to hold the hem of the clean sheet, if he can, while you remove the bath blanket, moving toward the foot of the bed. Do not expose the client.

30. Tuck the clean top sheet under the mattress at the foot of the bed. Make sure you leave enough room for the client to move his feet freely. Miter the corner of the sheet if the client likes this.

31. Spread the blanket over the top sheet. Be sure the middle of the blanket runs along the middle of the bed. The blanket should be high enough to cover the client's shoulders.

32. Tuck the blanket in at the foot of the bed if the client likes this. Make a mitered corner with the blanket.

33. Place the spread on the bed as the client prefers. Pull up the side rails.

34. Go to the other side of the bed. Put down the side rails, turn the top covers back and miter the top sheet, then miter the blanket. Be sure the top covers are loose enough that the client can move his feet.

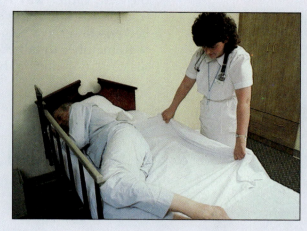

FIGURE 9.21 ■

35. To make the cuff:
    a. Fold the top hem edge of the spread over and under the top hem of the blanket.
    b. Fold the top hem of the top sheet back over the edge of the spread and blanket to form a cuff. The rough edge of the hem of the sheet must be turned down so the client does not come in contact with it.

36. Raise the backrest and knee rest to suit the client if this is allowed.

37. Lower the entire bed to its lowest horizontal position.

38. Put the side rails in place.

39. Make sure the client is comfortable.

40. Put all used linen in the proper place.

41. Wash your hands.

42. Chart any observations you made during this procedure.

SAMPLE CHARTING:	1/7/05 12:30 A.M. Patient incontinent of large amount of yellow urine. Entire bed changed and side rails replaced. Handbell placed within reach of client. Linen washed. Helen Marks H/HHA

Always keep the side rail up on the client's side. Usually, the occupied bed is made after giving the client a bed bath. The client should be covered with the bath blanket while you are making the bed. The sheets must be placed on the bed so the rough seam edges are kept facing the mattress and away from the client's skin.

Some clients prefer the pillow to be moved with them from side to side as the bed is being made. Some clients will ask you to remove the pillow while making

contraindication
condition that forbids
the use of a particular
treatment or drug

the bed. Either way is acceptable unless there is a medical **contraindication** (reason for not doing something). Your supervisor will tell you if a particular bed position must be maintained.

Remember to talk to your client while you make the bed. Continually notice his condition during the procedure.

SECTION 3

Safety and Fire Protection

OBJECTIVES

What You Will Learn to Do

1. List the general rules of home safety.
2. List special safety precautions to take with yourself and with older clients.
3. Explain what causes fire.
4. Explain what you can do to prevent fire.
5. Explain what to do in case of fire.
6. Describe the special safety precautions necessary when oxygen is being used.

Introduction: Safety

Safety is everyone's job. The rules that govern safety in a home must become part of every procedure and every decision you make while caring for your client. It is also important for you to remember that, by your actions, you are teaching family members. As they observe you practicing safety, they will be made aware of its importance.

It is your responsibility to protect your client and be continually aware of his safety. Make yourself aware of potential hazardous situations and their remedies in each home where you work.

It is also your responsibility to protect yourself. Be careful! Be aware! Be alert!

GENERAL SAFETY RULES

This section is designed to make you aware of the most common safety hazards in a home. More accidents occur in the home than in any other place. There are several reasons for this:

- We are careless.
- We do not have safety inspections in homes as we do in commercial buildings.
- We are not aware of the potential hazards that exist in homes.

General Safety Rules You Should Follow

- Discuss emergency communication with your supervisor. If no telephone is available, determine the best route of communicating.
- Report to your supervisor any unsafe conditions where you are working.
- When you see something on the floor that does not belong there, pick it up. If you see spilled liquid, wipe it up.

- Avoid slippery floors.
- If slippery floors cannot be avoided, walk on them carefully.
- Remove scatter rugs. If you cannot remove them, tack them down.
- Be sure to set the brakes on the wheelchair when a client is getting in or out.
- Use side rails on the bed if there is a chance the client will fall out.
- Do not work in poor light.
- Do not use any piece of equipment unless you are sure you know how it works.
- Keep the telephone numbers of the police, rescue squad, fire department, and poison control center near each telephone.
- Read labels. If a container does not have one, do not use the contents.
- Know how to leave the house in case of fire.
- Be aware of what accidents are most prevalent at different ages.
- Do not attempt a task if you have any doubt that you can do it.
- Do not reach into a garbage can or trash basket. You may hurt yourself on sharp objects.

Safety Precautions for Children

- Small children should never be left unattended when they are awake.
- Every child in a protective device should be checked frequently.
- Articles used in the child's care should be kept out of reach of a toddler when they are not being used. Watch especially for needles, water, safety pins, medications, matches, electrical equipment, syringes, and thermometers.
- Toys should never be left carelessly on the floor. Be especially alert to pick them up as they could cause someone to fall. Also, remember to clean up spills and messes such as food, urine, and feces.
- The sides of a child's crib should be up at all times except when someone is giving direct care to the child.
- Keep doors to stairways and the kitchen closed and locked.
- Keep venetian blind cords out of the reach of children.
- Be sure no small toys or objects are in the bed/crib that could be swallowed.
- Be sure no large objects on which the child could stand are in the bed or crib. The child might fall out of bed as a result.
- Keep all poisonous substances in a high place behind locked doors.

Safety Precautions for the Aged

Abilities change as we age. Unfortunately, few people realize this fact. Therefore, they attempt tasks that they can no longer do safely. As a homemaker/home health aide, be aware of the capabilities of your particular client. In addition, keep in mind these general rules:

- Ensure adequate lighting for every task.
- Be alert to sensory changes that may or may not have taken place.
- Protect your client from falling. Recovery from falls takes a long time.
- Protect your client from burns. Temperature sensation becomes less accurate as we age. Run cold water through a faucet after you run hot water so if your client touches the faucet, he will not burn himself. Test the bath water yourself.
- If a confused client tells you he is going to do something that you know to be harmful, take him seriously and protect him.

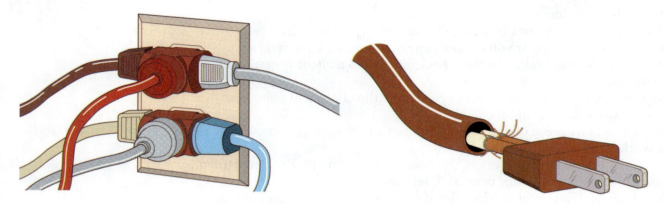

FIGURE 9.22 ■ Be familiar with misuses of electricity that exist in your client's home. Assist him with correcting them.

Electricity

Electricity is a great help in our lives. If we misuse it, however, it can cause a great deal of damage (Figure 9.22 ■).

■ Make sure all electrical equipment you use is in good condition.
■ Be sure the cords are not frayed and that you are using the proper tool for the job.
■ Do not put electrical cords under rugs. They may fray and go unnoticed under a rug. This is a perfect place for a fire to start.
■ Be sure your hands are dry before you use any electrical equipment.
■ Do not change fuses or touch circuit breakers unless you are sure you know what you are doing.
■ Do not run all household appliances at the same time in an effort to save time.

Smoking

Many clients smoke, as do many visitors. If a client permits smoking in his home—unless it is not allowed for medical reasons or because oxygen is present—you will be asked to tolerate it. If you are uncomfortable in a house with cigarette smoke, discuss this with your supervisor. Keep in mind these rules if people are smoking in the house.

■ Be sure ashtrays are provided and used.
■ Never empty warm ashtrays into plastic bags, plastic wastebaskets, or containers. When you empty ashtrays, be sure the contents are cool. Wet the ashes if you are in doubt.
■ A client who has been given a sedative should not smoke.
■ A confused client should not smoke.
■ A client in bed should not smoke unattended.
■ Check chairs, upholstery, and blankets for ashes or cigarettes if your client is smoking.
■ If a client has hand tremors, light his cigarette and assist him as he smokes.

Safety in the Kitchen

Some people cook in a hurry and think about many other things while they work. This leads to various types of accidents common to the kitchen area. Keep in mind basic safety rules when you are in the kitchen.

■ Keep a fire extinguisher in the kitchen.
■ Do not leave grease on the stove. Clean it up.
■ If you have a grease fire, do not put water on it. Use a chemical-type fire extinguisher or baking soda to smother it.

- Do not leave cooking pots unattended.
- Have good lighting in the kitchen.
- Be alert when carrying hot liquid.
- Keep paper towels, napkins, and potholders away from the burner.
- Keep the kitchen floor clean and free of clutter and spills.
- Store knives so that blades are protected.
- Electric cooking does not produce a visible flame, so be sure to check that the dial is at the setting you want or at OFF.
- If you or the client has a pacemaker, stay out of the kitchen when a microwave oven is working.

Safety in the Bathroom

Many accidents occur in the bathroom. Young and old alike have these accidents. You must be alert to potential hazards that exist due to conditions in the room and your client's abilities.

- Is the toilet secure to the floor? Is the seat secure to the toilet?
- Can your client get up and down safely? Can he sit without additional support?
- Are the hot and cold water faucets correctly marked?
- Is the tub deep, and can your client climb in and out safely?
- Does your client feel weak while bathing?
- Is there ventilation in the bathroom?
- Are the floor tiles slippery when wet? Is there a secure bathmat on the floor?
- If there are grab bars, are they secure in the wall? Towel bars were not designed to support weight. Special bars are necessary!
- If you must use electrical equipment such as hair dryers or shavers, be sure your hands, body, and feet are dry.

Proper Storage

Dispose of articles in well-ventilated containers. Do not keep used rags in closed containers. They can catch fire by a process called **spontaneous combustion.** This means they will burn as a result of their own heat. Get rid of the rags before this happens!

Do not store **flammable** liquids near any source of heat. Flammable liquids are those that can burn. Keep them in the garage but away from cars. Use flammable liquids in a well-ventilated area. This reduces the risk of fire and the risk of illness due to the fumes.

Do not keep piles and piles of newspapers. Make arrangements for them to be given to a recycling plant.

FIRE AND SAFETY PREVENTION

Fire safety means three things:

1. Preventing fires
2. Doing the right things if fire should occur
3. Protecting your client and yourself (Figure 9.23 ■)

Fires start because of:

- Smoking and matches
- Misuse of electricity
- Defects in heating systems
- Spontaneous combustion
- Improper rubbish disposal
- Improper cooking techniques
- Improper ventilation

spontaneous combustion
process of catching fire from the heat of chemicals burning

flammable
substance that will burn quickly

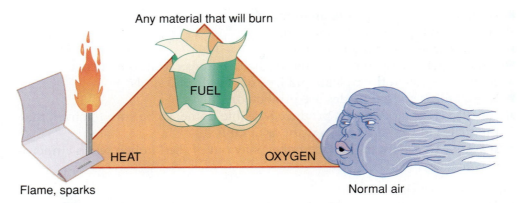

Any material that will burn

FUEL

HEAT

OXYGEN

Flame, sparks

Normal air

FIGURE 9.23 ■ By removing one of the needed elements, you can prevent a fire.

Making a Fire Plan

As you meet your client and learn the layout of the home, ask yourself the following questions:

- Where are the exits from this house in case of fire?
- How would I remove the client from this house in case of fire?
- If the client is bed-bound, how would I remove him from the fire scene?
- Are there fire extinguishers in this house—one for grease fires and one for other types of fires?
- Are there smoke detectors in this house? Do they work?
- Does the family have a fire evacuation plan?
- What special precautions, indicated by the town fire department, should be taken so they are aware of small children, bed-bound residents, or people dependent upon oxygen or ventilators?

What to Do in Case of Fire

Seal off the fire! If the fire is behind a closed door, do not open it (Figure 9.24a ■)! Take another route out of the building to safety. If you must go through a smoke-filled room, put a cloth (a wet one if possible) over your mouth and nose and one over those of your client. Crawl along the floor to safety or keep your client as low to the ground as possible (Figure 9.24b ■). Keeping in mind the word RACE will help you remember the steps to take in case of a fire (Figure 9.25 ■).

- Remove your client from the house.
- Call the fire department from a neighbor's house. Do not reenter the house for any reason.

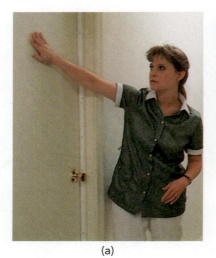

(a)

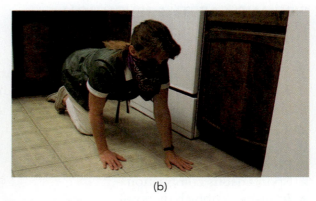

(b)

FIGURE 9.24 ■ (a) Feel the door BEFORE you open it. If it is hot, the fire is close. Stay in the room. (b) Heat and smoke rise. Crawling increases your ability to reach safety.

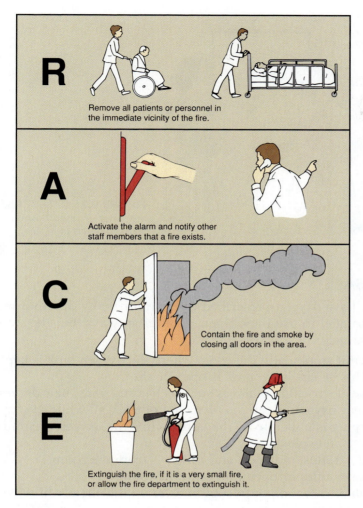

FIGURE 9.25 ■ In case of a fire, remember the word RACE.

- Keep your client warm and comfortable.
- Stay with your client.

POISONS

Children frequently swallow objects not meant to be swallowed. This is considered poisoning. Clients often forget that they took their medication and take additional doses of it. This, too, is considered poisoning. A confused client may take one medication when he really wanted another one. This, also, is considered poisoning.

Prevention is the best treatment for poisoning.

- Keep all poisons and medications locked away from children and confused clients.
- Never keep food products near poisons or cleaning products.
- Make it a habit to read labels each time you pick up any container.
- Call the poison control center for assistance if you have any suspicion a poisonous substance has been swallowed or an overdose of medication has been taken.
- Instructions for antidotes appear on the bottles of many potentially dangerous substances; unfortunately, these antidotes are not always correct. Do not use them. Call the poison control center and follow their instructions.

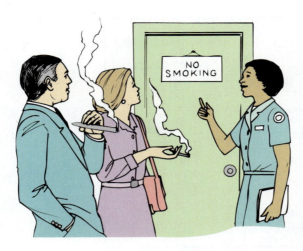

FIGURE 9.26 ■ NEVER allow smoking or open flame in the area when oxygen is in use.

OXYGEN SAFETY

Clients may have oxygen prescribed to them for many different reasons. They may be instructed to use the oxygen in different ways, but the safety rules are always the same.

- Never permit smoking in the room where the oxygen tank is kept (Figure 9.26 ■). This is true if the tank is open or shut.
- Do not use electrical appliances such as heating pads, hair dryers, or electric shavers near oxygen. Keep the plugs out of the wall while the oxygen is running. If a plug is pulled from the outlet while the oxygen is running, a spark could cause an explosion.
- Remove cigarettes, matches, and ashtrays from the room.
- Do not use candles or open flames in the room.
- Do not rub oil, alcohol, or talcum powder on the client while the oxygen is running.
- Avoid combing a client's hair while he is receiving oxygen. A spark of static electricity from his hair can set off an explosion.
- Wool blankets, nylon, and certain synthetic fabrics can cause **static electricity,** an electric spark sent into the air. Remove these from the client's room. Use cotton items when possible.
- Check the equipment regularly for leaks and proper functioning.
- Ask for careful instructions as to which valves you may touch and which valves should not be moved.
- All oxygen tanks are painted green.

static electricity
electrical discharges in the air

SECTION 4

Restraints

OBJECTIVES

What You Will Learn to Do

1. Recognize the difference between a restraint and a positioning device.

2. Discuss the rights of the client to be restraint-free.

3. Identify initiatives that should be explored prior to using restraints.

Introduction: Working with Restraints

A **restraint** is a device, prescribed by a physician, used to confine a client and prevent injury to that client or others. Every client has the right to a safe environment and to have his dignity and his rights as a person maintained. Tying a human being to a chair or bed does not support this. Restraint devices, while appearing to protect an individual, may actually violate his rights and could be identified as a form of abuse.

At times, a client may need to be restrained. This should always be for his protection and not the convenience of the caretaker. A client may not be restrained without a physician's order. Your supervisor will demonstrate the proper way to apply the restraint. Do not attempt to use restraints until you have been properly instructed. You will be expected to remain with the client while he is restrained and remove the restraint, reposition the client, and offer the client toileting and exercise at least every 2 hours. It is important that the family understand this routine. A family member is expected to remain with the client to remove the restraints and offer water and toileting after you have left. If, for any reason, you think the family is not adhering to the restraint release schedule, notify your supervisor immediately. Discontinue restraints as soon as possible. Documentation should include:

- Reason restraints were need
- Time and type of restraints were put on and by whom
- Position and status of client
- Time restraints removed and by whom
- Client status
- Position change, fluid/food offered, and toileting offered

A restraint should be the least-restrictive possible and used for the shortest length of time. Before using a restraint, be sure that alternative measures have been tried and proved futile. Be sure the following questions have all been answered:

- Can someone sit with the client to provide comfort, distraction, and direction?
- Has the medication regime been reviewed to be sure that the mediations are not contributing to the confusion?
- Can diversional activities be used, such as music, television, reading, and visitors?
- Can positional devices be used as reminders to clients instead of actual restraints (Figure 9.27 ■)?

restraint
a device prescribed by a physician to confine a client and prevent injury to that client or others

Clinical ALERT

Restraints
Restraints are the least desirable way to provide a safe environment for a client. They often frighten the client and the family. Explore with the family and your supervisor other methods of controlling and keeping the client safe. Try familiar music, soft radio sound, family members taking turns staying with the client, and talking to the client in his native language.

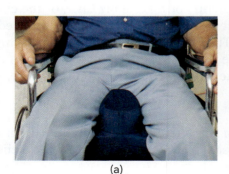
(a)

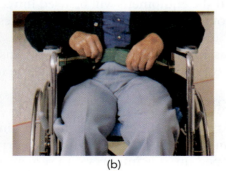
(b)

FIGURE 9.27 ■ Restraint alternatives: (a) saddle cushion, which prevents sliding forward; (b) self-releasing safety belt.

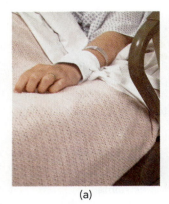
(a)

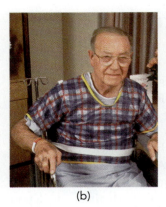
(b)

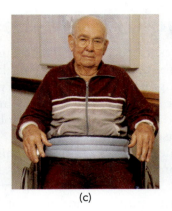
(c)

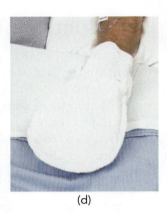
(d)

FIGURE 9.28 ■ Soft protective devices: (a) soft limb tie; (b) safety vest; (c) pelvic support; (d) soft cloth mitt.

Examples of restraints are seen in Figure 9.28 ■. When applying any of them:

■ Be sure the restraint is not too tight.
■ Be sure the client can still call for assistance.
■ Be sure the tie can be untied quickly in case of an emergency.
■ Be sure the family supports the restraint release schedule.

SECTION 5

Making Your Own Equipment

OBJECTIVES

What You Will Learn to Do

1. Improvise basic pieces of equipment.
2. Make a backrest.
3. Make a bed table.
4. Make a bed cradle.
5. Make a foot support.

Introduction: Making Your Own Equipment

At times you will want to make your client more comfortable or to provide him with items that will help him become more independent. Many of these items cost money and may be an expense the client cannot afford or does not want. Such items will not be used for long and therefore the family does not wish to buy them. If the equipment will be used infrequently or for a short time, or the client does not wish to purchase the item, suggest that you **improvise** and make needed items. The client may help in this task. The members of the family may help. Their assistance will be important because they will feel part of the client's care, and they will know how to construct the item when you are not in the house.

improvise
to make do with the tools or equipment at hand; to use an item for a task for which it was not originally designed

BACKREST

A backrest in a client's bed can prop him up when he eats, to take part in his care; and allow him to visit with people, read, or watch television. When a client is propped up, it is important to remember that:

■ He should be able to support himself in that position and not fall or slip out of bed or into an uncomfortable position.

- He should be able to call for help to change position.
- He should be comfortable in that position, and the position should be permitted by his physician.
- You will be able to secure the backrest so that it does not slip in the bed.

BED TABLE

The client can use a bed table during meal time, during personal care, and for recreation activities such as cards or reading. Having a light, easy-to-use bed table available encourages the client to be more independent. A table at the side of the bed, much like the ones in the hospital, can be improvised by standing an adjustable ironing board near the bed, adjusting the height, and locking it in place.

PROCEDURE 12

Making a Backrest

RATIONALE: A backrest promotes comfort and good body alignment while the client is in bed.

1. Gather the equipment you will need:
   A clean sturdy cardboard box about 24 inches by 24 inches by 18 inches
   A pair of scissors or sharp knife
   String, tape, or cord to secure the ends

2. Position the box on a flat surface with the wide side toward you.

3. Cut the right and left seams from the top to the bottom. The box will now be open and the front will be lying flat (Figure 9.29a ■).

4. Make a cut (score) through the inside layer of the cardboard on the side flaps as shown in the figure (Figure 9.29b ■).

5. Fold the ends toward the middle of the box along the scoring lines (Figure 9.29c ■).

6. Fold the front of the box (the part that has been laying flat) up to cover the triangles.

7. Fold the top down and tie or tape (Figure 9.29d and e ■).

SAMPLE CHARTING: 6/23/04   4:00 P.M.
Backrest made from a cardboard box and covered with a sheet. Client and daughter shown the proper way to use it. Client left in bed reading in good body alignment.
Sheryl Lobo H/HHA

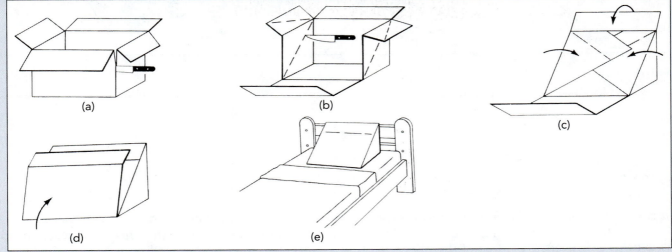

(a)   (b)   (c)   (d)   (e)

FIGURE 9.29 ■

PROCEDURE 13

Making a Bed Table

RATIONALE: A bed table helps the client safely take part in care and enjoy leisure activities such as reading, cards, or writing.

1. Gather the equipment you will need:
   A clean sturdy cardboard box about 10 inches by 12 inches by 24 inches
   A sharp knife or pair of scissors
   A pencil
2. Cut off the four top flaps of the box along the seams (Figure 9.30a ■).
3. Draw a curved opening on both wide sides of the box. Be sure the opening is large enough to fit over the client's legs. Be sure there is enough cardboard left on the side, at least 2 inches, to support the weight of the items you will put on the tray.
4. Cut out the opening along the lines you have drawn (Figure 9.30b ■).
5. Cut small openings in the side near the top for handholds.
6. Cover the table with adhesive-backed plastic or wallpaper to protect it and to make it more attractive (Figure 9.30c ■).

SAMPLE CHARTING: 2/7/04   3:00 P.M.
Bed table made from a cardboard box. Client ate lunch using it and was able to feed himself with ease. Client and family cautioned about placing heavy things on the table.
Jennifer Levine H/HHA

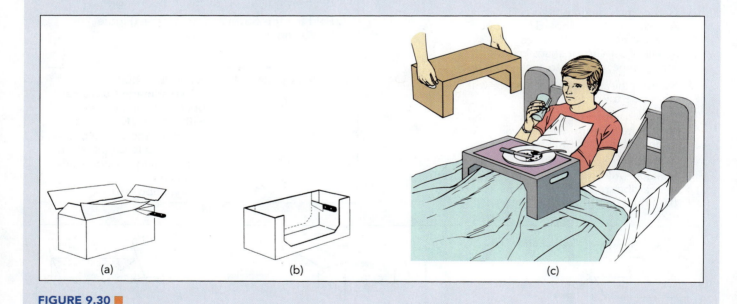

(a)	(b)	(c)

FIGURE 9.30 ■

BED CRADLE

bed cradle
frame placed over a body area to hold bed covers away from a body part

A **bed cradle** is used under the blankets and sheets and over the client's legs so that the covers do not touch the skin. This relieves the knees, the legs, and the feet of the pressure of the covers. Use the same procedure to make a bed cradle as you would to make a bed table. Be sure, however, that the box you choose is big enough to provide space for the client to move his legs.

PROCEDURE 14

Making a Footboard

> **RATIONALE:** Providing a footboard promotes good body alignment and prevents foot drop.

1. Gather the equipment you will need:
   A piece of wood just about as long as the bed is wide and high enough to keep the covers at least 2 inches off the client's feet
   Two blocks of wood for added support
   Sandpaper, nails or screws, hammer or screw-driver

2. Sand the edges of the boards so that they are smooth and will not cause splinters or tear the bed covers.

3. Secure the two pieces of wood at right angles to each other (Figure 9.31a ■).

4. Position the support on the bed under the bed covers (Figure 9.31b ■).

5. Instruct the client and family as to the function of the support.

> **SAMPLE CHARTING:** 4/5/05   2:30 P.M. Footboard made, with client's son, from two pieces of wood found in basement. The sides were sanded. Family instructed on the proper way to use the footboard. Client left in bed in proper body alignment with feet against the footboard.
> MaryEllen Caper   H/HHA

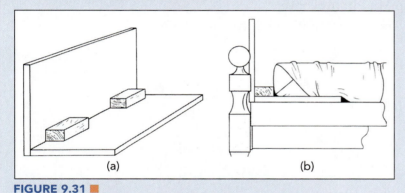

(a)   (b)

FIGURE 9.31 ■

FOOTBOARD

A **footboard** supports the covers so that they do not touch the client's toes and provides a place where the client can rest his foot. If the possibility of **foot drop** exists, this is a necessary piece of equipment.

footboard
a flat piece of wood or cardboard placed at the end of the bed, under the covers so that the client can rest his feet flatly against it and so that covers do not touch the client's toes

foot drop
a contraction of the foot due to a shortening of the muscles in the calf of the leg; the foot falls forward and cannot be held in proper position

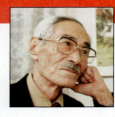

Case Study

Review the case study that appears on the first page of the chapter. Answer two sets of questions about the case study contained in the Explore and Apply sections.

EXPLORE

1. How do you feel about the fact that Mr. Phom is left alone, unable to communicate, and you are expected to help him with his personal hygiene and clean his room? Is the client safe? What makes you say so? What can you do to increase his safety without offending the family?

2. How do you know the client is in pain? Is it wise for the client to take both herbal medication and prescription drugs? What do you do?

APPLY

1. You have been assigned to assist Mr. Phom with changing his abdominal dressing. What do you note when you document the change? How can your notes and objective observations help Mr. Phom recover?

2. How do you provide diversion for Mr. Phom during the day?

Certification Exam Review Questions

Choose the best answer for each question or statement.

1. **You are responsible for keeping the home environment clean. You should**

   a. *request the cleaning supplies you like to use.*

   b. *use the supplies in the house whenever possible.*

   c. *bring your own cleaning supplies.*

   d. *get the supplies you think are needed as long as the house is clean.*

2. **Safety is everyone's job including the family.**

   a. *If the client does not care about safety in the household, you do not have to either.*

   b. *If the client does not care about household safety, you can tell him you will not return to care for him.*

   c. *Cats and dogs in the house keep the client company, so if they make a mess, it is worth it.*

   d. *You will make a list of what must be done and discuss it with the family, hoping that some of the more important problems can be rectified.*

3. **Safety is everyone's job, including yours. You should**

   a. *walk around and mentally plan an escape route for you and the client in case of fire.*

   b. *not check the oxygen equipment for a safety sticker because that is the responsibility of the company that supplies the oxygen.*

   c. *encourage the family to notify the local fire department if the client is bed bound only if they leave him alone.*

   d. *remove all the rugs so no one will slip on them.*

4. **Restraining a client**

   a. *is done to help the caregiver give good care to the client.*

   b. *is done only after all other avenues of care have been tried.*

   c. *can be done through the night so that everyone gets a good night's sleep.*

   d. *is never documented, as it is considered part of the general personal care.*

5. **Making your own equipment to be used while the client is in bed**

   a. *is silly. Insurance companies pay for the equipment anyway.*

   b. *will encourage the client to stay in bed.*

   c. *will provide a comfortable, safe environment for the client.*

   d. *is unnecessary because all clients should get out of bed at least once a day.*

CHAPTER 10

Planning, Purchasing, and Serving Food

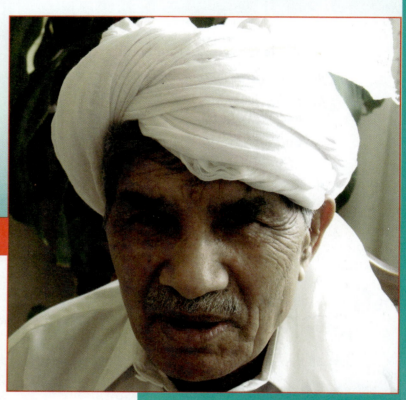

CASE STUDY

Mr. Patel has lived in the United States since he was a little boy. He is fluent in English and his native language. Although he lives in a primarily homogeneous neighborhood, he works in a big factory many miles away. Mr. Patel has developed a "heart condition" and has been placed on a salt- and calorie-restricted diet. He has been used to eating out each day or dining with friends at their house. He cooks only simple dishes and uses mostly canned food. He is sure that his condition will improve because he has no symptoms and takes his medications every day that he works. He is not receptive to suggestions about meal planning or taking his lunch to work.

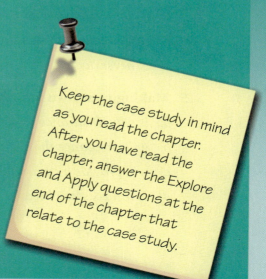

Keep the case study in mind as you read the chapter. After you have read the chapter, answer the Explore and Apply questions at the end of the chapter that relate to the case study.

SECTION 1

Basic Nutrition

OBJECTIVES

What You Will Learn to Do

1. Define a well-balanced diet.
2. Discuss the food pyramid and what it means.
3. List food sources of each nutrient.

Introduction: Basic Nutrition

Eating properly is important to all people. Good **nutrition** is especially important for a person whose body is in a weakened condition. Food gives us energy to carry out the day's activities and is necessary to rebuild body tissue. Eating is also a social activity. In some homes, it is the only time when all family members come together. Many family and personal preferences and practices associate with food. Do not assume that each family is the same.

Nutrients are substances that our bodies need to repair, maintain, and grow new cells. Each nutrient comes from many sources. It does not matter from which sources you get the nutrient as long as you get it in sufficient supply. A person unable to get the proper amount of a nutrient from food takes supplements. It is necessary for proper bodily function that a balance be kept among all nutrients—not too much of one or the other.

Dietary requirements differ at different stages of life. Children need more **protein** and **calories** than older persons need, but older persons need more of other nutrients.

All foods have been divided into basic **food groups:** milk, yogurt, and cheese; vegetables; meat, poultry, fish, eggs, dry beans, and nuts; breads, cereals, rice, and pasta; fruit; oils, fats, and sweets. The food groups are presented in a pyramid that indicates the recommended daily servings of each group (Figures 10.1 ■ and 10.2 ■). If you eat the correct number of servings from each food group, you will get the correct amount of each nutrient. Although diet will often be as important to the health of your client as medication or exercise, the client and his family may not understand this. Discuss with your supervisor ways to teach the family the importance of food and the proper diet while incorporating family and cultural preferences. If you do not understand certain practices, you may discuss them with the client or a family member in a respectful and nonjudgmental manner.

PERSONAL PREFERENCE

We all know foods we like and dislike or will not eat. Sometimes, a client will not eat a food for a cultural reason, a religious reason, or an unexplainable reason. You must respect these preferences and plan meals and diets taking these personal wishes into consideration. Discuss these situations with your supervisor so that you will be able to include all the nutrients in the client's meals and still adhere to his wishes. Your goal is to understand the client's and family's habits so that you can honor them when planning menus. Be observant as to what your client eats. Also note when he eats which foods.

nutrition
that which nourishes; food

nutrients
food substances required by the body to repair, maintain, and grow new cells

protein
one of the nutrients necessary to all animal life

calorie
unit for measuring the energy produced when food is oxidized in the body

food groups
the division of nutrients into four categories of dairy products, vegetables and fruits, meat and fish, and bread and cereal products

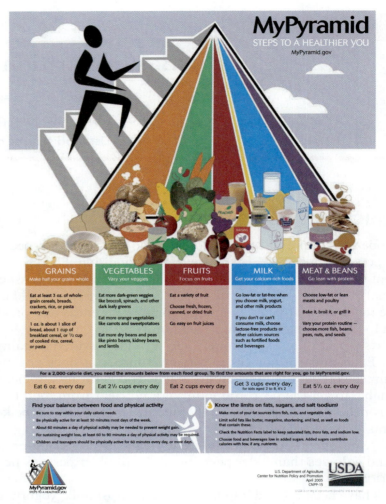

FIGURE 10.1 ■ The food guide pyramid. (*Source:* U.S. Department of Agriculture, www.nal.usda.gov, June 2004.)

Standards for a Healthy Diet

Various daily food guides have been developed to help healthy people meet the daily requirements of essential nutrients and to facilitate meal planning. Food group plans emphasize the general types or groups of foods rather than the specific foods, because related foods are similar in composition and often have similar nutrient values. For example, all grains, whether wheat or oats, are significant sources of carbohydrates, iron, and the B vitamin thiamine.

The new USDA food guide (Figure 10.1) has changed considerably from earlier versions of the food guide pyramid developed by the U.S. Department of Agriculture since 1992. Released in 2005, it reflects guidelines based on updated nutritional knowledge gained from research and data. The new food guide also allows people to personalize recommendations to their own body type and life style. Consult the U.S. Department of Agriculture Web site under the subject of Food and Nutrition for more information about MyPyramid.

As the U.S. population becomes more diverse, the nutrition and health needs of immigrant groups are being considered. Several variations have been made to adapt the food guide pyramid to ethnic diets (Figure 10.2).

ALTERNATE FOOD GUIDES

Several variations have been made to adapt the food guide pyramid to ethnic diets.

Asian Diet Pyramid

- A wide base of rice, rice products, noodles, breads, and grains; whole grains; and minimally processed foods
- A second level of fruits; vegetables; and legumes, nuts, and seeds
- Daily small amounts of vegetable oils; physical activity; and plant-based beverages (tea, sake, beer, or wine)
- Optional daily fish, shellfish, or dairy
- Weekly eggs or poultry and sweets
- Monthly meats.

(Although dairy products are largely absent, the plant-based diet of the Asians results in surprisingly low rates of osteoporosis.)

Mediterranean Diet Pyramid

- An abundance of food from plant sources, including fruits and vegetables, potatoes, breads and grains, beans, nuts, and seed
- Emphasis on a variety of minimally processed and, wherever possible, seasonally fresh and locally grown foods
- Olive oil as the principal fat, replacing other fats and oils
- Daily consumption of low to moderate amounts of cheese and yogurt
- Weekly consumption of low to moderate amounts of fish and from zero to four eggs per week (including those used in cooking and baking)
- Fresh fruit as the typical daily dessert; sweets with a significant amount of sugar (often as honey) and saturated fat consumed not more than a few times per week
- Red meat a few times per week

- Moderate consumption of wine, normally with meals
- Regular physical activity at a level that promotes a healthy weight, fitness, and well-being

Native American Food Pyramid

- Grain group is divided into bread and cereal group, and rice and pasta group (oats and wild rice) each group allows 6 to 11 servings per day
- Vegetables, 3 to 5 servings including corn, squash, and cactus
- Fruits, 2 to 4 servings fresh whole fruits
- Dairy, 2 to 3 servings including cheese, yogurt, and milk
- Meat, poultry, fish, dry beans, eggs, and nuts, 2 to 3 servings
- Fats and oils sparingly

Vegetarian Diet

Many ethnic diets are vegetarian based. The following make up a vegetarian food guide pyramid:

- Dairy intake may be 0 to 3 servings. Individuals who do not use dairy products need to find another source of calcium.
- Protein intake comes from dry beans, soy, and seeds (some do eat eggs).
- Grains and other sources of plant protein need to be varied to provide essential amino acids, which are all only found in animal protein sources.

(The eating patterns of vegetarians vary considerably. The lacto-ovo-vegetarian eating pattern is based on grains, vegetables, fruits, legumes, seeds, nuts, dairy products, and eggs, and excludes meat, fish, and fowl. The *vegan* (total vegetarian) eating pattern also excludes eggs, dairy, and other animal products. Individual assessment is required to evaluate the nutritional quality of a vegetarian's dietary intake.

FIGURE 10.2 ■ Cultural adaptations of the food pyramid.

RAMONT, ROBERTA PAVY; NEIDRINGHAUS, DEE MALDONADO, TOWLE, MARY ANN, COMPREHENSIVE NURSING CARE, 1st Edition, © 2005, p. 358. Reprinted by permission of Pearson Education, Inc., Upper Saddle River, NJ

Planning, Shopping, and Serving a Meal

OBJECTIVES

What You Will Learn to Do

1. List the factors a homemaker/home health aide must consider when purchasing food.
2. Become aware of ways to conserve energy when cooking.
3. List ways of making mealtime pleasant and therapeutic.

Clinical ALERT

PREPARING FOOD FOR CLIENTS

Including the client and the family in food preparation serves as an important social and learning activity and one in which the client can feel ownership of the process and the food. Preparing food that is familiar culturally entices the client to eat and gain strength and nutrients. Most foods can be included in a therapeutic diet in some way. If your client has specific food preferences, identify and communicate them to your supervisor.

Introduction: Planning

Mealtime is important. It should be a pleasant change in a client's day. The atmosphere, the place, and the way the food is served are important in stimulating an appetite. Try to serve a client in a room free from unpleasant odors and comfortable for the client. Keep the room at a comfortable temperature and a minimum of noise. It is often helpful to let the client decide what foods he wishes to eat and when he prefers to eat. Mealtime is more pleasant when a preferred food is served.

PLANNING A MENU

As the homemaker/home health aide, you may find it necessary to purchase food for the client. First, develop a menu of foods to prepare. Be sure the menu is planned from the client's diet and preferences. It is important to keep in mind the client's ability to chew and swallow as you prepare food. Consider the recommended servings from the food pyramid. Check the ingredients the client has on hand. Then make a shopping list. A list will help avoid unnecessary trips to the store for forgotten ingredients. It will also prevent duplicate buying of foods already on hand and, if grouped by types of food, avoid extra steps in the market. When planning a meal, remember:

- *Variety.* A well-balanced diet consists of nutrients from many different kinds of food. No one food is perfect.
- *Texture.* Combining crispy foods with smooth soft foods makes each texture seem more interesting. Unless the client is on a special diet and food texture is controlled, choose different types of texture within each meal served.
- *Flavors.* If all foods in the meal have a strong distinctive taste, they will compete with one another and overwhelm the client's taste buds. Keep the strong-flavored foods as the spotlight and milder-tasting foods as the background in a meal. Season food as the client prefers and his diet permits.
- *Temperature.* Cook food at the correct temperature. Ask the client at what temperature he prefers his food. Not everyone enjoys their food very hot or cold. Some people like ice. Some do not.
- *Taste.* Cook meals to the client's taste. Discuss with the family which spices they like and how they usually season their food.
- *Shape.* Prepare food with familiar shapes. Some families always slice their tomatoes, some cut them into chunks. Ask how food is prepared in this household.

■ *Color.* Give each meal eye appeal by keeping colors compatible. A sprig of parsley, radish roses, olives, or carrot curls may make an interesting dash of color to an otherwise drab-looking meal.

■ *Cost.* Few clients are free to spend an unlimited amount of money on their food. Plan meals within their budgets and do not cause waste.

Include all food eaten during a day in your planning. Food may be eaten at three traditional meals or as snacks throughout the day. Plan meals as close to the client's usual eating habits as possible.

When a client's diet is changed, special care could be taken to try to keep this new diet as close to the diet of the other family members as possible. For example, although food for a client on a salt-free diet should be separated from other family members' food before salt is added, the food may be the same.

Food habits can also be influenced by the client's religious beliefs or ethnic background. Jewish households may keep a kosher kitchen. This means that utensils and equipment used for meat products are kept separate from those used for dairy products. Meat and dairy products may or may not be eaten at the same meal. The degree to which a client keeps a kosher home should be discussed with the family. The impact of this upon the prescribed diet should be discussed with your supervisor.

Other ethnic groups may not eat pork, shellfish, or beef. Vegetarians eat no animal meat or by-products. Be alert that these foods or foods made from them are not included in any prepared foods you may purchase.

People who have strong bonds with their ethnic background may choose foods unfamiliar to the homemaker/home health aide. Clients often ignore a prescribed diet to eat foods more familiar to them. Encourage the client to stay on his therapeutic diet and notify the supervisor.

Most of the time your client's therapeutic diet can be adapted to his ethnic preferences. If you are unfamiliar with his dietary habits, discuss this with your supervisor. Then you will learn, and you will be able to help your client within his ethnic tradition.

FOOD ALLERGIES

Clients may have food allergies that can cause mild skin irritations or even severely affect his ability to breathe. Be sure to honor all of a person's allergies. Do not take it upon yourself to introduce any food even in small amounts. Sometimes children have food restrictions if one of their parents is highly allergic to a substance.

Purchasing Food Wisely

When purchasing packaged food, *read labels.* The ingredient lists on labels are critical to a person on a special diet. People on a salt-free diet should read the product label and see if salt was used in preparing the food item. Clients whose diet restricts sugar use can tell by reading the label if sugar has been used in the product. People sensitive to certain types of foods or chemicals will find the label's list of ingredients helpful in planning what to eat.

Labels also provide information on the amount in the container. Some labels list the number and amount of servings. Often, labels contain the calories per serving of the product. This information might be important to a client whose caloric intake is being monitored. The label may also list nutrients in the food and their amounts (Figure 10.3 ■).

Products that contain more than one ingredient, such as spaghetti in meat sauce, must list all ingredients used in making the product. The ingredient

Nutrition Facts

Serving Size 1 cup (49g)
Servings Per Container about 10

Amount Per Serving	Cereal	Cereal with 1/2 cup Skim Milk
Calories	170	210
Calories from Fat	5	5
	% Daily Value**	
Total Fat 0.5g*	1%	1%
Saturated Fat 0g	0%	0%
Polyunsaturated Fat 0g		
Monounsaturated Fat 0g		
Cholesterol 0mg	0%	0%
Sodium 0mg	0%	3%
Potassium 200mg	6%	11%
Total Carbohydrate 41g	14%	16%
Dietary Fiber 5g	21%	21%
Insoluble Fiber 5g		
Sugars 0g		
Other Carbohydrate 36g		
Protein 5g		
Vitamin A	0%	4%
Vitamin C	0%	2%
Calcium	2%	15%
Iron	8%	8%
Thiamin	8%	10%
Riboflavin	2%	10%
Niacin	15%	15%

FIGURE 10.3 ■
Learning to read labels will help you plan meals and budget money.

found in the greatest amount is listed first. In comparing two different brands of spaghetti in meat sauce, you can see that a can that listed meat first and flour last would have more meat than one that listed flour first and meat last.

SHOPPING FOR YOUR CLIENT

Before you go shopping for your client, be sure your supervisor knows that you are leaving the home. Usually, clients and their families will be encouraged to assume responsibility for shopping for themselves and managing their own budgets. Sometimes, however, you will be asked to help with shopping for a client within the family's budget.

Before you go shopping:

- Prepare a list and discuss it with the client.
- Discuss the size of the purchase, money available, likes and dislikes, and favorite stores.
- Be sure your client will be safe while you are out.

After you shop:

■ Save all receipts.
■ Carefully write down how much money you were given, how much you spent, and how much change you brought back.

UNIT PRICING

Unit pricing is another tool sometimes available to help make wise purchases. **Unit pricing** tells the customer what the cost is by a particular quantity. This can be determined by weight (for example, a box of cereal might read 72 cents per pound) or by pieces (for example, a bag of soap bars might read 25 cents per bar). This information is given in addition to the amount you will be charged for the product at the checkout counter.

The unit price can be displayed in a variety of ways. One way can be a poster that tells all the prices for the food in this section of the store. Another way might be a label on the edge of the shelf where the food is displayed. A third way might be on the price sticker that is put on each item.

Convenience foods (foods with some of the preparation already done) generally cost more than those made from scratch. But if only one or two people are eating the food, the ingredients for the scratch process might spoil before they are completely used. The decision as to which is most practical must be made individually by the client. You can share your opinion, but the client must make the final decision.

Purchasing larger quantities of an item is generally cheaper than buying small quantities. But if the item is rarely used or if storage is difficult, it may have to be discarded before it is finished. Discuss this with your client before you go to the store so you will not have to make this decision in the supermarket.

unit pricing
a system of showing the cost of food items in terms of common measurements such as ounces or pounds

Good Buys

Foods in season are almost always a good buy. Menus should be planned with seasonal foods in mind. The cost will be less and the selection greater.

In selecting foods, be aware that the best quality is not always necessary. In choosing tomatoes for a salad, the most attractive and usually the most costly would be desirable. However, in selecting tomatoes for tomato sauce, a less expensive product with perhaps a blemish on the skin might be considered a better buy. When buying foods high in protein, you can reduce the cost by:

■ Using poultry when it is cheaper than meat
■ Considering cuts of meat that may cost more per pound but give more servings per person
■ Learning to prepare less-tender cuts of meat in casseroles or pot roasts
■ Serving eggs or egg substitutes
■ Substituting dried bean and pea dishes for higher-cost meats
■ Using fillers such as bread crumbs or pasta to make a meat dish serve more people

STORING FOOD

After shopping for food economically, it is essential that you store it properly. Proper storage prevents loss of nutrients and possible food poisoning. If your client does not have good storage facilities, discuss this with your supervisor. Some people do not have sole use of a refrigerator or stove. Work with your client so that food can be stored appropriately and safely.

General Storage Hints

■ Do not buy more food than you can safely store.
■ Keep refrigerators operating properly by defrosting when needed.
■ Check the expiration date on food before purchasing it. Choose the food with the longest time before expiration.
■ Rotate food at home by using the most recently purchased food last.
■ Dry ingredients such as flour, sugar, cereal, and pasta products should be stored in tightly covered containers.

Tips for Specific Foods

■ *Meats.* Refrigerate all meats. Ground meat and variety meats spoil more quickly than others, so use them soon after purchase.
■ *Fruits and vegetables.* Keep most fresh fruits and vegetables in the refrigerator in plastic bags, tightly covered containers, or the crisper.
■ *Bread.* If wrapped properly, bread can be frozen to keep it most efficiently for a long time.
■ *Milk.* Instant nonfat dry milk can be used in many of the same ways as whole milk and can be stored for much longer periods without refrigeration.
■ *Canned foods.* Store in a cool, dry place.
■ *Frozen foods.* Keep in freezer at 0°F temperature.

Preparing a Meal

When preparing foods, be aware of the amount of energy you use. By doing this, you will save time and money, and indicate your concern for the client's resources.

■ Use the oven to prepare more than one food at a time.
■ Do not preheat the oven longer than necessary.
■ Put the pot on the correct-size burner. The burner should be as close to the size of the pan as possible. Too big a burner wastes fuel (Figure 10.4 ■).
■ Cover pots when they are cooking.
■ Make one-dish meals.
■ Make enough food for more than one meal and reheat the remaining servings.
■ If you are using an electric range, turn off the heat a few minutes before the food is ready.
■ Use the correct appliance for the job. Use a small toaster oven for small jobs and the big oven for big jobs.

Methods of Cooking

■ *Bake or roast:* cook with dry heat in a confined space, such as an oven.
■ *Boil:* cook in a liquid hot enough for bubbles to break on the surface.

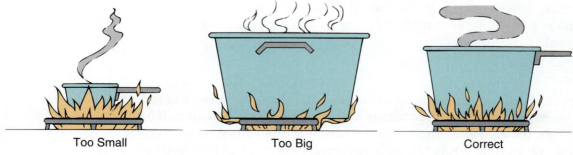

Too Small   Too Big   Correct

FIGURE 10.4 ■ Choosing the correct size pot is an important safety measure.

- *Braise:* a long, slow cooking method that makes use of moist heat in a tightly covered vessel at a temperature just below boiling. The cooking liquid should just barely cover the food to be braised. Braising is a good way to cook tough meats and vegetables as the long cooking breaks down their fibers.
- *Broil:* cook directly under or above a source of heat.
- *Fry:* cook food in fat or oil. When only a small amount of fat is used, the process is called pan frying or sautéing. When larger amounts of fat are used—enough to cover the food—the process is called deep frying or deep fat frying.
- *Poach:* a method of cooking used to preserve the delicate texture and prevent toughening foods. The food is covered by water or another liquid. Depending on the type of food being cooked, the liquid may be either boiling or at the boiling point.
- *Steam:* a method of cooking in which the food is exposed to the steam of boiling water. The food must be above the liquid, never in it. The container is kept closed during cooking to let the steam accumulate. Steaming keeps a high proportion of the original flavor and texture of the foods because the nutrients are not dissolved in the cooking liquid as is the case with boiling or poaching. Steaming is a more time-consuming way of cooking, however.
- *Stew:* a process of long, slow cooking of food in liquid in a covered pot with seasoning. Good for tougher cuts of meat.

PREPARING A CLIENT FOR A MEAL

Serve the client in an orderly and friendly fashion. Prepare small portions, especially if the client has a poor appetite. A great deal of food will only make him uncomfortable. Serve the meal as the client wants it. Some people want their soup first; some want their salad first. Accommodate the client unless there is a health reason why you may not. The place people eat is important. If a client enjoys eating in the living room, serve him there. If he would rather eat in his bedroom and you know of no reason not to, serve him there.

An important part of serving a client a meal are your observations about the client at mealtime:

- How is the client's appetite?
- Does he eat foods on his diet?
- What foods does the client avoid?
- Is there any discomfort associated with eating?
- Does the client drink fluids?
- Does the client eat several big meals, or does he eat all day long?
- Who serves the client when you are not there?

Serving a Meal

A poor appetite does not mean that the body's need for food is lowered. The sick person's body is in a weakened condition. The client needs as much food as ever—if not more—to return to health. The surroundings and the food served should be as cheerful, attractive, and appetizing as possible. The sight and aroma of food often make a person hungry. You can increase a client's appetite by showing him what he will be eating. Also, people have a better appetite for foods they especially like. Therefore, if a client asks for a particular food (and if he is permitted to have it), serve it to him.

Mealtime often is one of the highlights of the day for a convalescent client or a client who is not extremely sick. Mealtime is a break in the often boring routine. It gives the client something to look forward to.

- Tell the client you will be serving him a meal.
- Most people enjoy company during mealtime. Visitors and family members should be encouraged to remain with the client and even eat with the client if that is appropriate.
- Before or after the meal, offer the client the bedpan or urinal.
- After the meal, offer the client oral hygiene.

SECTION 3

Therapeutic Diets

OBJECTIVES

What You Will Learn to Do

1. Explain what is meant by therapeutic diet.
2. Describe various kinds of therapeutic diets.
3. Explain the purpose of each type of therapeutic diet.

therapeutic

an act that helps in the treatment of disease or discomfort

The type of diet will be determined by the doctor. The supervisor or dietitian will help the client plan his diet and work with you. The **therapeutic** diet will be planned to incorporate the client's likes and dislikes, his ethnic background, and his budget (Tables 10.1 ■ to 10.4 ■).

It is your responsibility to follow the diet plan when preparing the client's meals and to offer feedback to your supervisor. Assist the client and family with incorporating the therapeutic diet into the family's usual eating habits. If there are any questions about the diet or its preparation, call your supervisor. If the client is not eating the food on the diet, the supervisor should also be notified.

Table 10.1: Types of Patient Diets

Type of Diet	Description	Common Purpose	Foods Often Recommended	Foods to Avoid
Normal regular	Provides all essentials of good nourishment in normal forms	For clients who do not need special diets		
Soft (mechanical)	Same foods as on a normal diet, but chopped or strained	For clients who have difficulty chewing or swallowing		
Bland	Foods mild in flavor and easy to digest; omits spicy foods	Avoids irritation of the digestive tract, as with ulcer and colitis clients	Puddings, creamed dishes, milk, eggs, plain potatoes	Fried foods, raw vegetables or fruit, whole-grain products
Low-residue	Foods low in bulk: omits foods difficult to digest	Spares the lower digestive tract; for clients with rectal diseases		Whole-grain products, uncooked fruits and vegetables

Table 10.1: Types of Patient Diets (*continued*)

Type of Diet	Description	Common Purpose	Foods Often Recommended	Foods to Avoid
High-calorie	Foods high in protein, minerals, and vitamins	For underweight or malnourished clients	Eggnog, ice cream, frequent snacks, peanut butter, milk	
Low-calorie	Foods low in cream, butter, and fats; cereals; low-fat desserts	For clients who should lose weight	Skim milk, fresh fruit and vegetables, lean meat, fish	Fried foods, sauces, gravies, rich desserts
Low-fat	Limited amounts of butter, cream, fats, and eggs	For clients who have difficulty digesting fats and may have gall bladder, cardio-vascular, and liver disturbances	Veal, poultry, fish, skim milk, fresh fruits, and vegetables	Bacon, butter, cheese, fried foods, liver, whole milk, ice cream, chocolate
*Low-cholesterol	Low in eggs, whole milk, cheese, and meats	Helps regulate the amount of cholesterol in the blood	Fruits, vegetables, cereals, grains, nuts, vegetable oil	Brains, organ meats
*Diabetic	Balance of carbohydrates, protein, and fats, devised according to the needs of individual clients	For diabetic clients: matches food intake with insulin and nutritional requirements	Fresh fruits and vegetables, low-sugar products	High-sugar foods, alcohol, carbonated beverages
High-protein	Meals with high-protein foods, such as meat, fish, cheese, milk, and eggs	Assists in the growth and repair of tissues wasted by disease	Milk, meat, eggs, cheese, fish	
*Low-sodium (salt)	Limited amount of foods containing sodium; no salt allowed at the table	For clients whose circulation would be impaired by fluid retention; for clients with certain heart or kidney conditions	Puffed wheat/rice or shredded wheat, fruits, fruit juices	Canned vegetables, ham, luncheon meats, frankfurters, most cheeses
*Salt-free	Completely without salt		Most fresh or frozen vegetables	

*(See additional charts)

Table 10.2: Foods High in Cholesterol

Milk	whole milk, cream, soft cheeses, high fat cheeses, ice cream, sour cream
Breads/cereals	pastry, sweet rolls, snack crackers, doughnuts, egg noodles
Meat	prime meat, organ meat, animal fat, lard, sausage, bacon, luncheon meat
Eggs	egg yolks
Fats/oils	dressings with egg yolks, butter, lard, coconut oil, palm oil, margarines high in saturated fats
Desserts	ice cream, pies, cakes, milkshakes, frappes

Table 10.3: **Foods High in Potassium**

Apricots	Low-sodium baking soda
Avocado	Molasses
Bamboo shoots	Nuts
Bananas	Nectarines
Beet greens	Oranges
Bran	Potato with skin
Chocolate	Spinach
Coffee	Sweet potato
Low-sodium baking powder	Wheat germ

Table 10.4: **Foods High in Salt**

A-1 sauce	Anchovies	Bacon	Barbecue sauce
Bologna	Bouillon cubes or powders (regular)	Buttermilk	Canned gravies or sauces
Canned ravioli or spaghetti	Canned soups	Canned stews	Canned vegetables
Catsup	Caviar	Celery salt	Cheese doodles
Chili sauce	Corned beef	Cheese—regular, processed, and spreads	Chinese food, canned or restaurant
Frozen breaded meats and fish	Frozen TV dinners	Ham—smoked or cured	Hamburger Helper mix
Herring	Horseradish	Hot dogs/frankfurters	Kitchen Bouquet
Knockwurst	Kosher meats	Liverwurst	Lox
Luncheon meats	Malted milk	Meat tenderizers	Monosodium glutamate (Accent)
Mustard	Nuts—salted	Olives	Onion salt
Party spread and dips	Pastrami	Pickled pigs feet	Pickles
Popcorn—salted	Relishes	Salami	Salted snack foods—pretzels, potato chips, corn chips
Sardines	Sausage	Sauerkraut	Scrapple
Sea salt	Seasoned salt	Smoked salmon	Smoked tongue
Soy sauce	Tomato juice—regular	Worcestershire sauce	

MINESTRONE

Prep time: 30 minutes   *8 servings*
Cook time: 90 minutes

Ingredients

1 tablespoon olive or vegetable oil
1 ½ cups diced onion
1 cup diced celery
1 cup carrots, peeled and diced
2–4 leaves of green cabbage, shredded
  (optional)
4 cloves garlic, peeled and diced
10 cups water
1 bay leaf
1 teaspoon thyme

1 teaspoon basil
1 tablespoon parsley
1 14.5-ounce can tomatoes mashed into
  small pieces
1 15.5-ounce can garbanzo beans,
  drained
1 15.5-ounce can pinto, white, or kidney
  beans, drained
¾ cup macaroni, orzo, shells, or other
  small pasta

Instructions

1. Heat the oil in a soup pot. Add onions, celery, and carrots. Cook until limp, about 7
   minutes.
2. Add cabbage, garlic, water, bay leaf, thyme, basil, parsley, and tomatoes. Cook
   about 3 minutes.
3. Carefully add the water. Cover. Bring to a boil and simmer for 45 minutes.
4. Add the beans. Cook 20 minutes.
5. Add the pasta and cook until the pasta is soft, about 5–7 minutes.
6. Remove the bay leaf before serving.

Nutrient Content

Calories 81
Protein 3 g
14% calories from protein
Carbohydrates 14 g
Fat 2 g

22% calories from fat
Cholesterol 0 mg
Sodium 106 mg
Dietary fiber 3 g

Adaptations for Physical Limitations

• Adjust the consistency to the client's swallowing ability by pureeing before serving or
  adding thickening agent as needed.

Substitutions

• Use **chicken stock** instead of water.
• Vary the beans.
• Vary the greens, using spinach, dandelion greens, or collard greens.
• Add **sausage** or any leftover meat.
• Rice may be used in place of macaroni.
• Serve with a sprinkling of **grated cheese.**

FIGURE 10.5 ■ Is a recipe for a main dish that is versatile, nutritious, easy to prepare, and economical.

CAPRON, MARY ELLEN; ZUCKER, ELANA, ULTIMATE COOKING COMPANION FOR AT-HOME CAREGIVERS, 1st Edition, © 2003 pp. 62, 108, 116, 135, 163, 176, 239. Reprinted by permission of Pearson Education, Inc., Upper Saddle River, NJ

Figure 10.5 is a recipe for a main dish that is versatile, nutritious, easy to prepare, and economical. See additional recipes in Appendix B.

Introduction: Chemotherapy and Radiation

Many people who receive **chemotherapy** and **radiation therapy** change their eating habits due to periods of nausea, vomiting, appetite loss, and/or constipation. It is helpful to consult with your supervisor so that the best possible diet

chemotherapy
the regime of taking drugs to treat a malignancy

radiation therapy
the use of X-rays to treat a tumor or a condition

can be planned, taking nutrients from the four food groups and the minerals and vitamins.

Here are several helpful hints:

- Decrease intake of red meats; many people prefer fish, chicken, turkey, and other nonmeat foods high in protein.
- Use plastic utensils, as some people complain of a bitter taste from metal utensils.
- Maintain adequate fluid intake of cool, clear liquids.
- Eat small, frequent meals; chew food well; eat warm, not hot food.
- Decrease intake of sweets and fried or fatty foods; this will decrease nausea and decrease intake of empty calories.
- Remain in a sitting position for 2 hours after meals.
- Eat non–gas-producing foods.
- Discuss the fiber intake with your supervisor.
- Provide a pleasant, quiet atmosphere.
- Vary the diet.
- If the client has difficulty eating by himself or being neat as he eats, protect his clothes without making him feel like an infant.

SECTION 4

Feeding a Client

OBJECTIVES	
What You Will Learn to Do	1. List safety factors important in feeding a client.
	2. List emotional factors important in feeding a client.
	3. Know the proper technique for feeding a client.

Introduction: Why Clients Must Be Assisted with Eating

Some clients cannot feed themselves and therefore need to be fed. The reasons might be:

- The client cannot use his hands.
- The doctor wants the client to save his strength and to be on complete bed rest.
- The client may be too weak to feed himself.

Usually, it is hard for an adult to accept the idea of being unable to feed himself. A client who cannot feed himself may feel resentful and depressed. Be friendly and natural. Talk pleasantly but not too much. Encourage him to do as much as he can (Figure 10.6 ■).

WHEN YOU FEED A CLIENT

- Allow clients to feed themselves as much as possible; give assistance only as needed.
- Do not rush the feeding; sit if possible.
- Be gentle with forks and spoons; straws may help in feeding liquids.

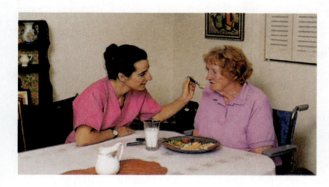

FIGURE 10.6 ■

Feed a client in a quiet atmosphere. Both you and the client should be comfortable.

- Keep the conversation pleasant and make the meal a highlight of the day.
- Feed foods separate rather than mixed together.
- When offering a glass or cup, first touch it to the lips.
- Record intake and output.
- Record your observations about the client when you were feeding him.

SAFETY FACTORS

Be sure a client can swallow before you put food in his mouth. Some clients will be able to swallow one food and not another. Pay special attention to the food temperature. If a food is hot, tell the client and then offer him a small amount. If the food is cold, do the same. Keep food on a table away from the client's bed so that the client can change position without spilling the food. If a client is blind, name each mouthful before you offer it to him.

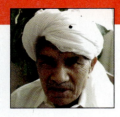

Case Study

Review the case study that appears on the first page of the chapter. Answer two sets of questions about the case study contained in the Explore and Apply sections below.

EXPLORE

1. Review the food pyramid and discuss the foods that Mr. Patel should be eating to adhere to the prescribed diet.

2. How would you find out which foods are of particular importance to Mr. Patel?

APPLY

1. What observations would you document after you leave the client? Why did you identify these in particular?

2. Mr. Patel has made it clear that he does not wish to change his dietary habits. They suit his lifestyle, and he can easily obtain food familiar to him. How do you feel about this and what will you do?

Certification Review Questions

Choose the best answer for each question or statement.

1. The Food Guide Pyramid is

   a. *a way to organize our shopping lists into like groups.*

   b. *an organization of food and vitamins.*

   c. *a guide of what we should include in our diet each day.*

   d. *a list that tells us which foods we should eliminate from our diet.*

2. When planning a menu, it is important to

   a. *consider the likes and dislikes of the client.*

   b. *follow the prescribed diet even if the client refuses to eat the food.*

   c. *always do the shopping before you go to the house to save time.*

   d. *borrow supplies from one client if you need the supplies elsewhere.*

3. Food allergies

   a. *are present at birth.*

   b. *never go away.*

   c. *will be outgrown.*

   d. *should be taken seriously by the client, his family, and the homemaker/home health aide.*

4. When shopping, it is always

   a. *best to buy the biggest size of an item because it is always most economical.*

   b. *wise to make a list and check it with the client before you shop.*

   c. *best to buy what you know you will need and get the money from the client later.*

   d. *best to buy brands with which you are familiar because you know they are good.*

5. A therapeutic diet

   a. *is only a suggestion. The client does not have to follow it all the time.*

   b. *can be changed only by a physician.*

   c. *is prescribed regardless of the medication a client takes.*

   d. *can usually be followed by the family with only slight changes.*

CHAPTER 11

Basic Body Movement and Positions

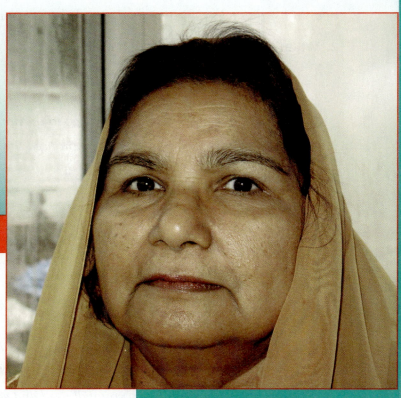

CASE STUDY

Mrs. Mahamoud suffered a broken hip in a fall in her kitchen. She was trying to retrieve a dish from a high shelf and slipped off a stool. Her sons are young adults and are in college and working. Prior to her fall, Mrs. Mahamoud was active in her neighborhood religious activities, but she is unable to drive now. Her husband works six days a week and spends his free time with his elderly father living nearby with his also elderly aunt. Mrs. Mahamoud exercises when she is reminded and when you are there to assist her, but she does not initiate the exercises. She remains in bed until everyone has left the house in the morning and then gets up using her own procedures. Her husband communicates with the doctor and the therapists via telephone. Mrs. Mahamoud manages to keep the house tidy and cook simple meals. She seldom eats with the family, preferring to eat after everyone is finished at the table. Shopping for food poses a serious problem as Mrs. Mahamoud cannot go herself and does not want to ask her family for help.

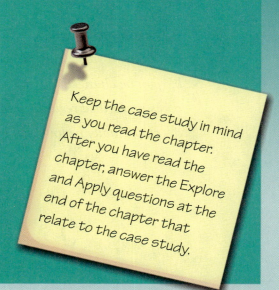

Keep the case study in mind as you read the chapter. After you have read the chapter, answer the Explore and Apply questions at the end of the chapter that relate to the case study.

SECTION 1

Body Mechanics

OBJECTIVES

What You Will Learn to Do

1. Discuss the basic ideas of good body mechanics.
2. Apply good body mechanics during activities on and off the job.
3. Explain to someone else (client or caregiver) how to use good body mechanics.

Introduction: Body Mechanics

The term ***body mechanics*** refers to the way of standing and moving one's body so as to prevent injury, avoid fatigue, and make the best use of strength. If you understand the rules of good body mechanics and apply them to your work and everyday life, you will be less tired and will feel better at the end of the day. Once you understand how to control and balance your body, you will understand how to control and balance your client's body. This is a major safety factor for both of you.

Remember, low-back problems are a leading cause of employee sick time. It is most important that you learn good body mechanics to protect your back and your job.

body mechanics
proper use of the human body to do work and to avoid injury and strain

BASE OF SUPPORT

The **base of support** determines how stable your balance will be. Try standing with both feet together. How far can you reach forward? Sideways? You probably lost your balance quickly. Now stand with your feet separated about 6 to 8 inches with one foot a half-step ahead of the other. Repeat reaching forward and sideways. You reach farther this time before losing your balance. That is because by separating your feet you made your base of support larger and your balance more stable (Figure 11.1 ■).

base of support
part of the body that bears the most weight

CENTER OF GRAVITY

The **center of gravity** of any object you hold is the point at which you have the greatest control over the object with the least amount of effort. A person's center of gravity is located around the pelvic area (Figure 11.2 ■). When moving or assisting a client, support him through his center of gravity. By holding a client close to his center of gravity and your center of gravity, you will have the

center of gravity
point at which you have the greatest control over an object you hold

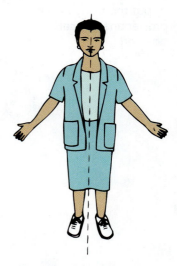

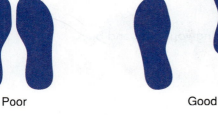

Poor   Good

FIGURE 11.1 ■
Providing the proper base of support for each activity will allow you to work in a safe manner and be less tired at the end of the day.

FIGURE 11.2 ■ Be aware of your center of gravity and your base of support as you work.

greatest amount of control with the least amount of effort. The client will also feel that you have control and will be more likely to trust you and follow your directions.

BALANCING

When you must lift heavy objects, spread your feet apart and bend your knees. This will lower your center of gravity, increase stability, and broaden your base of support. To balance yourself, your center of gravity must remain within your base of support. Getting up from a sitting position is one example: Some people have difficulty getting up from a sitting position because they are afraid to lean forward far enough. Their center of gravity is not balanced over their base of support. If you help them move their buttocks out over their feet (properly positioned), they will usually balance quite well and learn to lose their fear.

STRONGEST MUSCLES

Generally, muscles that flex (bend) joints are the strongest. In your arms, you have the greatest power and control when you lift with your palms facing up. In your legs, your hip flexors and your knee flexors are strongest. This is why you bend your hips and knees slightly when using good body mechanics. This puts the muscles in the best position to do heavy work. Your strongest muscles are not in your back, so do not expect your back to do heavy work.

align
to put the body into its proper anatomical position

◀ GUIDELINES

Good Body Mechanics

- When an action requires physical effort, use as many groups of muscles as possible. For example, use both hands rather than one hand to pick up a heavy piece of equipment.

- Use good posture. Keep your body properly **aligned.** Keep your back straight. Have your knees bent. Keep your weight evenly balanced on both feet.

- Check your feet when you lift something. They should be at least 12 inches apart. This will give you a broad base of support and good balance.

- If you think you may not be able to lift the load, or if it seems too large or heavy, find help.

- Lift smoothly to avoid strain. Always count "one, two, three" with both the client and with other helpers.

- If you must move or lift a heavy object or person, use a lumbar support. A support can be obtained from your agency, or you may prefer to purchase your own so it is always available to you.

- When you want to change the direction of movement:
  a. Pivot (turn) with your feet.
  b. Turn with short steps.
  c. Turn your whole body without twisting your neck and back.

- Get close to the load being lifted.

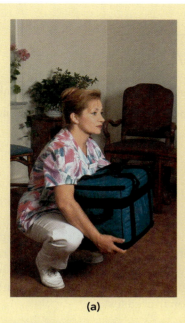 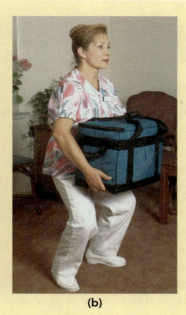

(a)   (b)

FIGURE 11.3 ■ (a) Use your longest and strongest muscles.
(b) Use your center of gravity and base of support as you lift
and move objects.

■ When you move a heavy object, it is better to push, pull, or roll it rather than
lift and carry it.

■ Use your arms to support the object. The muscles of your legs actually do the
job of lifting, not the muscles of your back (Figure 11.3 ■).

■ The muscles that bend your elbow are stronger than the ones that straighten
it out—your greatest lift power is in pulling.

■ When you do work such as giving a back rub, making a corner on a bed, or
exercising a client, work with the direction of your efforts, not against them.

■ When working with a client in a hospital bed (bathing, dressing, exercising,
etc.), raise the bed to a comfortable position for you. Also, move the client
close to the side of the bed where you are working.

■ When working with a client in a bed that does not raise up, if you must stand,
put one foot up on the lowered side rail or on a footstool to relieve the pressure on your lower back. Remember the same rules of a broad base of support: Use the strongest muscles for the work and keep your center of gravity
close to your work.

■ Avoid twisting your body (or your client's body).

Remember:

■ Knowing how your body balances means you will know how your client's
body balances.
■ Use proper body mechanics—protect your back, it is the only one
you have.
■ Use proper body mechanics *whenever* you stand or move. It cannot be an
only on-the-job behavior.
■ An injured back is painful, inconvenient, and costly.

Client's Daily Level of Ability

OBJECTIVES

What You Will Learn to Do

1. State why you must check your client's level of ability.
2. Demonstrate the proper technique to check daily level of ability.

Introduction: Daily Ability Level

daily ability level
the capability of the client to perform an activity on a given day

activity tolerance
the most activity the client will be able to do

Each client is different. Depending on many factors, such as age, disability, weather, and family pressures, a client may be totally or partially dependent on you, or he may be fully independent. Activities performed one day may be impossible the next. It is your responsibility to check the **daily ability level** of the client before you ask him to perform an activity. Observe the client's **activity tolerance** each day. Note if it decreases or increases.

CHECKLIST

- Can the client hear and understand you?
- Can the client follow directions?
- How much can the client do alone?
- How does the client look?
- What are his vital signs?
- Will pain be a factor in this activity?
- Are joint motions limited?
- Does the client tire easily?

Your role is to help the client complete the activity, not to do it for him. Because you are not in the house all the time, the client and his family must know how to give care when you are not there. They will learn from your supervisor and your example. By setting a good example, you will teach and you will assist the client and his family in accepting whatever limitations remain.

► GUIDELINES

Assisting Clients

- Expect the client to do as much as possible.
- Help only when needed.
- Work at the client's level and speed.
- Direct activity instead of asking for it. For example, say "It is time to stand, Mrs. N" instead of "Do you want to stand up, Mrs. N?" If Mrs. N says "No!" what do you do then?
- Plan ahead. Gather all equipment and put it in place before you begin the activity.
- Know your own capabilities.

- Give the client short, simple directions.

- Praise the client for following directions. If he does something incorrectly, stop the activity and redirect him until the correct activity is done. That way, the client will get used to doing the activity the correct way only.

- Your body language (your tone of voice, facial expression, the way you touch, etc.) will be more strongly received than the meaning of the words you use. Make sure your nonverbal messages fit the words you use.

- Touch is the most important of the senses. You will give your client contact care. If you are comfortable with this, they will be too.

- Always use smooth, steady motions with clients. Avoid sudden jerking movements.

SECTION 3

Positioning a Client in Bed

OBJECTIVES

What You Will Learn to Do

1. Be familiar with the words physical therapists use in their work.

2. Be familiar with the principles taken into consideration when positioning a client in bed.

3. Demonstrate the proper techniques for moving and positioning clients in bed.

Introduction: Body Support and Alignment

Many of your tasks require lifting and moving clients. Some clients will be able to help you. Some will not. A bedridden client must have his position changed at least once every 2 hours. Proper support and alignment of the client's body are important.

The client's body should be straight and properly supported; otherwise, his safety and comfort might be affected. The correct positioning of the client's body is referred to as **body alignment** or bed positioning. Arrangement or adjustment of the client's body is made so that all parts of the body are in their proper positions in relation to each other. Proper body alignment can be seen in proper standing posture. When people lie in bed, it is often necessary to use pillows and rolled-up towels to keep this alignment. Some conditions and injuries, as well as special client care treatments, make it difficult or even dangerous for a client to be in a certain position. You will be told as to any special positions that your client requires.

A client unable to move needs to have his position changed every 2 hours to:

- Minimize the possibility of muscle tightness
- Reduce the chance of skin breakdown
- Maintain proper body alignment
- Make the client comfortable
- Avoid delaying rehabilitation

body alignment
arrangement of the body in a straight line, placing of body parts in correct anatomical position

A client improperly positioned during the first part of his illness, can develop problems that must be taken care of before rehabilitation can begin. This often prevents or delays exercises and activities that would allow a client to function more fully. For example, if a client who is not properly positioned in bed develops a decubitus, or bedsore, this must heal before he can start exercises.

USING THE CORRECT TERMS

Clients who need physical therapy or any other types of assistance usually have some type of disability. They may have a weakness or an injury on one side. Do not refer to this side as the "bad side." There is nothing bad about it. Refer to it as the **involved** side. This means it is involved in the treatment. Refer to the other side as the **uninvolved** side. To continually call your client's weak side the bad side will only discourage him from using it.

If your client understands the concept of right and left, refer to his limbs in those terms. At times, you will have to touch the arm or leg you want him to move. You may also have to demonstrate the activity first.

You will hear the words *functional* and *nonfunctional*. **Functional** describes the usefulness of something. It may be an activity or a body part. An activity such as folding clothes, making salad, or combing one's hair is a functional activity because it produces a desired result. **Nonfunctional** body parts will not perform a useful activity.

You can see that words are important and that they describe the way you feel and the way you see the client and his disability.

MOVING CLIENTS IN BED

For good positioning, the client must be up at the head of the bed. If your client can stand, even briefly, have him sit over the edge of the bed. Help him to stand and move his buttocks up toward the head of the bed. Repeat the process until he is in a good position to lie back down with his head at the top of the bed. In this way, you not only have your client back where you want him, but he will have exercised his muscles, heart, balance system, and coordination system all at the same time. You also have taught him a valuable activity that he can use in the future when he is stronger.

When a client needs help to move, a **pull sheet** can help you move the client in bed. A regular extra sheet folded over many times and placed under the client serves as a pull sheet. The cotton draw sheet can also be used as a pull sheet. When moving the client, roll up the pull sheet tightly on each side next to the client's body. Grip the rolled portion underhand to slide the client into the desired position. By using the pull sheet, you avoid friction and irritation to the client's skin that touches the bedding.

COMMONLY USED POSITIONS

A client can be positioned on the back, stomach, or either side or in a position halfway between side lying and stomach lying. The client's diagnosis, condition, and comfort determine which one you choose to use. Also, remember that just because a client cannot move without help when asked does not mean that he will stay for 2 hours in the correct position. Keep checking your client for proper position.

---

involved
body part undergoing therapy or part of a disease process

uninvolved
body part not affected by the disease process

functional
able to be used

nonfunctional
having no use; not usable

pull sheet
a sheet or piece of cloth placed under the client and used by the caretaker to facilitate moving the client in the bed

GENERAL POSITIONING RULES

- A rolled-up washcloth makes an excellent support for the hand.
- If an arm or leg is swollen, try to keep the part higher than the heart. Gravity will help the extra fluid drain from the limb.
- Any open skin will heal more quickly if pressure is reduced and air is allowed to circulate around it.
- Position and support only nonfunctional parts of the body. The rest should be left free to move. This will help the blood to circulate.
- Proper positioning can help a client maintain or recover his best possible state of health.

POSITIONING A CLIENT ON HIS BACK

- Place:

  a small comfortable pillow under the client's head

  a small hand towel folded under the shoulder blade of the weak side

  a bath towel folded under the hip on the weak side

  a washcloth rolled up in the hand on the weak side

  a weak arm and elbow on a pillow higher than the heart

  a small pillow under the calf of the weak leg with the heel hanging off the mattress edge (Figure 11.4 ■).
- Loosen the top sheet so pressure is removed from the toes.

POSITIONING A CLIENT ON HIS UNINVOLVED SIDE

A. • Place a small pillow under the head. Keep the head in alignment with the spine.
- Roll a large pillow lengthwise, and tuck it in at the client's back to prevent him from rolling and to give him support.
- Place:

  a pillow in front to keep the arm the same height as the shoulder joint

  a medium pillow between the client's knees (the top knee may be slightly bent or both may be bent)

  a small pillow between the ankles and feet (Figure 11.5 ■)

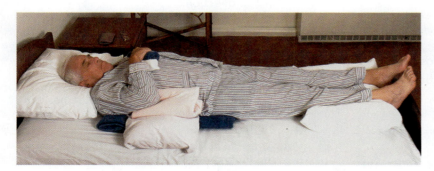

FIGURE 11.4 ■ Be sure the client is both safe and comfortable as you place the towels and pillows.

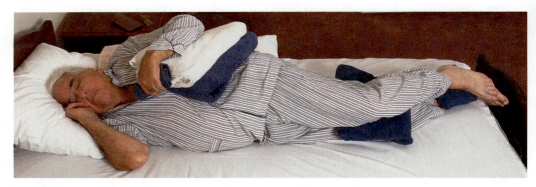

FIGURE 11.5 ■ Remember, the client also has a center of gravity and must be in proper alignment when he is in bed.

B.• Place:

a small pillow under the head

a large pillow under the involved arm to keep it level with the shoulder joint

a large pillow at the stomach area (if the client wishes) for the client to roll onto

POSITIONING A CLIENT ON HIS INVOLVED SIDE

The same principles of positioning are used as listed, plus:

■ The client's comfort will be the key to how and where support should be used.

■ Change the client's position more frequently than when he is positioned on the uninvolved side.

■ With disability can come a lessened sense of pain and pressure. Check the involved side for signs of pressure and skin irritation.

PROCEDURE 15

Moving a Client Up in Bed with His Help

RATIONALE: Keeping a client in good body alignment helps prevent decubiti, respiratory problems, and general discomfort. Working with the client prevents injury to both client and caretakers and allows the client to be an active participant in his care.

1. Wash your hands.
2. Tell the client you are going to help him move up in the bed.
3. Lock any wheels on the bed, if possible.
4. Raise the whole bed to a height best for you.
5. Remove the pillow. Put the pillow on a chair or at the foot of the bed.
6. Put the side rail in the up position on the far side of the bed.
7. Put one hand under the client's shoulder. Put your other hand under the client's buttocks.

8. Tell the client to bend his knees and brace his feet firmly on the mattress.
9. Tell the client to put his hands on the mattress to help push.
10. Have your feet 12 inches apart. The foot closest to the head of the bed should be pointed in that direction.
11. Bend your knees. Keep your back straight.
12. Facing the client and turned slightly toward the head of the bed, bend your body from your hips (Figure 11.6 ■).
13. At the signal "one, two, three," have the client pull with his hands toward the head of the bed and push with his feet against the mattress.
14. At the same time, help him to move toward the head of the bed by sliding him with your hands and arms.

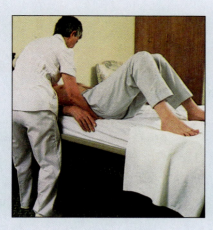

FIGURE 11.6 ∎

15. Put the pillow back in place. Reposition the client correctly.
16. Make the client comfortable. Lower the bed to the lowest horizontal position, if possible.
17. Wash your hands.
18. Chart your observations of the client during this procedure.

PROCEDURE 16

Moving a Client Up in Bed, Two People

RATIONALE: Keeping a client in good body alignment helps prevent decubiti, respiratory problems, and general discomfort. Asking for assistance when necessary helps prevent injury to client and caretakers.

1. Ask another person to work with you.
2. Wash your hands.
3. Tell the client you and your partner are going to move him up in bed. Say this even if he appears to be unconscious.
4. Remove the pillow from the bed. Place it on a chair.
5. Lock any wheels on the bed.
6. Raise the whole bed, if possible, to a height good for you.
7. Stand on one side of the bed. The person assisting will stand on the opposite side.
8. Both of you should stand slightly turned toward the head of the bed. Your feet should be about 12 to 14 inches apart. The foot closest to the head of the bed should be pointed in that direction. Bend your knees. Keep your back straight.
9. Use of a draw, pull, or turning sheet is always preferred for moving a client up in bed. This avoids friction between the client's skin and bedding. It will prevent irritation of the skin.
10. You will be sliding the client's body when you move him up in bed. Roll the draw sheet up to the client's body and grab underhand. Shift the weight of your body from your back leg to your front leg up near the head of the bed. By keeping your back and arms "locked" in position when you shift your weight, your legs will help you use your body weight to your advantage and pull the client up.

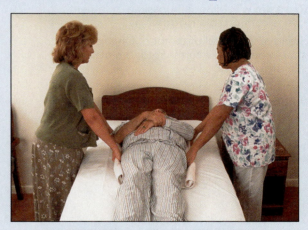

FIGURE 11.7 ∎ When a family member helps you, review the process together BEFORE you move the client.

11. Explain step 10 to both your assistant and the client. Count to three as prearranged. You and your partner will move together to slide the client gently toward the head of the bed (Figure 11.7 ∎).
12. Replace the pillow. Position the client correctly. Raise the side rails (if necessary). Replace the bed to the original horizontal position.
13. Wash your hands.
14. Chart any observations you may have made while doing this procedure.

PROCEDURE 17

Moving a Client Up in Bed, One Person

RATIONALE: Keeping a client in good body alignment helps prevent decubiti, respiratory problems, and general discomfort. Using aids to assist you will help prevent injury to client and caretaker.

1. Wash your hands.
2. Tell the client you are going to move him up in bed. Say this even if he appears unconscious.
3. Ask the visitors to leave, if appropriate.
4. Remove the pillow from the bed. Place it on a chair.
5. Lock any wheels on the bed.
6. Raise the whole bed, if possible, to a height that is comfortable for you.
7. Stand at the head of the bed. One foot should be in close to the bed, the other slightly behind.
8. Reach over the top of the draw sheet. Roll the edge and grab it.
9. On a count of three, "lock" your arms and back into one unbendable unit and shift your weight to your back leg. The client will slide easily to the top of the bed with the sheet. Make sure you do this slowly and use good body mechanics (Figure 11.8 ■).

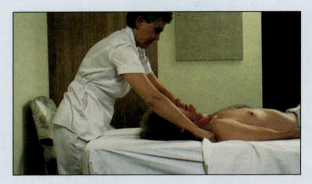

FIGURE 11.8 ■ Use the sheet and good body mechanics to move the client.

10. Replace the pillow. Position the client correctly. Raise the side rails. Replace the bed to its original horizontal position.
11. Wash your hands.
12. Chart your observation of the client during the procedure.

SAMPLE CHARTING: 2/9/05   10:30 A.M.
Client was at the bottom of bed. Repositioned correctly with the aid of a sheet. No discomfort noted. Client left watching television with call bell on his nightstand.
Sydney Blecher H/HHA

PROCEDURE 18

Moving a Client to One Side of the Bed on His Back

RATIONALE: Keeping a client in good body alignment helps prevent decubiti, respiratory problems, and general discomfort. When assistance is unavailable, using the correct procedure—even if it takes time—will prevent injury to client and caretaker.

1. Wash your hands.
2. Tell the client you are going to move him to one side of the bed on his back without turning him. Explain that this is a safety measure so that, when he is turned to his side, he'll be in the center of the bed.
3. Lock any wheels on the bed.

4. Raise the whole bed to the highest position best for you.
5. Lower the backrest and footrest, if this is allowed.
6. Put the side rail in the up position on the far side of the bed.
7. Loosen the top sheets but do not expose the client.
8. Place your feet in good position—one in close to the bed and one back. Slide both your arms under the client's back to his far shoulder, then slide the client's shoulders toward you by rocking your weight to your back foot (Figure 11.9 ■).

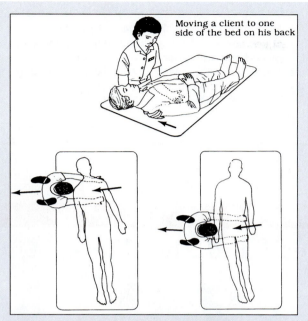

FIGURE 11.9 ■ As a safety measure, do this before turning the client so that when he is turned to his side, he'll be in the center of the bed.

9. Keep your knees bent and your back straight as you slide the client.

10. Slide both your arms as far as you can under the client's buttocks, and slide his buttocks toward you the same way. Use a pull (turning) sheet whenever possible for helpless clients.

11. Place both your arms under the client's feet and slide them toward you.

12. Replace and adjust the pillow, if necessary.

13. Remake the top of the bed.

14. Make the client comfortable. Lower the bed to its lowest horizontal position.

15. Wash your hands.

16. Chart your observations of the client during this procedure.

PROCEDURE 19

Rolling the Client (Log Rolling)

1. Wash your hands.

2. Tell the client you are going to roll him to his side as if he were a log.

3. Lock any wheels on the bed.

4. Raise the whole bed to the best height for you.

5. Raise the side rail on the far side of the bed.

6. Remove the pillow from under the client's head, if allowed.

7. Move the client to your side of the bed as in the previous procedure while moving a client to one side of the bed on his back.

8. Raise the side rail closest to the client, and go to the other side of the bed and lower that rail.

9. By holding the client at his hip and shoulder, roll the client toward you onto his side. Turn him gently (Figure 11.10a ■ and 11.10b ■).

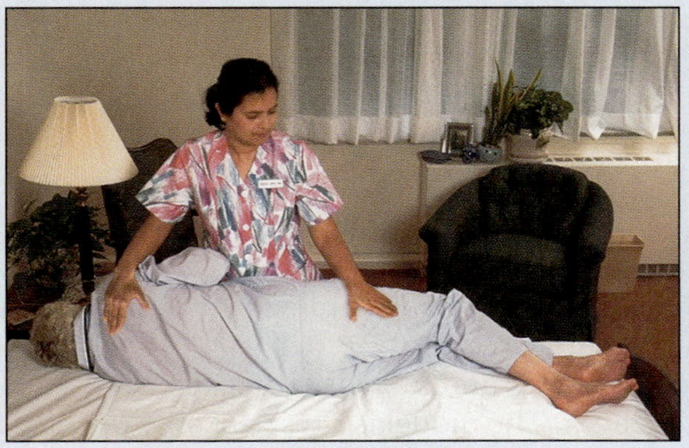

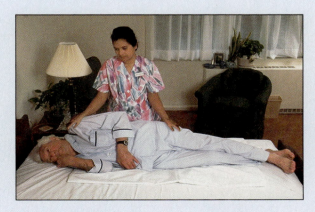

FIGURE 11.10a ■

FIGURE 11.10b ■

continued

10. Place the client in a good bed position, and remake the top covers of the bed.
11. Wash your hands.
12. Chart your observations of the client during this procedure.

SAMPLE CHARTING: 7/15/04   1:50 P.M.
Client positioned in bed using log-rolling method. Pillow placed behind his back to ensure his proper alignment. Call bell within reach on his pillow. Daughter in the house. Client position to be changed by her at 3:45 or before if needed.
Dana Jenkins H/HHA

PROCEDURE 20

Raising the Client's Head and Shoulders

RATIONALE: Keeping a client in good body alignment helps prevent decubiti, respiratory problems, and general discomfort. Some clients require assistance to sit up. Sitting up comfortably and safely prevents poor body alignment. Using correct procedures prevents injury to client and caretaker.

1. Never pull on a client's arm to lift him up. If assistance is required, slide your arm under the shoulder blade to lift. Or raise the head of the bed, if possible.

2. If a client has some strength in one or both arms, "plant" your feet in the proper position, hold your arm out steady, and let the client pull up on you. That way you remain stationary while the client does the work. You then have one hand free to adjust the pillow, and so on (Figure 11.11 ■).

3. Remember, good body mechanics are important to your success.

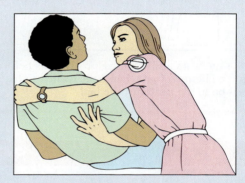

FIGURE 11.11 ■ Client's hand should be under your armpit and placed on your shoulder or across his waist.

SAMPLE CHARTING: 6/7/05   11:30 A.M.
Client left sitting in bed watching television with side rails in position. Pillows placed on either side to assist with maintaining correct position. His wife will check on him frequently and reposition the pillows or change his position before lunch. Affected left arm supported on a pillow.
Brian Smith H/HHA

ELASTIC SUPPORT STOCKINGS

Elastic support hose are often prescribed by the physician or improve the client's circulation and blood return to the heart. This is accomplished when stockings exert pressure on the leg veins. Stockings may be ordered postoperatively or at any time during the client's care.

Elastic stockings come in various sizes and models. Some are up to the knee, and some may be up to the groin area. The model is prescribed by the physician and usually sized by the company or a technician. Stockings may also vary in weight and color and may be made to order.

GUIDELINES

Using Elastic Support Stockings

■ Always use clean, dry stockings that have been prescribed for the client. Do not switch stockings with anyone else.

■ Ask when the client should wear the stockings. Should they be left on when he sleeps, is in bed, walking?

■ Always remove stockings before bathing.

■ Remove stockings at least twice a day to check the skin and toes for reddened areas or edema of the feet and/or ankle.

■ Check the client's entire leg frequently to be sure stockings are not twisted or bunched up. This can hurt and cause decreased circulation.

■ Always put on stockings before the client leaves the bed.

■ Be sure the client's leg is dry before putting on the stockings.

■ Never roll the stocking down or wear a garter to hold it up. This drastically decreases circulation to the limb.

■ Wash and dry stockings according to manufacturer directions. Do not use bleach.

PROCEDURE 21

Applying Support Stockings

RATIONALE: Correctly applied support stockings will increase circulation and provide comfort and support to the client.

1. Assemble equipment

   Clean, dry support stockings

2. Wash your hands.

3. Have the client assume a supine position in the bed with his legs exposed.

4. Gather the stocking in your hands from the top until you reach the toe.

5. Standing with your back to the client and using good body mechanics, insert the client's toe into the toe of the stocking.

6. Pull the stocking up the leg. Be sure it is smooth and not twisted.

7. Repeat the procedure on the second leg.

8. Assist the client into a safe, comfortable position.

9. Wash your hands.

SAMPLE CHARTING: 2/18/05   11:00 A.M. Knee-high support stockings put on both legs. Skin appeared intact. Client assisted to chair for his lunch. Daughter will remove stockings when she visits this afternoon.

To remove stockings, roll them down and carefully pull away from the client's toes. Never pull stocking toes while the whole stocking is still on the foot. Be sure to inspect the foot and the leg when you remove the stockings. Report any red, tender, or puffy areas immediately to your supervisor.

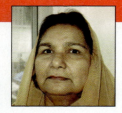

Case Study

Review the case study that appears on the first page of the chapter. Answer two sets of questions about the case study contained in the Explore and Apply sections below.

EXPLORE

1. Discuss how you think a client feels when he is being moved. Does he feel helpless? Does he feel embarrassed? Does he feel that he deserves to be cared for? What could you do to help the client accept assistance?

2. Some clients choose to remain alone rather than ask for assistance with exercise or activities of daily living. How would you encourage her to ask for help so that she can become more independent?

APPLY

1. What would you do if you were unable to move a client by yourself and nobody was available to help you?

2. What activities would you complete to ensure Mrs. Mahamoud's safety? Would you enlist the help of others? Who?

Certification Exam Review Questions

Choose the best answer for each question or statement.

1. Good body mechanics means

   a. taking into account only how your body works.

   b. taking into account only the proper position of the client's body.

   c. using the proper muscles to move a client or an object.

   d. using only the proper muscles when you are working.

2. A client's ability to move

   a. is always the same regardless of the time of day.

   b. varies with the time of day.

   c. is prescribed by the physician.

   d. is delegated to you by the physical therapist.

3. The client's position in bed

   a. is always prescribed by the physician.

   b. is always prescribed by the physical therapist.

   c. is a combination of the client preferences, client safety, and the client's medical condition.

   d. should always be the same so the client becomes used to it.

4. Client's position should be changed and toileting and water offered

   a. when you think the client needs the change.

   b. at the minimum every two hours.

   c. before you leave the client.

   d. when you arrive in the house.

5. Restraints

   a. should be used whenever you think the client will hurt himself.

   b. should be put on by the family and left until you can take them off.

   c. are used when all other avenues of calming and protecting the client have failed.

   d. should be used before you try other avenues as it is the safest and most time-efficient method of calming the client.

CHAPTER 12

Skin Care

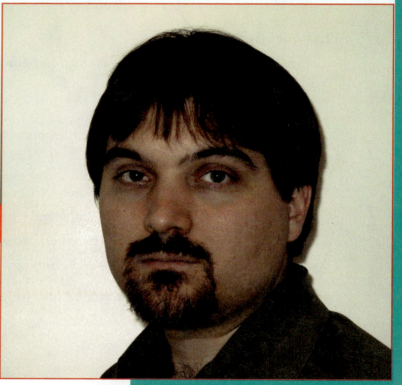

CASE STUDY

Mr. Flannery has always been active in sports. He is now in a full leg cast following his recent skiing accident. He lives alone and talks on the phone most of the day. His social life, which centered on his sports life, decreased, and he seldom has visitors. His work friends call during the day but do not see him. He is confident that he will return to his job as a supervisor at a local tree service. Mr. Flannery has no regular eating schedule and drinks about 6 cans of soda a day but says he does not like water, and besides, if he doesn't drink a great deal, he will not have to get up to go the bathroom. Mr. Flannery says his cast itches, and he has red areas on his back near his shoulders.

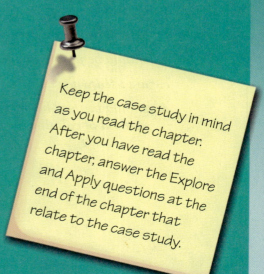

Keep the case study in mind as you read the chapter. After you have read the chapter, answer the Explore and Apply questions at the end of the chapter that relate to the case study.

SECTION 1

Basic Skin Care

OBJECTIVES	
What You Will Learn to Do	**1.** List the basics of good skin care.
	2. List conditions that increase the risk of skin breakdown.
	3. Discuss the effects of aging on the skin.
	4. Demonstrate special considerations when caring for an elderly client.
	5. Demonstrate ways of decreasing pressure to body areas.
	6. Discuss the effects of medication and chemotherapy on the skin.

Introduction: Providing an Environment for Good Skin Care

Good skin care is one of the prime responsibilities of the homemaker/home health aide. It is much easier to prevent skin deterioration than to heal a decubitus ulcer. The skin must be inspected daily for changes, reddened areas, tender places, sore areas, or areas of breakdown. It is important to recognize the client who is at risk of skin breakdown and protect him from the danger of the formation of decubiti. Besides being observant of your client's skin condition, you must provide a safe environment for your client. By protecting him, you prevent injury to his skin. Be alert to your activities.

GENERAL FACTORS AFFECTING SKIN

Many conditions working together affect the health of your client and the condition of his skin. These conditions include the following:

- Disease process
- Medication
- Nutrition
- Assistance in his home when you are not with him
- Exercise and mobility
- Health habits
- Financial resources

When you accept your assignment, discuss with your supervisor how these factors will affect your client's skin and how your care will be affected by them.

HIGH-RISK FACTORS

The primary cause of skin breakdown is pressure on body parts, especially the **bony prominences.** These are places where the bones are close to the skin. Pressure on these areas decreases the circulation, leading to **decubitus**

bony prominences
areas of the body where the bones are close to the skin surface and subject to decubiti

decubitus ulcer
bedsore; open wound that occurs from lack of blood supply to an area usually located on a bony prominence

ulcer formation. These areas are the shoulder blades, elbows, knees, heels, ankles, and backbone. Because these areas are covered by thin layers of skin that receive a smaller blood supply than other areas, they are at high risk of decubiti.

Obese clients tend to develop decubiti where skin surfaces rub together, causing friction in areas such as under the breasts, between the folds of the buttocks, and between the thighs.

Shearing is another force that can cause skin breakdown. Shearing occurs when the skin moves one way and the bone and tissue under the skin moves another. When this happens, the skin is pinched, the tiny blood vessels are pinched, and the blood supply to the skin is decreased. This leads to skin damage. Cornstarch placed directly on the sheets decreases friction and allows the client to move more easily.

shearing
the action of skin being moved in one direction while underlying tissue and/or bone is moved in another direction

SKIN CARE OF THE ELDERLY

Skin care of the elderly client is an important aspect of your daily care. The elderly are especially susceptible to skin problems. Aging brings a gradual loss of skin tone. This includes loss of the natural oils, leading to dry, itchy, scaly, or rough skin. As the skin loses its underlayer of fat, the skin becomes thin, fragile, and unable to sense or maintain temperature accurately. With aging, there is also a decrease in circulation to the skin. Protecting a client from heat and cold becomes one of your responsibilities.

WAYS OF DECREASING PRESSURE TO BODY AREAS

You may be instructed to reduce the pressure to the back under the base of the spine or leg using an air cushion. If you use an air cushion, do not fill it more than half-full.

You may also use sheepskin. These special pads should be placed against the skin and should be washed and dried frequently. An egg-crate mattress placed on the mattress and under the sheet will also decrease the pressure on the back and permit air to circulate. An air mattress or a water-filled mattress redistributes the weight of a patient and is placed over the regular mattress and under a loosely fitting sheet (Figure 12.1 ■). Do not use safety pins to anchor the mattress. If your client has a special mattress, be sure to ask how you should care for the equipment.

Sheepskin booties and elbow pads can help reduce pressure on the heel and elbows. Bed cradles used under blankets and sheets and over the client's legs make sure that the covers do not touch the client's skin (Figure 12.2 ■).

GENERAL OBSERVATIONS

Observe the condition of the skin each time you visit (Figure 12.3 ■). Be sure to note the temperature, cleanliness, and dryness. Any difference between two extremities is important and should be reported immediately. Observe for bruises and scratches. A bruise could indicate a reaction to a medication, a change in diet, a change in the client's ability to complete certain tasks, a safety issue, or abuse. Try to determine when the bruise appeared, note how big it is, how long it lasts, and if it becomes worse or improves. Document all observations and discuss them with your supervisor.

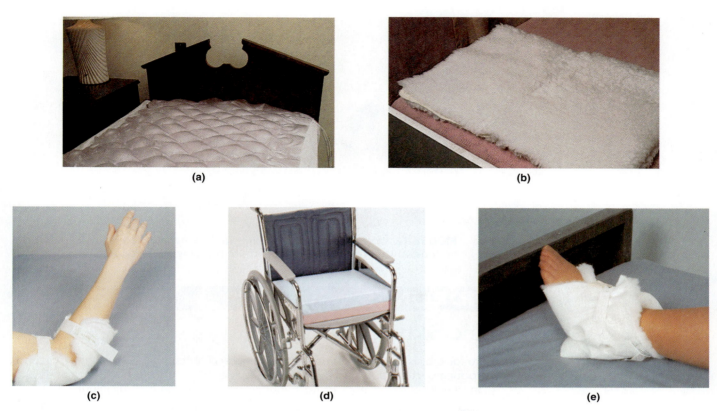

FIGURE 12.1 ■ Special mattresses: (a) water-filled mattress; (b) sheep skin pad; (c) elbow protector; (d) wheelchair cushion; (e) heel protector

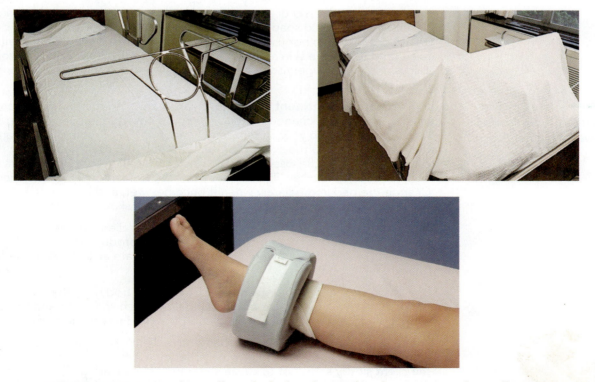

FIGURE 12.2 ■ Secure the cradle to the bed so that neither the covers nor the cradle touch the client's toes and feet.

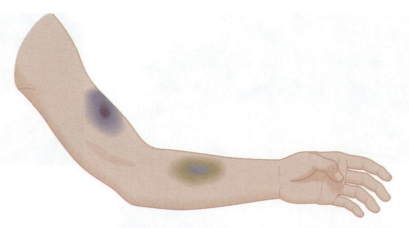

FIGURE 12.3 ■ Bruises on the skin may indicate one of several situations. Always document and report your findings immediately.

◄ GUIDELINES

Basic Skin Care

■ Care for the skin gently. A simple act, such as accidentally scratching the skin, can introduce bacteria and lead to infection. Accidentally stubbing a toe can cause many weeks of discomfort. Protect your client and his skin from all injuries.

■ Protect your client from exposure to the sun and the elements, such as wind, cold, or rain. If your client insists on sitting in the sun, encourage him to use a protective lotion with a sunscreen in it.

■ Keep the client's body as clean and dry as possible. A client need not bathe daily unless he exercises heavily or perspires heavily. It is important to keep his perineum clean and dry, but a complete bath on a daily basis is often unnecessary. Use a mild soap to wash the client, and be sure to dry each body area thoroughly. Do not use perfumes, bubble-bath crystals, or bath salts. They tend to dry the skin and make the tub slippery. If itchy skin is a problem, discuss with your supervisor what can be added to the bath water or put on the client's skin.

incontinence
the inability to control one's bowel movements or urination

■ If the client is **incontinent,** keep him clean and dry no matter how often you must wash him and change the bed. If you do not have enough linen in the house, report this to your supervisor. Do not put the client in rubber pants, as they are irritating to the skin. To protect the bed and to make cleaning the client easier, use a disposable bed protector. This allows the soiled area to be cleaned easily and often. These pads protect the linen on which the client lies. Change the bed immediately when it becomes wet, and be sure that the plastic side of the protector never touches the client's skin.

■ Many new types of disposable products support a client who is incontinent. Before you request that your client purchase any product, discuss with your supervisor which product would be most appropriate and fit within the family budget.

■ Use lotion on the skin to prevent contact with any bodily discharges or drainage from a wound. Use powder and cornstarch sparingly, and be sure to wash it all off when you bathe the client. Both tend to cake in body creases.

■ Turn the client often. You should change the client's position at least every 2 hours. The family should follow this schedule when you are not there. Move the client slowly so as not to cause sheet burns or shearing.

■ Be careful when using bedpans. Pressure from sitting on the rim causes friction when getting on and off the pan, and this can worsen the skin condition. Never leave your client on the bedpan longer than necessary. Use care when removing the bedpan. Avoid spilling urine on the skin, as urine can irritate and cause skin damage. Padding the rim of the bedpan can reduce some pressure. Powdering the rim will also minimize friction.

■ Keep linen wrinkle-free and dry at all times.

■ Remove crumbs, hairpins, and any other hard objects from the bed promptly.

■ Do not let the client lie on catheters or any type of tubing.

■ Be alert to the effects of medications on the skin.

■ Do not rub the skin hard. Always rub the skin with lotion and in a circular motion. Rubbing stimulates the circulation of blood to the skin, but hard rubbing can damage fragile skin.

■ Keep walkways clear of furniture so the client will not bump his toes or legs.

■ Encourage good eating habits and the adequate intake of fluids.

SECTION 2

Decubitus Ulcers (Bedsores)

OBJECTIVES	
What You Will Learn to Do	1. Recognize signs of decubiti.
	2. Demonstrate ways to prevent further skin breakdown after decubiti formation.
	3. Discuss your role as a homemaker/home health aide once decubiti have formed.

Introduction: Decubitus Ulcers

Decubitus ulcers—**bedsores**, or **pressure sores**—occur where the skin has broken because of pressure. Both external and internal factors affect the skin's breakdown. External factors may be abrasions, scratches, burns, or chemicals. Internal factors may be swelling, abscesses, or allergic reactions. Disease may also cause skin breakdown. An elderly or ill client may have poor circulation as part of his disease process, which leads easily to decubitus formation. The pressure can also come from the weight of the body lying in one position too long or from splints, casts, or bandages. Even wrinkles in the bed linen can cause a decubitus ulcer. Decubiti are often made worse by continued pressure, heat, moisture, and lack of cleanliness. Irritating substances on the skin, such as perspiration, urine, feces, wound drainage, or even soap, tend to make decubiti worse. If a decubitus ulcer is not treated, it will quickly become larger, very painful, and even infected.

A decubitus ulcer is the responsibility of the entire health team. Therefore, as the homemaker/home health aide, you have to know how to recognize decubiti

bedsores
decubiti

pressure sore
decubitus

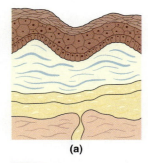

Inflammation or redness of the skin that does not return to normal after 15 minutes of removal of pressure. Edema is present and involves the epidermis. Skin may or may not be broken.

(a)

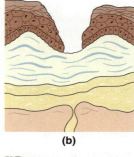

Skin blister or shallow skin ulcer. Involves the epidermis and dermis. Looks like a shallow crater. Area is red and warm and may or may not have drainage.

(b)

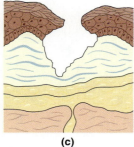

Full thickness skin loss exposing subcutaneous tissue; may extend into next layer. Edema, inflammation, and necrosis present. Drainage present that may or may not have an odor.

(c)

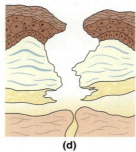

Full thickness ulcer. Muscle and/or bone can be seen. Infection and necrosis present. Drainage present that may or may not have an odor.

(d)

FIGURE 12.4 ■ Stages of skin breakdown.

when they occur. Report the first sign of decubiti to your supervisor so that steps can be taken to prevent further damage.

SIGNS OF DECUBITI

The signs of a decubitus are a warm area of skin, redness, tenderness, discomfort, and a feeling of burning. After this, the skin often becomes gray in color. This means that the blood supply to the area is greatly decreased. If the condition is allowed to continue, a blister will form, and finally the skin will actually break and a wound will appear (Figure 12.4 ■). If you notice any one of these signs, alert your supervisor and remove the pressure to the area. By doing this, you may well prevent further skin breakdown. When the skin is broken, a decubitus ulcer has formed.

CARE OF A DECUBITIS ULCER

Specific treatment for a decubitus is prescribed by a doctor. The wound, however, must be kept clean and the rules of asepsis followed. The client must be positioned so that pressure is removed from the decubitus. If care is a simple, nonsterile dressing, you may be assigned to clean the area and cover it. Be sure you understand the procedure. Ask your supervisor to advise you of the way to fasten the dressing. If tape is used, alternate the site so the tape doesn't cause irritation. Be gentle when removing the tape.

If the client is incontinent, so that urine and feces continue to drain into the wound, discuss alternatives with your supervisor. The client's care plan may have to be changed so that the decubitus remains dry and can heal.

Encourage all the practices of good basic skin care to prevent further skin deterioration and improve the healing climate. Often, even with good practices, clients suffer from skin breakdown. It is important for you to feel that you have done all you could to prevent this. But do not feel guilty if the client, despite your efforts, forms a bedsore. Sometimes, other contributing factors occur over which you have no control.

Once in a while, a decubitus ulcer does not heal with conservative care and the client must be placed on medication and even hospitalized. It is the goal of your good care to prevent this from happening.

CARE OF CLIENT BY THE FAMILY

A decubitus will have to be cared for 24 hours each day. Your supervisor will establish a plan of care. You, as the homemaker/home health aide, will perform the care while you are in the house. The client's family will assume the care the rest of the time. It is important to the healing of the decubitus that the care be done on a regular basis. If the care is not carried out throughout the day, healing will either be delayed or not take place at all.

You may notice that no healing is occurring. If you believe the client's family is unable to care for the wound in your absence, or you find out the family is definitely not caring for the decubitus, report this. Skin care is a 24-hour concern and must be shared by all caregivers.

SECTION 3

Basic Foot Care

OBJECTIVES

What You Will Learn to Do

1. List several causes of foot problems.
2. Demonstrate ways to maintain proper foot hygiene.
3. Discuss your role in correcting practices that contribute to poor foot care.

Introduction: Basic Foot Care

Feet are often the site of many problems because of decreased circulation, infection, poor nutrition, and poor care. Although you will not be able to help your client reverse all conditions, you will be able to help prevent further deterioration.

Many chronic diseases predispose people to foot problems. Diseases such as diabetes, arthritis, COPD, and hypertension often cause foot problems because of lack of circulation, poor nutrition, and decreased physical ability to care for the feet.

Clients may not notice changes in their feet. You will have to observe and report changes on the following conditions:

- Pain either while resting or during exercise
- Changes in sensation on skin or in the feet, either tingling, "pins and needles," or lack of feeling
- Change in color, such as to blue or dark red
- Decreased temperature sensation—sensitivity to cold
- Increased fluid—edema or swelling
- Dry, cracked skin
- Presence of open areas, such as ulcers or blisters

- Toenails that are thick and curling into the toes
- Absence of toenails

BASIC FOOT CARE

If you notice any such changes in your client's feet, report these to your supervisor, who will help you establish a foot care regime for your client. Remember, do not cut your client's toenails or apply any over-the-counter medication to open areas! The basic guidelines for foot care are the following:

1. Inspect the feet each day for changes before you wash them.
2. Wash and dry feet daily. Feet should be washed with mild soap in warm water and dried well, especially between toes. Soaking is not desirable or needed. If the skin is dry, a lubricant or cream can be applied. Check to see if this is permitted. Use of heavily scented soaps or lotions may cause skin irritation.
3. Do not cut nails, corns, or bunions. Observe these and report changes or pain.
4. Help your client choose proper shoes. They should fit well and give support. They should be proper for the time of year and the activity he will be doing. Going barefooted is not advised, as this decreases support and permits injuries to toes and feet. Socks or stockings should be worn. Certain socks are the best because they "breathe" and absorb perspiration. Socks and stockings should be the proper size: Ones that are too big cause irritation and ones that are too small constrict circulation. Do not use garters or rubber bands to hold up socks or stockings.
5. Check the temperature of bath water. If a client has decreased temperature sensation, he may not notice that the water is too hot. The client should not use heating pads to keep warm but rather cotton socks and down slippers inside and insulated boots out of doors. Walk in well-lit and clear areas. Do not try to walk in areas with trash or other debris. In warm weather, keep feet protected from hot sand, boardwalks, objects on the beach, and the sun.
6. Encourage your client to wear the correct shoes for each activity.
7. Diet is important for the health of the entire body. A client should consult a nutritionist for specific foods that will affect his feet. For example, if circulation is a problem, discuss the use of caffeine.

If you notice the following problems, call your supervisor immediately.

Problem	Immediate Action
Swollen legs and feet	Elevate the legs and feet on a chair or couch and report this.
Pain	Stop exercise or activity, rest, and call your supervisor.
Open areas	Do not put on socks or bandage with tape. Cover with clean dressing and call your supervisor.
Temperature variations: hot and cold	Cover lightly with blanket and report this. Do not use a hot water bottle or ice.

SECTION 4

Radiation and Chemotherapy: Effects on the Skin

OBJECTIVES

What You Will Learn to Do

1. List the possible effects of radiation on the skin.
2. Discuss ways of decreasing possible skin breakdown during radiation treatment.
3. Demonstrate the usual care of the radiation site.
4. Discuss possible effects on the skin of chemotherapeutic agents.
5. List actions to decrease skin discomfort during chemotherapy.

Introduction: Radiation Therapy

Radiation therapy uses a specialized type of energy ray to stop the growth of cancer cells by destroying the cells' ability to grow and reproduce. Radiation is used at various times in the treatment of cancer.

During the first visit to the radiation center, lines are drawn on the skin to indicate the target for the radiation. It is important not to wash off these marks. The skin within these marks may appear red or burned. Should the skin break, contact your supervisor immediately. Care for the skin gently with cool water. Do not wash the area with soaps or lotions.

Protect the radiation site from sunlight. Cover it with loose-fitting clothing that will not scratch or irritate it.

Should the client need to shave in the radiation site, use only electric razors. Check with your supervisor as to the type of shaving cream to be used, and make sure it is specific for electric razors. Do not use hair-removal chemicals or lotions.

radiation therapy
the use of X-rays to treat a tumor or a condition

Introduction: Chemotherapy

Chemotherapy is a general term used to describe the use of drugs to treat cancer. There are many differences in the way drugs are given, how often they are given, and how each person responds. Be sure to follow the plan of care for your client and do not change it without consulting your supervisor.

Chemotherapy works by destroying cancer cells' ability to reproduce. Unfortunately, normal cells also pick up some chemicals, and this can cause side effects.

- Sometimes, a dry mouth and throat is a problem. The client can eat moist foods and drink fluids. Also, eating cold, soft foods is easier. Bland foods help avoid further irritation.
- Mouth care is important. Gently use a soft-bristle toothbrush followed by a nonirritating mouthwash with salt or alcohol. Check with your supervisor before the client uses either salt or alcohol.
- Keep lips moist and lubricated.
- Discuss a dental consult with your supervisor.
- Hair follicles frequently are affected by drugs, and hair falls out. Often the hair grows back when the drugs are stopped. It is important to help your

chemotherapy
the regime of taking drugs to treat a malignancy

client feel as attractive as possible at this time. Wigs are often used. Men may wear hairpieces. Some women wear turbans or hats. It is important to keep the scalp clean and free of irritations during this time.

■ Skin rashes often occur generally over the body or in specific areas. A nonirritating lotion or cornstarch-based powder can be used. Contact your supervisor if the itching becomes severe or if the skin is broken.

Clients receiving radiation and/or chemotherapy are under a great deal of stress. Their skin condition is important because it is a visible sign to them and their family that they are ill and having side effects from the treatments. It is your role as a homemaker/home health aide to assist these clients in maintaining a clean body and one that minimizes the skin side effects of the treatments.

CHAPTER REVIEW

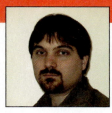

Case Study

Review the case study that appears on the first page of the chapter. Answer two sets of questions about the case study contained in the Explore and Apply sections below.

EXPLORE

1. You are assigned to visit Mr. Flannery twice a week to assist with personal care, shopping, and nutritional supervision. What basic safety precautions would you establish for him?

2. Although you are visiting twice a week, how might you increase assistance with nutrition? Why are these activities so important for the maintenance of good skin care?

APPLY

1. How would you position the client so as to decrease the pressure on the red areas he already has? What would you advise the client do so that new ones do not form?

2. You notice after several visits to Mr. Flannery that his bed linen have not been changed and the chair in which he usually sits has a slight odor. What additional information would you have to gather before you called your supervisor? How would you explain to Mr. Flannery what you are doing and why you are asking so many questions?

Certification Exam Review Questions

Choose the best answer for each question or statement.

1. **Good skin care is**

   a. the result of good nutrition, exercise, and proper amounts of fluid intake.

   b. the responsibility of the client and not the homemaker/home health aide.

   c. a special part of the assignment, and if it is not assigned, it does not have to be done.

   d. not possible in older people with fragile skin.

2. **When a homemaker/home health aide sees a red area on a client, the first action is to**

   a. document this immediately.

   b. remove pressure from the area.

   c. call the supervisor.

   d. call the doctor.

3. **If a client is incontinent, you should**

   a. put him in diapers for the whole night to protect his skin.

   b. limit the amount of fluid intake to decrease the amount of urine, which will protect his skin.

   c. put waterproof pants on the client to protect the linen and the client's skin.

   d. change the bed immediately after each incontinent episode and explore the use of a catheter and diapers to protect the client's skin.

4. **When a client develops a decubiti ulcer, you should**

   a. always blame the homemaker/home health aide.

   b. put cream on the area.

   c. treat it with good nutrition, removal of pressure, and frequent turning.

   d. cover the area with a dressing soaked in alcohol.

5. **When a client develops a decubitus ulcer, you should tell**

   a. the family to never touch it but wait until the nurse comes.

   b. the family how to care for the area.

   c. the client that he will heal with no change in care but oral medication.

   d. the doctor, as he is the first person to call.

CHAPTER 13

Personal Care

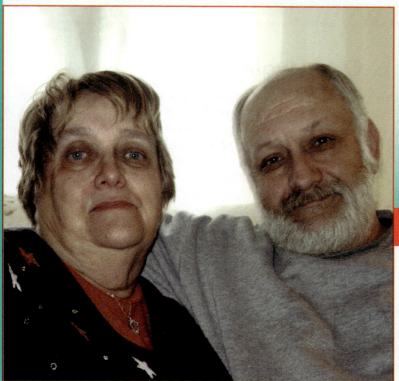

CASE STUDY

Mr. Ricci lives with his wife, tends his garden, and makes his own wine in the basement each year. He takes medication, but his wife is unable to say what it is. "He takes care of himself," she says. Mr. Ricci is a retired steel worker and is very independent. He continues to care for his personal needs, although his wife says that he is often unable to thoroughly wash himself. The family, which is large and lives nearby, visits each weekend, and Mrs. Ricci takes great pride in the fact that she cooks for all 13 of them. She says the children stop by during the week on their way home from work. "They think we do not know they are checking up on us," Mrs. Ricci says, "but at least they come."

Keep the case study in mind as you read the chapter. After you have read the chapter, answer the Explore and Apply questions at the end of the chapter that relate to the case study.

Oral Hygiene

OBJECTIVES

What You Will Learn to Do

1. Discuss the reasons for giving oral hygiene.
2. Demonstrate the proper way to give oral hygiene.
3. Demonstrate the proper way to clean dentures.
4. Demonstrate the proper way to give oral hygiene to an unconscious client.

Introduction: Oral Hygiene

People who are ill need frequent oral hygiene. They may have a bad taste in their mouth. The tongue may become coated or they may have sore gums. A clean, fresh-feeling mouth improves appetite, communication, general appearance, and dental health. It gives a feeling of well-being and decreases mouth odor.

oral hygiene
cleanliness of the mouth

Oral hygiene includes the cleansing of the mouth, gums, and teeth or dentures. This procedure should be done twice a day and after meals whenever possible.

Oral hygiene is part of every client's care, whether he is conscious or unconscious, eating or not eating, self-sufficient or partially dependent. Unconscious clients cannot respond to you or tell you they need oral hygiene. It is your responsibility to see that each client receives oral hygiene. If the client can be responsible for cleaning his teeth and mouth, encourage this. However, if he is unable, you as the homemaker/home health aide must do it for him.

PROCEDURE 22

Oral Hygiene

RATIONALE: A clean mouth and clean teeth help prevent oral problems and promote fresh breath and a general feeling of well-being.

Be sure that your client can spit out water before you allow him to take it.

1. Assemble your equipment:
   Fresh water
   Cup
   Straw, if necessary
   Toothbrush and toothpaste
   Emesis basin (or sink) or small basin
   Face towel and disposable gloves
   Mouthwash (optional)
2. Wash your hands.
3. Ask visitors to step out of the room, if appropriate.

4. Explain the procedure to the client.
5. Have the client sit up or assist him to the sink. (If the client goes to the sink, omit any unnecessary steps.)
6. Spread the towel across the client's chest to protect him. Put on gloves.
7. Offer the client water to rinse his mouth.
8. Hold the emesis basin under the client's chin so he can spit out the water (Figure 13.1 ▪).
9. Put toothpaste on the wet toothbrush.
10. Offer the toothbrush to the client if he can brush his own teeth. If he is unable, you must do it. Use a gentle motion, starting above the gum line and going down the teeth. Repeat this until you have brushed all the teeth.

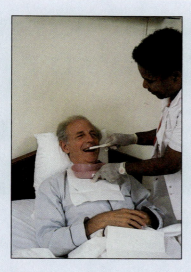

FIGURE 13.1 ■

11. Offer the client water to rinse his mouth.
12. Offer the client mouthwash if he likes it.
13. Make the client comfortable.
14. Clean and put away the equipment. Remove your gloves.
15. Wash your hands.
16. Make a notation on the client's chart that you have completed this procedure. Also note anything you observed about the client during this procedure.

SAMPLE CHARTING: 5/5/04   7:30 A.M.
Client brushed his teeth with minimal assistance.
Carol Smith H/HHA

ORAL HYGIENE FOR CLIENTS WHO WEAR DENTURES

Clients who wear **dentures** (false teeth) also require oral hygiene. Pieces of food must be removed from gums and the tongue. The gums must also be stimulated to ensure good circulation. Gums should be stimulated with a soft toothbrush whenever dentures are removed. Dentures need not be cleaned each time they are removed if the client removes them several times a day. They can, however, be soaked in a cleansing solution each time. They should be brushed thoroughly at least once every 12 hours.

Be careful while you are handling dentures. They are expensive and difficult to replace. Always put them in a carefully marked denture cup. Do not wrap them up in tissue, put them under a pillow, or leave them on a night table. They could be thrown out by accident.

dentures
false teeth

PROCEDURE 23

Oral Hygiene for Clients Who Wear Dentures

RATIONALE: Food and bacteria that collect under dentures cause discomfort and mouth odor. Clean dentures promote general well-being and help prevent oral problems.

1. Assemble your equipment:
   Tissues
   Denture cup
   Small basin or emesis basin
   Toothbrush or denture brush
   Denture-soaking solution
   Towel and disposable gloves
   Denture toothpaste

2. Wash your hands.
3. Ask visitors to step out of the room, if appropriate.
4. Tell the client you wish to clean his dentures.
5. Spread the towel across the client's chest to protect his bedclothes. Put on gloves.
6. Ask the client to remove his dentures. Have tissue in the emesis basin ready to receive the dentures. Help the client if he cannot remove them himself.
7. Take the dentures to the sink in the basin. Hold them securely.

continued

8. Line the sink with a paper towel or washcloth so that if the dentures slip out of your hand, they will be cushioned as they fall. Fill the sink with water.

9. Apply toothpaste or denture cleanser to the dentures. With the dentures in the palm of your hand, brush them until they are clean. *Do not use kitchen cleanser or abrasive cleansers* (Figure 13.2 ■).

10. Rinse the dentures thoroughly under cool water.

11. Fill the denture cup with denture soaking solution, cool water, or mouthwash and water. Place the dentures in the cup, and cover it.

12. Help the client rinse his mouth with water and/or mouthwash.

13. Have the client replace the dentures in his mouth if that is what he wants. Be sure the dentures are moist before replacing them. Ask the client if he uses denture adhesive.

14. Leave the labeled denture cup with the clean solution where the client can easily place the dentures if he takes them out between cleanings.

15. Clean your equipment and replace it in the proper place.

16. Remove gloves and wash your hands.

17. Make a notation on the client's chart that you have completed this procedure. Also note

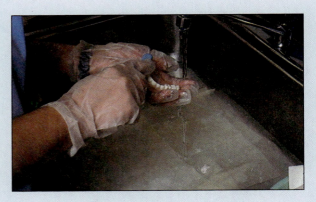

FIGURE 13.2 ■

anything you have observed about the client during this procedure.

Note: It is a safety precaution to label a denture cup so that no one throws the dentures out accidentally.

SAMPLE CHARTING:	10/30/04 10:30 A.M. Cleaned dentures, which had been soaking overnight. Oral care given. Client reminded to cover denture cup to prevent spilling contents. Elaine Frank H/HHA

Oral Hygiene for the Unconscious Client

Be careful not to overlook mouth care of a client who is unconscious. A responsible homemaker/home health aide always remembers to give frequent and thorough oral hygiene to unconscious clients. By doing this, you will prevent the oral tissues from cracking and bleeding. If you share the care of a client with family members, be sure they observe you giving oral hygiene. This way they will learn, by your example, the necessity of this procedure.

PROCEDURE 24

Oral Hygiene for the Unconscious Client

RATIONALE: Unconscious clients often breathe through their mouths, which dries lips and mucous membranes. Careful, frequent care and observation are necessary to prevent oral problems.

Do not put water into the client's mouth.

1. Assemble your equipment:
   Towel and disposable gloves

Small basin or emesis basin
Special disposable mouth care kit—if such a kit is not available, you will need:
Tongue depressor, padded with several gauze squares. (Be sure they are securely fastened to the tongue depressor.)
Lubricant, such as glycerine or a solution of glycerine and lemon juice.

2. Wash your hands.

3. Ask visitors to step out of the room, if appropriate.

4. Tell the client what you are going to do. Even though the client seems unconscious, he may hear you.

5. Stand at the bedside and turn the client's face toward you. Put on gloves.

6. Support the client's face on a pillow covered by a towel.

7. Put a small basin on the towel under the client's chin.

8. Place the mouth care equipment near you so you do not have to move.

9. Wipe the client's entire mouth (roof, tongue, and inside the lips and cheeks) with the swab or the tongue depressor dipped in solution. *Do not put your fingers in the client's mouth. He may close his mouth and injure you.*

10. Put used swabs in the basin. The swabs will leave a coating of glycerine solution on the entire mouth and tongue. This will protect and lubricate the oral tissues.

11. Dry the client's face with a towel.

12. Using a clean applicator, put a small amount of lubricant on the client's lips.

13. Make the client safe and comfortable.

14. Clean your equipment and put it in the proper place.

15. Remove your gloves and wash your hands.

16. Make a notation on the client's chart that you have completed this procedure. Note your observations of the client during the procedure.

SAMPLE CHARTING: 4/4/05   3:30 P.M.
Gave complete oral care. Lips dry. Small area on left lower lip is cracked. Discussed with his mother. She will apply lip moisturizer every two hours while she is awake.
Sally Hansen H/HHA

SECTION 2

Assisting a Client to Dress

OBJECTIVE
What You Will Learn to Do

1. Demonstrate the proper way to assist a client with dressing and undressing.

Introduction: Assisting a Client to Dress and Undress

Allow a client to choose his own clothes if he wishes to do so. If a client is in his bed most of the day, bedclothes are preferred (be sure they are not wrinkled). If a client spends most of the day out of bed, encourage him to dress in street clothes.

If a client has a method of dressing himself that suits him and is safe, allow him to continue using his personal method. For example, some clients may not zip up their dresses all the way or always leave the top button on a shirt unbuttoned. The following procedure is a guide. Individualization is always necessary.

Remember not to expose the client unnecessarily as you assist him. In this way, you will avoid chilling the client and embarrassing him.

Remember: An injured or **inflexible** (rigid) arm or leg is first into the garment and last out.

inflexible
unbending, rigid

PROCEDURE 25

Assisting a Client to Dress and Undress

RATIONALE: Dressing in familiar street clothes assists the client to a feeling of well-being and inclusion in the family. Assisting rather than dressing the client reinforces independence and control.

1. Assemble your equipment:
   Clean clothes

2. Wash your hands.

3. Ask visitors to leave the room, if appropriate.

4. If the client can sit on the edge of the bed, assist him into this position. Avoid exposing him. If the client must remain in bed, assist him into a flat position on his back.

5. Put on underwear and trousers or pajamas. If a leg is injured, place it into underwear or pajamas first, followed by the other leg.

6. Ask the client to stand up, if possible, and pull the pants to his waist. If the client is in bed, have him lift his buttocks as you pull up his pants.

7. To put on an over-the-head type shirt (or other garment), place an injured arm into the shirt first. Then put the neck of the shirt over the client's head. Finally, guide the other arm into the shirt.

8. To put on a button-type shirt, place the sleeve over an injured arm first. Bring the shirt to the back of the client and guide the other arm into the sleeve (Figure 13.3 ■).

9. Assist the client with socks or stockings. Do not use round garters, as they decrease circulation.

10. Assist the client with shoes. Be sure they fit well and give support. Look for any blisters or red areas on the feet.

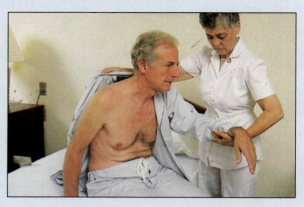

FIGURE 13.3 ■

11. Make the client comfortable.

12. Wash your hands.

13. Make a notation on the client's chart that you have completed this procedure. Also note anything you have observed about the client during this procedure.

SAMPLE CHARTING:	1/1/05 11:30 A.M. Minimally assisted client to dress in street clothes. Several shirts appear very large for him now. Mentioned this to his daughter, who says she will discuss buying him the correct size clothing. Katherine Magee H/HHA

SECTION 3

Bathing a Client

OBJECTIVES

What You Will Learn to Do

1. Discuss the reasons for bathing a client.

2. Demonstrate a complete bed bath.

3. Demonstrate a partial bath.

4. Demonstrate the proper technique for assisting a client with a shower or tub bath.

Introduction: Helping a Client to Bathe

There are several important reasons for bathing a client:

- Bathing takes waste products off the skin.
- Bathing cools and refreshes the client.
- Bathing stimulates the skin and improves circulation.
- Bathing requires movement of the muscles.
- Bathing provides a good opportunity for the homemaker/home health aide to observe the client.
- Bathing provides an opportunity to talk with the client.

Clients at home may not need to have a complete bath each day. They may prefer to have a partial bath at times. Most people are used to bathing themselves privately. Some clients are embarrassed by having another person do this for them. Demonstrate your understanding of the client's feelings by keeping him covered and not exposing him, and by bathing him in a professional and reassuring manner. Clients who tire easily may prefer to have a different part of the body bathed each day. The frequency of your client's bath will depend on climate, need, skin condition, and the client's diagnosis. Discuss your client's preferences with your supervisor, and try to meet the client's preferences.

There are four types of baths. When you are given your assignment, your supervisor will indicate which type of bath to give. Do not change the type of bath unless you check with your supervisor and discuss the change.

1. *The complete bath.* This is usually given in bed. If the client is weak or unable to bathe himself, it is your responsibility to bathe him. When you are giving the bath, the client will usually give you little or no assistance.
2. *The partial bath.* A client may take care of some of his own bathing requirements. When this is the case, you will be responsible for bathing only the areas that are hard for him to reach (back, feet, or genitalia).
3. *The tub bath.* This is given in a tub and requires a special order from the doctor. Do not give a client a tub bath until you have checked with your supervisor. Sometimes, you will be asked to help the client with a bath into which he puts medication. Be sure that the client or his family can assume responsibility for the medication.
4. *The shower.* The client is bathed under running water. This, too, requires a special order from the doctor.

▸ GUIDELINES

Bathing a Client

- Usually, the complete bath is given as part of morning care. However, if your client enjoys his bath at another time of day, try to follow his request.
- Take everything to the bedside *before* you start the bath.
- Always cover the client with a bath blanket before giving the complete bath. If you do not have a bath blanket, use a thin blanket, big towel, or terry cloth bathrobe.
- Use good body mechanics. Keep your feet separated, stand firmly, bend your knees, and keep your back straight.

continued

▪ GUIDELINES (continued)

Bathing a Client

- ▪ When you use soap, keep it in the soap dish, not the basin of water.

- ▪ Observe safety rules.

- ▪ Use lotions and creams the client usually uses. Do not ask him to buy the one you prefer. Deodorant is used only if the client requests it and after the entire bath is completed.

- ▪ Check the client's bedclothes for personal items before putting them in the laundry.

- ▪ Talk to the client as you bathe him.

- ▪ Keep the client's body in proper alignment.

- ▪ Change the water as often as you need to so that you have warm, clean water at all times.

- ▪ Continually observe the client for distress. If he appears tired or uncomfortable, stop the bath.

PROCEDURE 26

The Complete Bed Bath

RATIONALE: Giving a bed bath improves circulation, provides a general feeling of well-being, and provides an opportunity to examine the client's skin and body. This is an opportune time to interact with the client.

1. Assemble your equipment:
   Soap in a soap dish
   Washcloth and disposable gloves
   Several bath towels
   Wash basin
   Powder, deodorant
   Clean gown or pajamas
   Bath blanket/large towel
   Orange stick for nail care if used by
      your agency
   Lotion for back rub
   Comb and hairbrush

2. Wash your hands.

3. Ask visitors to step out of the room, if appropriate.

4. Tell the client you are going to give him a complete bed bath.

5. Offer the bedpan or urinal. (See *Procedures 34 and 35, pp. 244–246.*)

6. Assist the client with oral hygiene. (See *Procedure 22, pp. 226–227.*)

7. Take the bedspread and regular blanket off the bed. Fold them loosely over the back of a chair, leaving the client covered with the top sheet.

8. Place the bath blanket over the top sheet. Ask the client to hold the blanket in place.

9. Remove the top sheet from underneath without uncovering (exposing) the client (Figure 13.4 ▪). Fold the sheet loosely over the back of the chair if it is to be used again; if not, put it in the laundry bag.

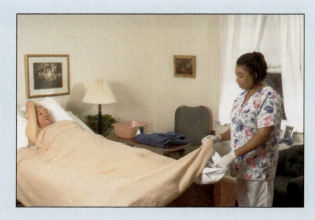

FIGURE 13.4 ▪

10. Lower the headrest and knee rest of the bed, if possible and if permitted. The client should be in a flat position, as flat as is comfortable for him.

11. Raise the bed to its highest horizontal position, if possible.

12. Remove the client's nightclothes and jewelry. Keep the client covered with the bath blanket. Place the gown in the laundry bag, and put the jewelry in a safe place.

13. Fill the wash basin two-thirds full of water. Ask your client how he likes the water—hot, warm, or cool. Test it with your whole hand. Then let him test it with the inside of his hand.

14. Help the client to move to the side of the bed closest to you. Use good body mechanics. Put on gloves.

15. Put a towel across the client's chest and make a mitten with the washcloth (Figure 13.5 ■). Wash the client's eyes from the nose to the outside of the face. Be careful not to get soap in his eyes. Rinse and dry by patting gently with the bath towel.

16. Put a towel lengthwise under the client's arm farthest from you. This will keep the bed from getting wet. Support the arm with the palm of your hand under his elbow. Then wash his shoulder, armpit (axilla), and arm. Use long, firm strokes. Rinse and dry the area well.

17. Place the basin of water on the towel. Put the client's hand into the water and let it soak. Be sure to support the arm and the basin. Wash, rinse, and dry the hand well. Place it under the bath blanket.

18. Wash, rinse, and dry the arm, hand, axilla, and shoulder closest to you in the same way.

19. Clean the client's fingernails with an orange stick if used by your agency.

20. Place a towel across the client's chest. Fold the bath blanket down to the client's

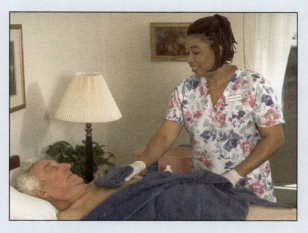

FIGURE 13.6 ■

abdomen. Wash and rinse the client's ears, neck, and chest. Take note of the condition of the skin under the female client's breasts. Dry the area thoroughly.

21. Cover the client's entire chest with the towel (Figure 13.6 ■). Fold the bath blanket down to the pubic area. Wash the client's abdomen. Be sure to wash the umbilicus (navel) and in any creases of the skin. Dry the client's abdomen. Then pull the bath blanket up over the abdomen and chest and remove the towels.

22. Empty the dirty water. Rinse the basin and refill it.

23. Fold the bath blanket back from the client's leg farthest from you.

24. Put a towel lengthwise under that leg and foot.

25. Bend the knee and wash, rinse, and dry the leg and foot (Figure 13.7 ■). Support the leg if the client is unable to do so. Take hold of the heel for more support when flexing the knee.

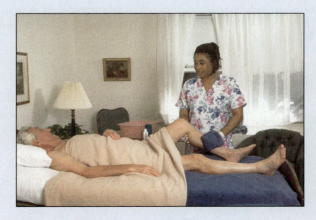

FIGURE 13.7 ■

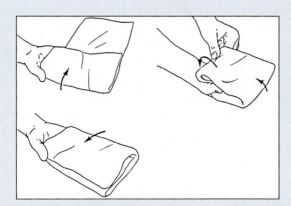

FIGURE 13.5 ■

continued

26. If the client can easily bend his knee, put the wash basin on the towel. Then put the client's foot directly into the basin to wash it. Support his leg and the basin. Protect the ankle area from too much pressure on the basin.

27. Observe the toenails and the skin between the toes for general appearance and condition. Look especially for redness and cracking of the skin. Take away the basin. Dry the client's leg and foot and between the toes. Cover the leg and foot with the bath blanket and remove the towel.

28. Repeat the entire procedure for the leg and foot closest to you. Empty the basin, and rinse and refill it with clean water.

29. Ask the client to turn on his side with his back toward you. If he needs help in turning, assist him.

30. Put the towel lengthwise on the bottom sheet near the client's back. Wash, rinse, and dry the back of the neck, back, and buttocks with long, firm, circular strokes. Give the client a back rub with warm lotion. The client's back should be rubbed for at least a minute and a half. Give special attention to bony areas (for example, shoulder blades, hips, and elbows). Look for red areas. Dry the client's back, remove the towel, and turn him on his back.

31. Offer the client a soapy washcloth to wash his genital area. Give him a clean, wet washcloth to rinse himself well. Give him a dry towel for drying himself. If he is unable to do this for himself, it is your responsibility to wash the client's genital area. Provide for privacy at all times.

32. Put a clean gown or pajamas on the client. *Note:* Usually, the client's hair is combed and the bed is changed; however, this depends on the needs of *your* client.

33. Arrange the bed so that your client is comfortable and safe.

34. Clean your equipment and put it in its proper place.

35. Remove gloves and wash your hands.

36. Make a notation on the client's chart that you have completed this procedure. Note your observations of the client during this procedure.

SAMPLE CHARTING: 7/30/04 7:30 A.M. Complete bath given. Small red area noted on left hip. Client left turned on right side. Note left for his daughter to turn client at least every two hours to decrease pressure on right hip area. Supervisor alerted via phone. Esther Simms H/HHA

The Partial Bath

Your clients should be encouraged to take as active a part in their care as their medical condition allows. It may be easier, faster, and more efficient for *you* to bathe your client, but do not let the client know how you feel. Remember, as a homemaker/home health aide, you will have to leave the client after a period of service. It is your responsibility to help him gain his independence so he can function when you are gone. He will gain this independence and self-confidence only if you encourage him to take an active part in his care. A partial bath routine must be individualized to suit the needs of your client. However, there are certain rules to always keep in mind—safety and client ability.

- Assist the client with establishing a bathing routine to save his energy.
- Allow the client to bathe as much of his body as he can safely reach.
- Bring a basin to his bed, or assist the client to the bathroom.
- Take a chair into the bathroom or have the client sit on the toilet covered by a towel (Figure 13.8 ■).
- Be observant of safety while the client is bathing.
- Give the client privacy as he bathes.

The Tub Bath and Shower

Several of your clients will want a tub bath. Some houses do not have showers. Some clients are used to taking baths rather than showers. Some baths are prescribed for therapeutic reasons. Remember, you must have specific instructions

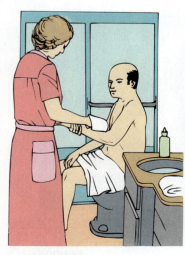

FIGURE 13.8 ■ Assisting a client with a partial bath

from your supervisor to give a client a tub bath, and you, as the homemaker/home health aide, must be sure that you can carry out this procedure.

Handheld Showers

Some clients may have a handheld shower in their bathroom, attached to their tub or their shower. These allow the user to direct the water to a single place on the body or head. Apply the same safety precautions you would use for a regular shower. There are a few additional considerations.

■ Remember to keep the client covered and warm when using this appliance. This will protect his privacy and maintain his body temperature.

■ Test the water temperature away from the client so neither too hot nor too cold water touches him.

■ Be extra careful when changing water-flow direction so neither you nor the bathroom gets an unexpected shower.

■ Remember to turn off all water after you are finished using the appliance.

PROCEDURE 27

The Tub Bath

RATIONALE: Tub bathing provides a relaxing atmosphere for the client and an opportunity for observing the client's skin.

1. Assemble your equipment:
   Bath towels
   Nonskid bathmat on the bathroom floor
   Washcloths and disposable gloves
   Soap
   Nonskid bathmat to be used in the tub
   Chair for client to sit on, or use the commode
   Clean gown or pajamas
   Equipment to wash the tub before and after
      your client's bath

2. Check the tub. Wash it if necessary.

3. Wash your hands.

4. Ask visitors to leave the room, if appropriate.

5. Tell the client that you would like to assist him with his tub bath.

6. Assist the client to the bathroom.

7. For safety, remove all electric appliances from the bathroom. Check grab bars. Check to see that there is proper ventilation.

8. Fill the bathtub half full with water. Ask your client how he likes the bath water—warm, hot, or cool. Run cold water through the faucet last so it will be cool if the client should touch it. Test the water for temperature. Have the client test the water.

9. Assist the client in undressing and getting into the bathtub (Figure 13.9 ■).

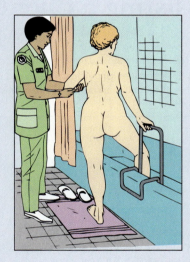

FIGURE 13.9 ■

10. Let the client stay in the bathtub as long as permitted, according to your instructions. Give him privacy as is safely permitted.

11. Help the client wash himself as needed. Wear gloves.

12. Empty the tub. It is easier to exit an empty tub than a full one.

13. Put one towel across the chair or the commode. Have the client sit on this.

continued

14. Allow the client to dry as much of his body as he can. Assist him with putting on clean bed-clothes or street clothes.

15. Assist the client out of the bathroom to his bed or chair. Make him comfortable.

16. Return to the bathroom. Clean the tub and bathroom as necessary.

17. Remove all used linen and put them in the proper place.

18. Wash your hands.

19. Make a notation on the client's chart that you have completed this procedure. Also note anything you have observed about the client during this procedure.

SAMPLE CHARTING:	1/09/05 2:30 P.M. Assisted client with tub bath. No skin problems noted. No problems getting in or out of tub. Client able to dress herself except for tying her shoes. Ray Tanner H/HHA

PROCEDURE 28

Assisting a Client with a Shower with/without a Shower Chair

RATIONALE: A shower provides a relaxing atmosphere for the client and an opportunity for observing the client's skin.

1. Assemble your equipment:
   Bath towels
   Nonskid bathmat on the bathroom floor
   Soap
   Shower cap (optional)
   Washcloth and gloves
   Nonskid bathmat in the shower
   Clean pajamas or street clothes
   Equipment to clean the shower before and
       after your client's shower
   A shower chair (optional)

2. Check the shower. Wash it if necessary.

3. Wash your hands.

4. Ask visitors to leave the room, if appropriate.

5. Tell the client that you would like to assist him with his shower.

6. Assist the client to the bathroom.

7. For safety, remove all electrical appliances from the bathroom. Check grab bars. Check ventilation.

8. Position the shower chair in the shower or tub.

9. Turn on the shower and adjust the water temperature. Ask your client how he likes the water—hot, warm, or cool.

10. Assist the client into the shower.

11. Give the client as much privacy as is safely permitted.

12. When the client is finished washing, turn off the water and assist the client out of the shower. Assist the client with washing and drying those body areas he finds difficult to reach. Wear gloves when washing or drying the client.

13. Help the client to dress as needed. Assist the client out of the bathroom to his bed or a chair. Make him comfortable.

14. Return to the bathroom. Clean the shower and bathroom as necessary.

15. Remove all used linen and put in the proper place.

16. Wash your hands.

17. Make a notation on the client's chart that you have completed this procedure. Also note anything you have observed about the client during this procedure.

SAMPLE CHARTING:	3/27/05 8:30 A.M. Assisted client with shower following breakfast. No skin problems noted. Client dressed himself for doctor's visit later in morning. Tina Lee H/HHA

Giving a Back Rub

OBJECTIVES	1. List the reasons for giving a back rub.
What You Will Learn to Do	2. Demonstrate the correct technique for giving a back rub.

Introduction: The Back Rub

Rubbing a client's back refreshes him, relaxes his muscles, and stimulates circulation. Because of pressure caused by the bedclothes and lack of movement to stimulate circulation, the skin of a client who spends a great deal of time in bed needs special attention.

Back rubs are usually given as part of morning care after the client's bath. They are also given in the evening before a client goes to sleep and during the day whenever a client changes position or requires this procedure.

Sometimes, a client does not enjoy having his back rubbed. Respect his wishes unless this procedure is ordered to increase circulation. Then discuss this problem with your supervisor. Do not take it personally if a client refuses a back rub. He just may not enjoy this.

PROCEDURE 29

Giving a Client a Back Rub

RATIONALE: Giving a back rub promotes circulation and provides an opportunity to help the client relax and to check his back and arms for any skin changes.

1. Assemble your equipment:
   Towels and disposable gloves
   Lotion of the client's choice
   Basin of warm water (optional)

2. Wash your hands.

3. Ask visitors to leave the room, if appropriate.

4. Tell the client you are going to give him a back rub.

5. Raise the bed to its highest horizontal position, if possible. Ask the client to turn on his side or abdomen so that you can easily reach his back. Have him positioned as close to the side of the bed where you are working as possible.

6. If the client's bed has side rails, keep the side rail up on the far side of the bed, but lower it on the side of the bed where you are working.

7. Warm the lotion by placing it in a basin of warm water. Put on gloves.

8. Expose the client's back and buttocks. Do not overexpose him.

9. Pour a small amount of lotion into the palm of your hand.

10. Rub your hands together, using friction to warm the lotion.

11. Apply lotion to the entire back with the palms of your hands. Use firm long strokes from the buttocks to the shoulders and the back of the neck and shoulders.

12. Use proper body mechanics. Keep your knees slightly bent and your back straight.

13. Exert firm pressure as you stroke upward from the buttocks toward the shoulders. Use gentle pressure as you move your hands down the back. Do not lift up your hands as you massage.

14. Use a circular motion on each bony area. Continue this rhythmic rubbing motion 1 to 3 minutes (Figure 13.10 ■).

continued

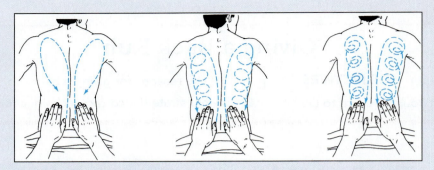

FIGURE 13.10 ■

15. Dry the client's back by patting it with a towel.
16. Assist the client in putting on a gown or pajamas.
17. Reposition the client. Make him comfortable.
18. Arrange the top sheet of the bed neatly.
19. Arrange the bed so that your client is safe and comfortable.
20. Put your equipment back in its proper place.
21. Remove gloves and wash your hands.

22. Make a notation on the client's chart that you have completed this procedure. Also note anything you have observed about the client during this procedure.

SAMPLE CHARTING:	10/14/04 8:30 P.M. Backrub given before client retired for night. Noted elbows were dry. Skin moisturizer applied. Linda Pham H/HHA

SECTION 5

Hair Care

OBJECTIVES

What You Will Learn to Do

1. Demonstrate the proper technique for a bed shampoo.
2. Demonstrate the proper technique for a sink shampoo.
3. Demonstrate the proper technique for combing a client's hair.

Introduction: Shampooing a Client's Hair

It is important to keep your client's hair neat and clean. This prevents scalp and hair breakdown, improves the client's appearance, improves circulation to the scalp, and improves the client's general feeling about himself.

There are various methods of washing a client's hair:

■ Bed shampoo
■ Shampoo at the sink
■ Shampoo in the shower (usually done by the client)
■ Dry shampoo

Before you wash a client's hair, consider two important points:

■ Has your supervisor given you specific instructions to wash the client's hair?
■ Can the client safely remain in the required position during the procedure?

╋ GUIDELINES

Hair Care

◼ Keep the client free of drafts.

◼ Never cut a client's hair.

◼ Never color a client's hair.

◼ Never give a client a permanent.

◼ Never use a hot comb or curling iron on a client's hair.

◼ Style the client's hair as he or she is accustomed to have it.

PROCEDURE 30

Giving a Shampoo in Bed

RATIONALE: Clean hair promotes general health and well-being. Being well groomed promotes self-esteem.

1. Assemble your equipment:
   Client's comb and brush
   Client's shampoo
   Conditioner (optional)
   Several containers of warm to hot water, as client prefers
   Chair
   Pitcher
   Large basin or pail to collect dirty water
   Bed protectors
   Several large bath towels
   Wash cloth and disposable gloves
   Water trough or 1½ yards of 60-inch-wide plastic to make one
   Cotton balls (optional)
   Bath blanket
   Waterproof pillow (optional)
   Electric blow dryer (optional)
   Curlers (optional)

2. Wash your hands.

3. Ask visitors to leave the room, if appropriate.

4. Tell the client that you are going to shampoo his hair in bed.

5. Raise the bed to the highest horizontal position, if possible. Lower the headrest and the side rail on the side you are working, if possible. Ask the client what water temperature he prefers.

6. Place a chair at the side of the bed near the client's head. The chair should be lower than the mattress. Put on gloves.

7. Inspect the client's hair for knots and lice. If the client has knots, carefully comb them out. If the client has lice, stop the procedure and report this to your supervisor. Lice are tiny black insects that live on hair and scalp.

8. Place a towel on the chair. Place the large basin or pail on the towel.

9. (Optional) Remove the pillow from under the client's head. Cover the pillow with a waterproof case. Have the pillow under the small of the client's back so when he lies on it his head is tilted backward.

10. Put the bath blanket on the client. Fanfold the top sheets to the foot of the bed without exposing the client.

11. Ask the client to move across the bed so that his head is close to where you are standing.

12. Place the bed protectors on the mattress under the client's head.

13. Put small amounts of cotton in the client's ears for protection.

14. Place the shampoo trough under the client's head. A trough can be made by rolling up the sides of the plastic sheet. This makes a channel for the water to run into the pail. Three sides must be rolled to make the channel. The top edge should be rolled around a rolled bath towel. Place the edge with the rolled towel in it under the client's neck and head. Have the open edge hanging into the pail on the chair.

15. Loosen the pajamas so the client is comfortable and no clothing is in the trough.

continued

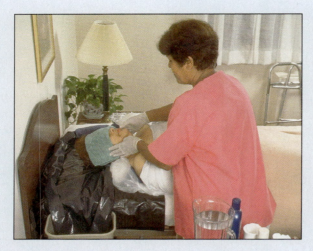

FIGURE 13.11 ■

16. Ask the client to hold the washcloth over his eyes (Figure 13.11 ■).

17. Pour some water over the client's hair. Use a pitcher or a cup. Repeat until the hair is completely wet.

18. Apply shampoo and, using both hands, wash the hair and massage the scalp with your fingertips. Avoid using your fingernails as they could scratch the client's scalp.

19. Rinse the shampoo off by pouring water over the hair. Have the client turn from side to side. Repeat this until the hair is free of soap.

20. If the client uses a conditioner, apply it after reading the directions.

21. Dry the client's forehead and ears.

22. Remove the cotton from the client's ears.

23. Raise the client's head and wrap it in a bath towel.

24. Rub the client's hair with a towel to dry it as much as possible.

25. Remove the equipment from the bedside. Be sure the client is in a safe, comfortable position before you leave.

26. Comb the client's hair as he is accustomed to having it done. You may leave a towel spread over the pillow under the client's head as his hair dries or you may set the client's hair. If an electric blow dryer is available, use it on cool.

27. Remove the bath blanket and, at the same time, bring up the top sheets to cover the client.

28. If possible, lower the bed to its lowest horizontal position and raise the side rails.

29. Make the client comfortable.

30. Clean your equipment and put it in its proper place.

31. Remove gloves and wash your hands.

32. Make a notation on the client's chart that you have completed this procedure. Also note anything that you have observed about the client during this procedure.

SAMPLE CHARTING: 1/30/05   3:00 P.M.
Hair washed while in bed. No evidence of scratches or redden areas. Hair styled as per client's request. Lee Ham H/HHA

Shampooing a Client's Hair at the Sink

If a client can sit with his head over the sink, this procedure is preferable to a bed shampoo. It is faster and easier.

PROCEDURE 31

Shampooing a Client's Hair at the Sink

RATIONALE: Clean hair promotes general health and well-being. Being well groomed promotes self-esteem.

1. Assemble your equipment:
   Client's comb and brush
   Client's shampoo
   Pitcher for water (optional)
   Chair that allows the client to sit comfortably facing the sink
   Several towels
   Washcloth and disposable gloves
   Cotton balls (optional)
   Electric blow dryer (optional)
   Curlers (optional)

2. Wash your hands.

3. Ask visitors to leave the room, if appropriate.

4. Assist the client to the sink. Be sure a chair is available for him to sit on if he tires.

5. Place a towel around the client's shoulders. Put on gloves.

6. Inspect a client's hair for knots and lice. If the client has knots, carefully comb them out. If the client has lice, stop the procedure and report this to your supervisor.

7. Put a small amount of cotton in the client's ears for protection.

8. Give the client a washcloth to cover his eyes.

9. Ask the client what temperature he prefers the water. Adjust it.

10. Ask the client to lean forward so that his head is over the sink.

11. Wet his head thoroughly.

12. Apply shampoo and, using both hands, wash the hair and massage the scalp with your fingertips. Avoid using your fingernails as they may scratch the client's scalp.

13. Rinse the shampoo off by pouring water over the hair.

14. Dry the client's forehead and ears. Have him assume a comfortable position. Raise the client's head and wrap it in a towel.

15. Remove the cotton from the client's ears.

16. Rub the client's hair with a towel to dry it as much as possible.

17. Comb the client's hair as he is accustomed to having it done. You may leave a towel around the client's shoulders while his hair is drying. Leave a towel under the client's head if he prefers to lie down as his hair dries. You may also set curlers in a client's hair and use the electric blow dryer set on cool.

18. Make sure that the client is comfortable and safe following this procedure.

19. Clean your equipment and the area you used.

20. Remove gloves and wash your hands.

21. Make a notation on the client's chart that you have completed this procedure. Also note anything you have observed about the client during this procedure.

SAMPLE CHARTING: 7/14/05   10:00 A.M. Client's hair washed at her kitchen sink. No redden areas noted on scalp. Hair combed as per client's request. Client left sitting on patio.
Rose Rodriquez H/HHA

Combing a Client's Hair

As with other types of personal care, a client may be unable to take care of his own hair. When this is the case, it is your responsibility to comb and brush his hair. This almost always makes him look better and feel better.

PROCEDURE 32

Combing a Client's Hair

RATIONALE: A client's appearance plays a role in his self-image. Combing and styling hair is usually done according to client's personal preference. This should be respected regardless of the client's age or health status.

1. Assemble your equipment on the bedside table:
   Towel
   Comb or brush
   Any hair preparation the client usually uses
   Hand mirror, if available

2. Wash your hands.

3. Ask visitors to leave the room, if appropriate.

4. Tell the client you are going to brush or comb his hair.

5. If possible, comb the client's hair after the bath and before you make the bed. Some clients prefer to have their hair combed while sitting in a chair.

6. Lay a towel across the pillow, under the client's head. If the client can sit up in bed, drape the towel around his shoulders.

7. If the client wears glasses, ask him to take them off before you begin, unless this makes

continued

the client uncomfortable. Be sure to put the glasses in a safe place.

8. Part the hair down the middle to make it easier to comb.

9. Brush or comb the client's hair carefully, gently, and thoroughly in his usual style.

10. For the client who cannot sit up, separate the hair into small sections. Then comb each section separately, using a downward motion, starting at the loose end and working up toward the head. Ask the client to turn his head from side to side. Or turn it for him so that you can reach the entire head.

11. Arrange the client's hair the way he wants it.

12. If the client has long hair, suggest braiding it to keep it from tangling.

13. Be sure you brush the back of the head.

14. Remove the towel when you are finished.

15. Let the client use the mirror.

16. Make the client comfortable.

17. Wash your hands.

18. Make a notation on the client's chart that you have completed this procedure. Also note anything you have observed about the client during this procedure.

SAMPLE CHARTING: 9/25/05   9:00 P.M.
Client requested her hair be left loose today. Her daughter will braid it before she returns to bed.
Jana Shaid H/HHA

SECTION 6

Shaving a Client

OBJECTIVE

What You Will Learn to Do

1. Demonstrate the proper technique for shaving a client's beard.

Introduction: Shaving a Client's Beard

A regular morning activity for most men is shaving the beard. A client is often well enough to shave himself. In this case, you will give him any help necessary, such as being sure he has the equipment he needs. Sometimes, however, clients cannot shave themselves. In such cases, you will do it. Before shaving any client's face, be sure you have been instructed to do so by your supervisor. Certain clients may not be permitted to shave or be shaved.

Shaving can be done only with an electric razor or a **safety razor.** Never use an electric razor if the client is receiving oxygen.

safety razor
razor provided with a guard to prevent cutting the skin

PROCEDURE 33

Shaving a Client's Beard

RATIONALE: A client's appearance plays a role in his self-image. Shaving facial hair is a key part of daily grooming for many men.

1. Assemble your equipment at the bedside:
   Basin of water, very warm to hot
   Shaving cream

Safety razor
Face towel and disposable gloves
Mirror
Tissues
Aftershave lotion (optional)
Face powder (optional)
Washcloth

2. Wash your hands.

3. Ask visitors to leave the room, if appropriate.

4. Tell the client that you are going to shave his beard.

5. Adjust a light so that it shines on the client's face but not in his eyes.

6. Raise the head of the bed if possible and if allowed. Put on gloves.

7. Spread the face towel under the client's chin. If the client has dentures, be sure they are in his mouth.

8. Put some warm water on the client's face, or use a damp warm washcloth, to soften his beard.

9. If using a razor, apply shaving cream generously to the face.

10. With the fingers of one hand, hold the skin taut (tight) as you shave in the direction that the hair grows. Start under the sideburns and work downward over the cheeks. Continue carefully over the chin. Work upward on the neck under the chin. Use short firm strokes.

11. If using a razor, rinse it often in the basin of water.

12. Areas under the nose and around the lips are sensitive. Take special care in these areas.

13. If you nick the client's skin, wash the area and report this to your supervisor. Do not put any medication on the area.

14. If you used a razor, wash off the remaining shaving cream when you have finished.

15. Apply aftershave lotion or powder as the client prefers.

16. Make the client comfortable.

17. Clean your equipment and put it in its proper place.

18. Remove gloves and wash your hands.

19. Make a notation on the client's chart that you have completed this procedure. Also note anything you have observed about the client during this procedure.

SAMPLE CHARTING: 6/18/05   4:00 P.M. Nephew visited this afternoon and shaved his uncle with a safety razor. Both seemed to enjoy the experience. No skin irritation noted.
Maria Tomo H/HHA

SECTION 7

Assisting a Client with Toileting

OBJECTIVES

What You Will Learn to Do

1. Demonstrate the proper technique for assisting a client with a bedpan.

2. Demonstrate the proper technique for assisting a client with a urinal.

3. Demonstrate the proper technique for assisting a client with a bedside commode.

Introduction: Assisting a Client with Toileting

Toileting is usually a private activity and one not openly discussed. The clients you care for must perform this activity with varying amounts of assistance. They may be embarrassed. You may be embarrassed. Your role is to assist the client with this important and normal bodily function in a way both acceptable to him and safe to you both. People often associate special words with elimination. Knowing these words may make the communication between you and your client easier. Try to keep to the schedule and way the client usually toilets, as this will help when you are not there.

Body waste elimination is important if the body is to maintain its health and function. You will be asked to report on your client's eliminations. Often, this

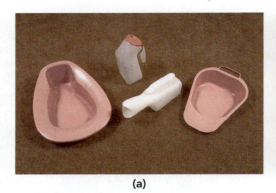 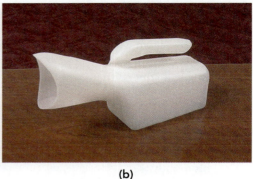

(a)   (b)

FIGURE 13.12 ■ (a) Two different types of bedpans and male and female urinals (b) female urinal

information will provide an indication of your client's health status. Report the following:

- Frequency of elimination
- Color
- Odor
- Any pain with elimination
- Ability to control elimination
- Any foreign material, such as blood or mucous

Some clients cannot leave bed to use the bathroom. These clients require a urinal and a bedpan (Figure 13.12 ■). The **urinal** is a container into which the male client urinates. The **bedpan** is a pan into which he **defecates** (moves his bowels). The female client uses the bedpan for urination and defecation. There are times, however, when a female urinal must be used. You should always cover the bedpan and remove it from the client's bedside to the bathroom as quickly as possible after use. At this time, you would collect a specimen, if required. You would also measure the urine, if necessary.

Some clients can climb out of bed but cannot walk to the bathroom. For these clients, your supervisor will arrange to have a portable **commode** brought to the house. Whenever the client uses it, you will be responsible for cleaning it just as if he had used the bedpan or urinal.

When a client is told he may go to the bathroom, you will be responsible for assisting him to the bathroom and observing all the rules of safety you have been taught. Do not take a client to the bathroom unless your supervisor says that you may do so.

urinal
container into which male clients can urinate; women use female urinals

bedpan
container into which a person defecates or urinates while in bed

defecate
to have a bowel movement

commode
a portable frame, with pan or pail, into which a client urinates and/or defecates

PROCEDURE 34

Offering the Bedpan

RATIONALE: Carefully and skillfully placing the bedpan prevents discomfort and increases the client's comfort with needing assistance for this intimate task.

1. Assemble your equipment:
   Bedpan and cover, or fracture bedpan and cover
   Toilet tissue

   Wash basin with water or wet washcloth
   Soap
   Talcum powder or cornstarch
   Hand towel and disposable gloves

2. Wash your hands.

3. Ask visitors to leave the room, if appropriate. You may, however, wish to demonstrate this procedure to the family members.

4. Ask the client if he would like to use the bedpan. Put on gloves.

5. Warm the bedpan by running warm water inside it and along the rim. Dry the outside of the bedpan with paper towels and put talcum powder or corn starch on the part that will touch the client. If the client is going to move his bowels and a specimen is not needed, place several sheets of toilet tissue or a slight bit of water in the bedpan. This will make cleaning it easier.

6. Raise the bed to the highest horizontal position, if possible.

7. Lower the side rail on the side where you are standing, if possible.

8. Fold back the top sheets so that they are out of the way.

9. Raise the client's gown, but keep the lower part of his body covered with the top sheets.

10. Ask the client to bend his knees and put his feet flat on the mattress. Then ask the client to raise his hips. If necessary, help the client to raise his buttocks by slipping your hand under the lower part of his back. Place the bedpan in position with the seat of the bedpan under the buttocks (Figure 13.13 ■).

11. Sometimes a client cannot lift his buttocks to get on or off the bedpan. In this case, turn the client on his side with his back to you. Put the bedpan against the buttocks. Then turn the client back onto the bedpan (Figure 13.14 ■).

12. Replace the covers over the client.

13. Raise the backrest and knee rest, if allowed, so the client is in a sitting position.

14. Put toilet tissue where the client can reach it easily.

15. Ask the client to signal when he is finished.

16. Raise the side rails to the up position.

17. Leave the room to give the client privacy. Remove gloves and wash your hands if you are going to do another task.

18. When the client signals, return to the room.

19. Wash your hands and put on gloves.

20. Help the client to raise his hips so you can remove the bedpan.

21. Help the client if he cannot clean himself. Turn the client on his side. Clean the anal area with toilet tissue.

22. Raise the side rails, if possible. Cover the bedpan immediately. You can use a disposable pad or a paper towel if no cover is available.

23. Take the bedpan to the client's bathroom. Remove gloves and wash your hands.

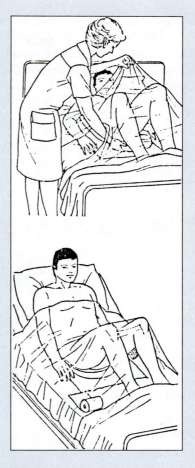

FIGURE 13.13 ■

24. Return to the client. Offer the client the opportunity to wash his hands in the basin of water.

25. Make the client comfortable.

26. Put on gloves and note the excreta (feces or urine) for amount, odor, and color.

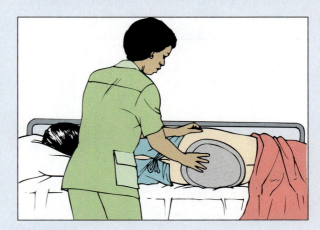

FIGURE 13.14 ■

continued

27. If a specimen or sample is required, collect it at this time. Measure the urine, if necessary.

28. Empty the bedpan into the client's toilet.

29. Clean the bedpan and put it in the proper place. Cold water is always used to clean the bedpan. You may also use a toilet brush, if available.

30. Remove gloves and wash your hands.

31. Make a notation on the client's chart that the client has used the bedpan. Also note anything you have observed about the client during this procedure.

> **SAMPLE CHARTING:**   12/14/04   6:00 A.M.
> Small amount of yellow urine. Large dark-brown bowel movement. No skin irritation noted.
> Lisa Gutierrez H/HHA

PROCEDURE 35

Offering the Urinal

> **RATIONALE:** Carefully and skillfully placing the urinal prevents discomfort and increases the client's comfort with needing assistance for this intimate task.

1. Assemble your equipment:
   Urinal and cover
   Basin of water or wet washcloth
   Soap
   Towels
   Disposable gloves

2. Wash your hands.

3. Ask visitors to leave the room, if appropriate. You may, however, wish to demonstrate this procedure to family members.

4. Ask the client if he wishes to use the urinal. Put on gloves.

5. Give the client the urinal. If the client is unable to put the urinal in place, put his penis into the opening as far as it goes (Figure 13.15 ■). If the client cannot hold it in place, you will do so. Raise the head of the bed if the client prefers, if possible.

6. Ask the client to signal when he is finished.

7. Leave the room to give the client privacy. Remove gloves and wash your hands.

8. When the client signals, return to the room. Wash your hands and put on gloves.

9. Take the urinal. Be careful not to spill it. Cover it and take it to the client's bathroom. Remove gloves and wash your hands.

10. Return to the client. Put on gloves. Help him wash his hands in the basin of water or with a wet washcloth. Remove gloves and wash your hands.

11. Make the client comfortable.

12. Put on gloves. Check the urine for color, odor, and amount.

13. Measure the urine, if necessary. Collect a specimen or sample at this time, if necessary.

14. Empty the urinal into the toilet. Rinse the urinal with cold water.

15. Clean it as is your agency policy and return it to the proper place.

16. Remove gloves and wash your hands.

17. Make a notation on the client's chart that he has used the urinal. Also note anything you have observed about the client during this procedure.

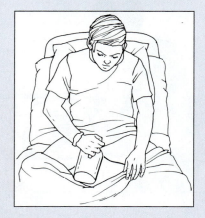

FIGURE 13.15 ■

> **SAMPLE CHARTING:**   7/19/04   7:00 P.M.
> Voided large amount of yellow urine. No problems noted.
> Pamela Susowitz H/HHA

PROCEDURE 36

Assisting the Client with a Portable Commode

RATIONALE: Using a commode in a safe and private manner is more comfortable and familiar than using a bedpan or urinal.

1. Assemble your equipment:
   Portable bedside commode
   Toilet tissue
   Basin of water or wet washcloth
   Soap
   Towel and gloves

2. Wash your hands.

3. Ask visitors to leave the room, if appropriate. However, you may want to demonstrate the procedure to family members.

4. Tell the client you are going to assist him onto the commode (Figure 13.16 ■). Put on gloves.

5. Put the commode next to the client's bed in a position to which he can safely transfer.

6. Using proper body mechanics and transfer techniques, assist the client onto the commode.

7. If you do not have to collect a specimen, leave a small amount of water in the bottom of the pail. This will make cleaning it easier.

8. If the client is safe, leave the room to give him privacy.

9. Remove gloves and wash your hands if you are going to do another task.

10. When the client signals you that he is finished, return and wash your hands. Put on gloves.

11. Offer the client toilet tissue to clean himself. If he is unable to do so, it is your responsibility to clean him. After doing so, remove gloves and wash your hands.

12. Assist the client back to his bed.

13. Offer the client the basin of water or wet washcloth to wash his hands.

14. Make the client comfortable. Put on gloves.

15. Remove the pail from the commode. Cover it and carry it to the bathroom.

16. Check the excreta (feces or urine) for color, amount, and odor.

17. Measure output if that is ordered. If a specimen or sample is required, collect it at this time.

18. Empty the pail into the toilet and clean it according to your agency policy.

19. Put the pail back into the commode.

20. Remove gloves and wash your hands.

21. Make a notation on the client's chart that he has used the commode. Also note anything that you observed about the client during this procedure.

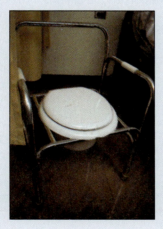

FIGURE 13.16 ■

SAMPLE CHARTING: 9/30/05   11:00 P.M.
Patient transferred to commode. Large amount of brown, formed stool and small amount of urine eliminated. Client transferred to chair to watch television.
Sonja Antonio H/HHA

SECTION 8

Perineal Care

OBJECTIVES

What You Will Learn to Do

1. List reasons why you will be asked to give a client peri-care.

2. Demonstrate the correct procedure for giving peri-care.

Introduction: Care of the Perineal Area

perineal care
cleansing of the perineal area; peri-care

perineum
area between the anus and the external genital organs

Perineal care or peri-care is the gentle cleansing of the perineal area or **perineum.** This may be necessary following the birth of a child, following surgery, or when a female client does not take a full bath but wishes to clean the genital area. This procedure promotes healing, helps prevent infection, and refreshes the client. The use of a squeeze bottle—or peribottle—is encouraged, rather than cleansing the area with a washcloth. The bottle directs a stream of water so that it removes waste or drainage without damaging the skin. The use of the bottle also enables clients to clean themselves even if they cannot reach the area with their hands.

PROCEDURE 37

Care of the Perineal Area

RATIONALE: Keeping the perineum clean and free of discharge and bacteria is an important part of personal care and contributes to general health and well-being.

1. Assemble your equipment:
   2 peribottles or squeeze bottles
   Mild soap
   Clean dressings or peripads and undergarments
   Towels and gloves
   Garbage bag for soiled dressings
   Warm water

2. Wash your hands.

3. Ask visitors to leave the room, if appropriate.

4. Tell the client what you are going to do and what you expect. Put on gloves.

5. Remove old peripads or dressings and discard in a paper or plastic bag. Note the drainage, color, amount, and odor.

6. Assist client onto commode, toilet, or bedpan.

7. Fill one bottle with warm, soapy water and the other with warm, clean water.

8. Place the bottle filled with soapy water parallel to the perineum. Let the water drain over the perineum. Move the bottle so that the whole

perineal area is cleansed. Do this for at least 2 minutes. You may have to refill the bottle.

9. Rinse the perineum with plain warm water.

10. Assist the client to stand up or to move off the bedpan.

11. Pat the area dry.

12. Assist the client with clean dressings and undergarments. Make the client comfortable.

13. Clean the equipment and commode.

14. Remove gloves and wash your hands.

15. Make a notation on the client's chart that you have completed this procedure. Also note anything you observed about the client during this procedure.

SAMPLE CHARTING: 8/28/04   10:00 A.M. Perineal care given. A dime-sized red area noted inside of left thigh. Skin moisturizer applied. Daughter-in-law alerted. Client positioned so that area is open to the air and not touching other leg. Jacqueline Dupris H/HHA

SECTION 9

Postpartum Care

OBJECTIVES

What You Will Learn to Do

1. Recognize the first physical changes that occur after childbirth.

2. Discuss emotional changes experienced by women after childbirth.

3. List the changes that would require medical attention.

4. Discuss changes families experience after the birth of a child.

Introduction: The Postpartum Period

The first several weeks after childbirth are considered the postpartum period. This is the time when a woman is getting used to being a mother for the first time or getting used to this baby. She is bonding with the child and getting acquainted with it. Her body is changing rapidly. Women also experience emotional changes as their role changes, as their hormones change, and as their bodies return to their prepregnancy state.

Families react to the addition of a new child in many ways. Families have cultural practices that dictate how they react to the new mother. Some families react differently when the child is a girl or when the child is a boy. Some families lavish gifts and attention on the child. Some lavish gifts and attention on the mother. Some do neither.

CHANGES FOR FAMILY MEMBERS

Changes affect all members of the family. Husbands or significant others either become fathers for the first time or learn to balance emotions for one more child. Sometimes, the new responsibility is assumed with ease. Sometimes, the man becomes frightened and does not know how to respond. It takes time to learn the role of father. Be patient. Refer to role models the man may have had as he grew up. He will be able to identify those behaviors he liked as a child and those he did not. Thinking about those things will help him pattern his behavior to support his child.

Learning to relate to a woman who has become a mother also takes time. Encourage the new mother and father to talk about their needs and feelings with each other. If they need professional assistance, contact your supervisor for a referral.

Children adjust to a new sibling, too. The presence of a new brother or sister can affect each child differently. Respect each child's way of adjusting to the new family member. If you have any questions about the meaning of behaviors, discuss it with your supervisor. Remember, children are all individuals. Do not compare one child with another.

- Some children assume extra responsibility.
- Some children return to childish behaviors such as baby talk, thumb sucking, or even bedwetting.
- Some children may refuse to go to school, leave their house, or leave their parents.
- Some children ignore the new baby.
- Some children are anxious to take part in the care of the new baby.

EMOTIONAL CHANGES FOR THE NEW MOTHER

It is difficult to predict how a woman will react to a new baby. Each woman is different, and each birth experience is different. Usually, however, there are several shared experiences. When emotional concerns prevent the woman from taking part in care of the new baby or from having any interest in her family, report this to your supervisor so that a complete assessment can be made and a plan of care formulated that will help the woman through this difficult time.

- Women usually experience some mood swings. This occurs as a result of the hormonal changes and the fact that the woman is assessing her new role and planning how to adjust. Some women are weepy. Some are euphoric and have a great deal of energy.

■ Women may want friends around or they may want to be alone. Be sensitive to the wish of your client. If she wants to be alone, gently tell friends and family that perhaps they should call before coming to visit or they should come and stay for short periods of time. Designating a time to visit is helpful so that the client and the visitor know the time frame set for the visit.

■ Getting used to a body that is continuously changing is difficult for some women. It takes about 6 weeks until the internal organs return to prenatal status. It may take 6 months for the woman to lose weight and regain her prenatal appearance. Support her as she tries to exercise, change diet, and become familiar with her changing needs. Encourage her to discuss exercise regimes with her physician before any new activity is started.

PHYSICAL CHANGES

During the first 6 weeks after birth, a woman's body is continuously changing. During the first 2 to 3 days, a reddish, bloody discharge from the vagina is to be expected. This is called lochia. About the fourth day, this discharge changes to yellowish and continues for another week. Usually, all discharge stops about the twenty-first day. The discharge is normal, and the woman should wear whatever peripads she wishes. It is usually recommended that they be deodorant-free. Tampons are not worn. Dispose of the used pads as you would any dressing in a paper or plastic bag. The perineum should be cleaned and washed with warm soapy water after each bowel movement and voiding. The peripads should be changed at that time, too.

Usually, the woman loses the fluid she accumulates during pregnancy between the second and fifth day postpartum. Encourage her to continue to drink fluids throughout this period as water and fruit juices will help with the process and prevent dehydration.

It is important that bowel function be regular during this time. Because the perineal area may be sore, bowel movements may be uncomfortable. If this is the case, encourage your client to discuss this with her physician so that stool softeners can be prescribed. A diet that has sufficient fiber and fluid usually prevents most discomfort. If you have concerns that regular bowel function is not occurring, discuss this with your supervisor.

Diet

During this period, a balanced diet is important. It helps with maintaining a feeling of well-being, regulating bowel and bladder function, and helping the body return to prenatal status. A woman who is nursing requires additional calories and fluids. During the postpartum period, a woman should be encouraged to eat regularly and enjoy her food. This is not the time to start crash diets or decrease fluids in an attempt to lose weight.

Contraception

Sexual relations following the birth of a child are a deeply personal activity. Sometimes, a change occurs in the pattern of sexual activity. This change will be discussed between the client and her partner. Often, if questions or concerns remain, she should be encouraged to discuss these with her physician.

Remind your client that pregnancy can occur shortly after the birth of a child. Pregnancy can occur while a women is nursing a child. Pregnancy can also occur before normal menstrual periods have resumed. Contraception or abstinence is recommended if another pregnacy is to be avoided.

Breast Care

The decision to breast-feed a baby is a personal one. If your client has made a decision different from the one you would have made, respect her decision and support her. Sometimes, even when a woman decides not to breast-feed, her breasts fill with milk. Encourage her to call her physician if this happens. Breasts should always be supported with a good bra until they return to prenatal size. They should be kept clean at all times.

Your Role as a Homemaker/Home Health Aide

You will be asked to support the client during this time of change. The way in which you respond to her emotional needs and her physical changes will signal to the client and her family whether her actions are normal and acceptable. Every family reacts to childbirth differently. You will be asked to reinforce the family's culture and their customs in dealing with the new baby and the new mother. If you do not understand some of the actions, ask your supervisor to explain them. If you believe some actions are unsafe or are contrary to your assignment, discuss them with your supervisor immediately. You may suggest a change in routine or an action that in your experience has worked. Do not be offended if the family chooses not to adopt your suggestions. There are often many ways to accomplish the same goal, and each family must set up a system that is comfortable for them when you leave.

GUIDELINES

Postpartum Care

Document the normal activities of the household including:

- activity level
- client sleep patterns
- emotional status
- diet and fluid intake
- lochia: amount, color, odor
- bowel and bladder function
- family dynamics

Call your supervisor if:

- The client experiences temperature and/or chills.
- There is any discomfort, pain, or discoloration of limbs or abdomen.
- There is any difficulty breathing or speaking, or general anxiety.
- The lochia is excessive and/or foul-smelling.
- The client has difficulty urinating or voiding is painful.
- There is a sudden change in the client.

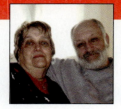

Case Study

Review the case study that appears on the first page of the chapter. Answer two sets of questions about the case study contained in the Explore and Apply sections below.

EXPLORE

1. You have been sent to Mr. Ricci's home to assist with his bath. The plan is for you to visit twice a week. Discuss the questions you will ask your supervisor before you visit. Discuss the way in which you will introduce yourself to the client and how you will complete your assignment.

2. What will you do if Mr. Ricci refuses your assistance?

APPLY

1. Discuss the proper order for offering complete care to a client who is bedbound.

2. What would you do if you did not have the following equipment to give personal care?
   - a basin
   - a bath blanket
   - hot water
   - clean sheets
   - soap

Certification Exam Review Questions

Choose the best answer for each question or statement.

1. **Giving a client oral hygiene**

   a. *is done once in the morning.*

   b. *may be done several times a day depending on the client's need.*

   c. *is the responsibility of the family and not the homemaker/home health aide.*

   d. *is always done in the bathroom.*

2. **Many clients dress in layers that are difficult to take off when they must use the bathroom or commode. You would**

   a. *dress the client in clean clothes that are easy to maintain.*

   b. *take all the dirty clothes and hide them.*

   c. *discuss with the client the problem and come to an understanding.*

   d. *call the client's daughter and tell her to bring more clothes.*

3. **Bathing a client is important because it**

   a. *provides time to talk to the client privately, allows you to observe the client's skin and body movement, and feels good to the client.*

   b. *is always on the list of things to do when you receive your assignment.*

   c. *is a state law that all clients must be bathed each day.*

   d. *is the one activity the families of clients dislike doing.*

4. **Shaving a male client is**

   a. *always done with the shaving implement the client likes best.*

   b. *usually left for a male family member to do.*

   c. *always done with a safety razor or an electric razor.*

   d. *always done after a bath.*

5. **Perineal care is**

   a. *done because the area is dark and moist and can easily breed bacteria.*

   b. *never the responsibility of the family.*

   c. *never the responsibility of the client.*

   d. *an activity the family is not permitted to do.*

CHAPTER 14

Rehabilitation of the Client

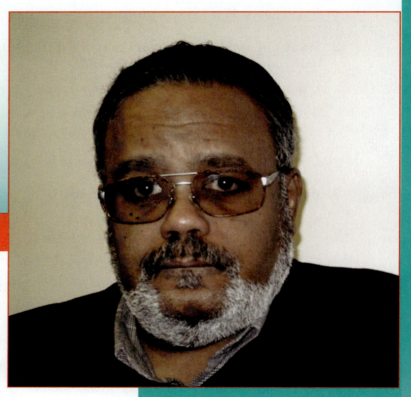

CASE STUDY

Mr. Robinson lives in a small basement apartment. He has lived all his life in this neighborhood and knows all the nearby families. Although he has never married and has no family of his own, he is included in many of his neighbors' activities. Prior to his retirement, Mr. Robinson worked as a railroad conductor. He now goes for walks and spends time in the playground watching the children. Recently, he fell in the street and broke his wrist. It is still in a splint. Mr. Robinson usually remembers his physical therapy appointments, but he lately missed two, stating that he forgot them. The physical therapist has given Mr. Robinson daily exercises, but he admits he does not do them regularly. The neighbors are concerned; they think Mr. Robinson has not been as visible as usual, and when they do see him he does not look as neat and clean as he has in the past. They are also sure he has lost weight.

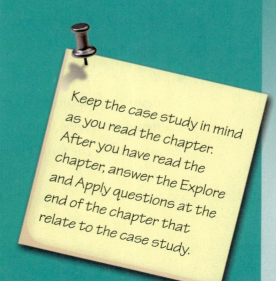

Keep the case study in mind as you read the chapter. After you have read the chapter, answer the Explore and Apply questions at the end of the chapter that relate to the case study.

Introduction to Rehabilitation

OBJECTIVES
What You Will Learn to Do

1. Define rehabilitation.
2. Discuss the many issues therapists consider when they establish a program for your client.

Introduction: What Is Rehabilitation?

Rehabilitation is the process of relearning how to function, in the best possible way, as an independent person despite a disability. Rehabilitation is not easy and not always pleasant but, with proper direction and encouragement, the client can accomplish his goals. Sometimes, a client will use a brace or support for an injured body part. Be sure you completely understand the care and use of this piece of equipment. The way in which you assist the client will communicate to him if you really believe he will succeed or if you believe his attempts are useless. Be alert to your verbal and nonverbal communications.

rehabilitation
process by which people who have been disabled by injury or sickness are helped to recover as many as possible of their original abilities and live with the remaining disabilities

ESTABLISHING A REHABILITATION ROUTINE

Before a therapist establishes a routine for the client, she reviews the whole client profile, including his environment. Your objective reporting during this assessment will help establish a useful individualized program for your client. Factors considered during this assessment include:

- How much active motion does the client have?
- How much passive motion does the client have?
- Symptoms of all medical diagnoses that may affect function.
- Sensory deficits in vision, hearing, speech, touch, balance, or proprioception (knowledge of limb position in space with eyes covered).
- How does the client see his situation? his disability?
- *Attitude.* Is he depressed, euphoric, angry, cooperative, resentful, or frustrated? Is he motivated: Does he want to try to do things for himself?
- *Ability.* What can he do for himself? What does he attempt to do?
- *Previous level of function.* Which limb is **dominant** (used for most activities)? What did he do before he became disabled? If a person did not want to do something before an illness, he may not be motivated to do it afterward.
- *Priorities.* A **priority** is something the client wants to do. Often, the priority might not seem important, but achieving it makes the client feel less handicapped. It could be a little thing like putting on makeup, setting hair, shaving, tying shoes, using the telephone, or signing checks.
- *Equipment.* What is the client using now, and what does he need to help him function (hospital bed, commode, crutches, catheter, walker, cane, brace, splints, or adaptive equipment such as built-up spoons or dressing sticks)?
- *Environmental barrier.* Objects and structures in the client's home that make it difficult for him to care for himself: a second-floor bathroom when a client cannot climb stairs, throw rugs that can trip him, narrow doorways that prevent him from moving from room to room in a wheelchair, heavy furniture that he cannot pass in a walker or with crutches or a cane, or a bed without side rails to help him sit up.

dominant
stronger half of a pair

priority
giving one thing more importance than another

■ *Support system.* The people involved in the care of a client. Besides the homemaker/home health aide, will family members or friends help him regain functional independence?

Working with a Physical Therapist

OBJECTIVES	
What You Will Learn to Do	1. Explain the principles of range-of-motion exercise.
	2. Demonstrate the proper techniques for complete or partial range-of-motion with a client.
	3. Lift, hold, or transfer a client using good body mechanics.
	4. Demonstrate several types of client transfers.
	5. Discuss the proper type of chair for client use.
	6. Demonstrate various ways of assisting your client with ambulation.

Introduction: Muscles, Joints, Movement

Joints are where two or more bones meet to form a movable area of the skeletal frame. Muscles move the bones. Unused muscles can shorten and tighten. This makes the joint motion painful and limited. Muscle shortening can happen in a short time. Therefore, it is important that clients are helped to use their muscles by encouraging them to do normal daily activities and their prescribed exercises (Figure 14.1 ■).

You may be instructed by your supervisor to place your hands in a position different from that indicated in the photo. This is acceptable, provided the patient's head is supported and the rules of safety and good body mechanics are observed (Figure 14.2 ■).

RANGE-OF-MOTION EXERCISES

range-of-motion (ROM) exercises

exercises that take a body part through its entire ability of motion

There are four types of **range-of-motion (ROM)** exercises. Each is ordered for a specific purpose.

Type	Client	Helper
Passive		Takes client through ROM Client does not help
Active/assist	Active motion	Helps make motion easier; moves part farther than client can
Active	Done totally by client	
Resistive	Active motion	Makes exercise harder by providing resistance to motion but allows completion of motion

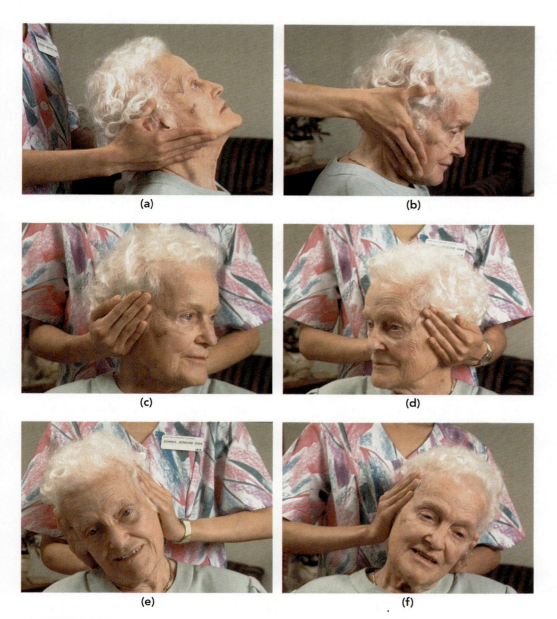

(a)

(b)

(c)

(d)

(e)

(f)

FIGURE 14.1 ■ Assist clients with proper exercises to keep muscles flexible.

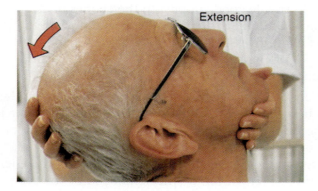

Extension

FIGURE 14.2 ■ Depending on the client's condition and comfort, alternate hand positions may be used.

GUIDELINES

Assisting with ROM

- Do not start ROM exercises until you have received specific instructions for your particular client.
- Never take a client beyond the point of pain. Pain is a warning sign and should be heeded. Report client pain to your supervisor.
- Report to the supervisor if the client does not do the exercises when you are not in the house.
- Report to the supervisor if the client is finding the exercises harder to do rather than easier.
- Use the flat part of your hand and fingers to hold the client's body parts. Do not grip with your fingertips. Some people are sensitive to pressure. Some people are ticklish.
- If you forget what to do, think of your own body and how it works.
- Talk to the client. Explain what is being done and why. Even if the person does not appear to understand, the tone of your voice and touch of your hands can help you communicate.
- Better communication greatly improves your chances for client cooperation.
- Do each exercise three to five times or as you have been instructed.
- Follow a logical sequence during the exercises so that each joint and muscle is exercised. For example, start at the head and work down to the feet.
- Be gentle—never bend or straighten a body part farther than it will go.
- Slow, steady movement of a tight muscle will help the muscle relax and so increase the joint range.
- Include the family or caregivers in the activity so they can learn and continue the exercises when you are not there.

Choosing a Chair for a Client

A client usually spends all or at least part of the day out of bed. But where is "out of bed"? Sometimes a client will sit in a wheelchair, a favorite reclining chair, the sofa, or a kitchen chair. Which is best? Here are several guidelines to follow when choosing a chair:

- The chair should provide good support to the client's back.
- A reclining chair is difficult to get out of, especially when the client is tired.
- The best type of chair gives the client the most independence.
- Consider the types of chairs available.
- Use the safest chairs.

A dining room chair or straight-back chair provides a great deal of support. One with arms is best, if it is available. The client should be able to sit with his feet resting on the floor or to place his feet on the floor comfortably without straining. Otherwise, he will not be able to rise safely.

A wheelchair can provide good support while allowing the client freedom to move around the house. However, a wheelchair is not for every client. If you think a wheelchair might be useful to your client, discuss this with the therapist or your supervisor before you suggest it to the client.

PROCEDURE 38

Range-of-Motion

RATIONALE: Correct movement of joint and muscles assists the client to remain independent, contracture free, and mobile. It also contributes to increased strength and sense of well-being.

1. Wash your hands.

2. Explain to the client that you are going to help him exercise his muscles and joints.

3. Ask visitors to leave, if appropriate.

4. Offer the client the bedpan or urinal.

5. Drape the client for modesty.

6. Raise the bed to the highest horizontal position, if possible.

7. Lower the side rail on the side you are working, if possible. Move the client close to you.

8. Proceed with the exercises as you have been instructed (Figure 14.3 ■).

9. Make the client comfortable.

10. Wash your hands.

11. Chart that you have completed the exercises. Also note anything you observed about the client during the procedure.

SAMPLE CHARTING: 12/13/04   11:00 A.M. Passive range of motion to neck and hips. Some discomfort noted in left hip with adduction. Reported to supervisor via telephone at 11:30 A.M. She will visit this afternoon. Client remains in bed awaiting lunch. Karen Caspernot H/HHA

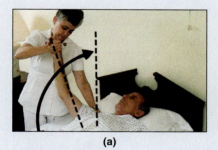

(a)

Shoulder flexion
With elbow straight, raise arm over head, then lower, keeping arm in front of you the whole time.

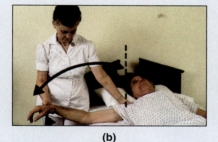

(b)

Shoulder abduction and adduction
With elbow straight, raise arm over head, then lower, keeping arm out to the side the whole time.

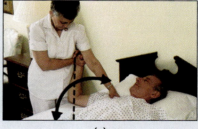

(c)

Shoulder internal and external rotation
Bring arm out to the side. Do NOT bring elbow out to shoulder level. Turn arm back and forth so forearm points down toward feet, then up toward head. With arm alongside body and elbow bent at 90° angle, turn arm so forearm points across stomach, then out to the side.

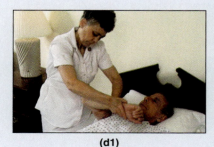

(d1)

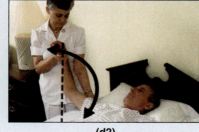

(d2)

Shoulder horizontal abduction and adduction
Keeping arm at shoulder level, reach across chest past opposite shoulder, then reach out to the side.

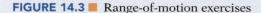

(e)

Elbow flexion and extension
With arm alongside body, bend elbow to touch shoulder, then straighten elbow out again.

FIGURE 14.3 ■ Range-of-motion exercises

continued

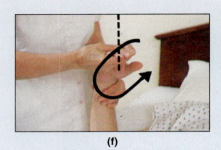

(f)

Forearm pronation and supination
With arm alongside the body and elbow bent to 90° (a right angle), turn forearm so palm faces first toward head, then toward feet.

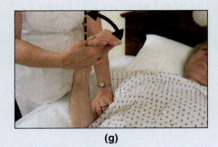

(g)

Wrist flexion and extension
Bend wrist up and down.

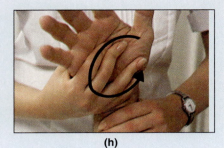

(h)

Wrist flexion and extension
Bend wrist back and forth and in a circle.

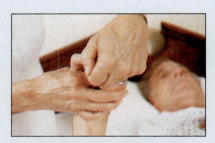

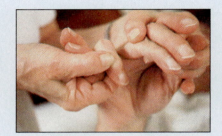

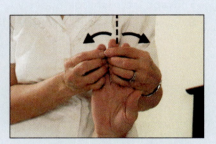

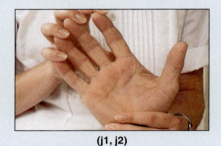

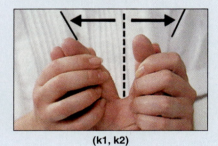

(i1, i2)

Finger flexion and extension
Make a fist, then straighten fingers out together.

(j1, j2)

Finger flexion and extension
Touch tip of each finger to its base, then straighten each finger in turn.

(k1, k2)

Finger adduction and abduction
With fingers straight, squeeze fingers together, then spread them apart.

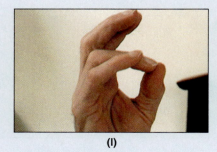

(l)

Finger/thumb opposition
Touch thumb to the tip of each finger to make a circle. Open hand fully between touching each finger.

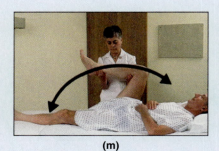

(m)

Hip/knee flexion and extension
Bend knee and bring it up toward chest, keeping foot off bed. Lower leg to bed, straightening knee as it goes down.

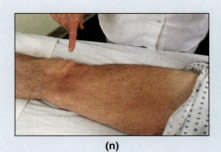

(n)

Quad sets
With leg flat on bed, tighten thigh muscles to straighten the knee, *hard,* pushing it into the bed. Hold for count of five, then relax. Repeat exercise with rolled towel under the knee.

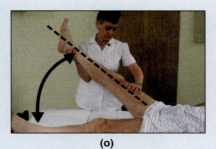

(o)

Straight leg raising
Keeping the knee straight, raise leg up off the bed. Return slowly to the bed, keeping the knee straight.

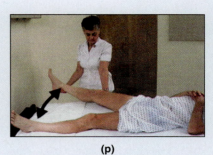

(p)

Hip abduction and adduction
With leg flat on bed and knee pointing to the ceiling, slide leg out to the side. Then slide it back to touch the other leg.

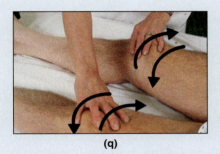

(q)

Hip internal and external rotation
With legs flat on bed and feet apart, turn both legs so knees face outward. Then turn them in so knees face each other.

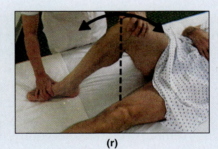

(r)

Hip internal and external rotation (variation) With one knee bent and foot flat on the bed, turn leg so knee moves out to the side, then inward across the other leg. Do each leg separately.

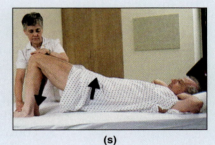

(s)

Bridging
With both knees bent up, feet flat on bed, push on bed with feet to raise hips (as in lifting for a bedpan). Hold for count of five, then relax.

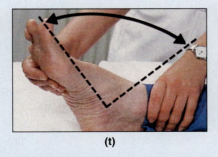

(t)

Ankle dorsiflexion and extension
Bend ankles up, down, and side to side.

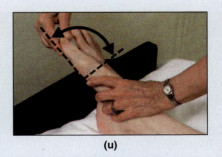

(u)

Toe flexion and extension
Bend and straighten toes.

FIGURE 14.3 ■ Range-of-motion exercises (continued)

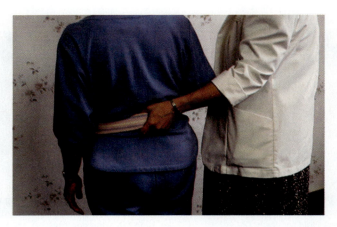

FIGURE 14.4 ■ Assisting a client wearing a guarding belt.

If using a wheelchair, always have the brakes locked when standing the client up or sitting him down. Never leave a confused client restrained in a wheelchair with his feet on the foot pedals. The client may think his feet are on the floor and try to stand up.

Transferring Clients from Place to Place

To transfer a client means to help him move from one place to another (for example, from his bed to a chair and back again). How well the transfer goes depends on how much confidence your client has in you. *Know yourself. Know your capabilities. Always stay within your capabilities.* If you feel confident, your client will sense this and have confidence in you, too.

When a person loses the use of a body part, it becomes important to him to control what remains. Use this to your advantage. Observe the client's abilities and do not help him more than necessary. A **guarding belt** (any leather belt buckled around the midsection) can help you with a large client and give you better control over his center of gravity (Figure 14.4 ■).

Before a person can move from bed to another place, he or she must come to a sitting position with legs over the side of the bed. You can help a client by raising the head of the bed, if possible. This gives him extra assistance. Raise the bed to a high horizontal position so the client is almost standing when he slides off the bed. Be sure the bed is locked and anchored against a wall so it does not move.

guarding belt
device placed around the waist, used to assist a client during ambulation

---

PROCEDURE 39

Helping a Client to Sit Up

RATIONALE: Clients who are too weak to adjust their position themselves require assistance. Good body alignment promotes a sense of well-being and prevents fatigue and injury.

1. Wash your hands.
2. Ask any visitor to step out of the room, if appropriate.

3. Tell the client what you are going to do.
4. Roll the client on his side, facing you. Bend his knees.
5. Reach one arm over to hold him in back of his knees.
6. Place your other arm under the neck and shoulder area (Figure 14.5a ■).

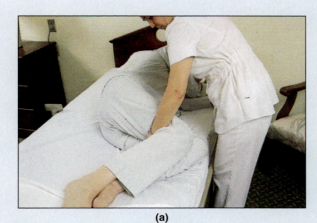

(a)

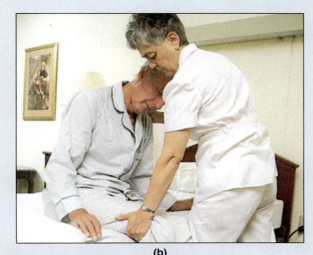

(b)

FIGURE 14.5 ■

7. Position your feet with a wide base of support and your center of gravity close to the bed.

8. On the count of "one, two, three," shift your weight to your back leg. While you are doing this, swing the client's legs over the edge of the bed while pulling his shoulders to a sitting position (Figure 14.5b ■).

9. Remain in front of the client with both your hands on him for support. Do not leave him until you are sure he is stable.

10. Proceed with the remainder of the transfer. (For a client who requires only a little assistance, the procedure remains the same. Direct the client through the steps above and support him when necessary. Be sure to remain with him in the sitting position until he is stable.)

SAMPLE CHARTING:	7/15/04 12:45 A.M. Helped client to sitting position. No complaints noted. Remained in this position for 10 minutes while I combed her hair. Left in bed with side rails up. Barbara Schuster H/HHA

TAKING CARE OF BUSINESS

Taking care of business (TCOB) is necessary as you are moving, transferring, and directing clients. Concentrate on what you are doing and be aware of what is going on around you. Dizzy spells, sudden weakness, or loud noises can cause lapses in concentration that could cause a client to fall or lose his balance. If you are TCOB, you will usually be able to prevent serious injury to the client and yourself.

Using a Mechanical Lift

Some clients are too weak or too heavy to be transferred by another person. Such cases require a **mechanical lift**. Practice using the model you have available. Some of them differ slightly, but the principles of operation are the same (Figure 14.6 ■).

mechanical lift
machine used to lift a client from one place to another

Helping a Client to Stand and Sit

The procedure to help a client stand up can be used with clients who need a great deal of assistance and with those who need little. By using the same sequence of actions each time, you teach the person how to stand up by himself.

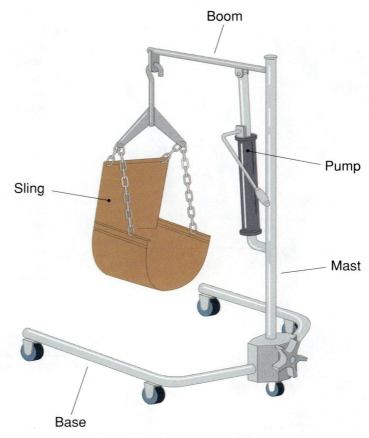

Boom

Sling

Pump

Mast

Base

FIGURE 14.6 ■ A mechanical lift.

PROCEDURE 40

Using a Portable Mechanical Client Lift

RATIONALE: Some clients may require mechanical assistance to leave bed. Having this assistance available ensures that all clients, regardless of size or condition, can be maintained in good body alignment and moved safely from place to place when needed.

1. Assemble your equipment:
   Mechanical lift
   Sling

2. Wash your hands.

3. Tell the client that you are going to help him out of bed using the portable mechanical client lift. (You may need the help of a second person as a partner.)

4. Position the chair next to the bed with the back of the chair in line with the headboard of the bed.

5. Cover the chair with a blanket or sheet.

6. Turn the client from side to side on the bed as you slide the sling under him.

7. Attach the sling to the mechanical lift with the hooks in place through the metal frame facing out.

8. Have the client fold both arms across his chest, if possible.

9. Using the crank, lift the client from the bed.

10. Guide the client's legs.

11. Lower the client into the chair.

12. Remove the hooks from the frame of the portable mechanical lift.

13. Leave the client safe and comfortable in the chair for the proper amount of time according to your instructions.

14. To return the client to bed, put the hooks facing out through the metal frame of the sling, which is still under the client.

15. Raise the client by using the crank on the mechanical client lift. Lift him from the chair into the bed. Have your partner guide the client's legs.

16. Lower the client into the center of the bed.

17. Remove the hooks from the frame.

18. Remove the sling from under the client by having him turn from side to side on the bed.

19. Put a pillow under the client's head. Properly position the client.

20. Remake the top of the bed.

21. Raise the side rails to the up position.

22. Lower the bed to its lowest horizontal position.

23. Wash your hands.

24. Chart your observations about the client during this procedure.

SAMPLE CHARTING:	4/7/05 12:12 P.M.
	Client moved to new bed via mechanical lift with H/HHA and husband in attendance. Tolerated the procedure well. Left in new bed on her back in proper body alignment supported by two pillows on either side.
	Lynne Piper H/HHA

PROCEDURE 41

Helping a Client to Stand

RATIONALE: Some clients require assistance to stand up and find their balance. Providing this assistance contributes to their independence and sense of well-being.

1. "Move to the front of your chair or bed. Put your hands on the arms of the chair." This client is sitting over the edge of the chair or bed. Place one of your knees between his knees. Your feet should be in good position and you should be close to the chair or bed. If the client has a weak knee, brace it with your knee (Figure 14.7a ■).

2. "Put one foot in under you." This should be the strongest leg. Bend your knees and lean onto your forward foot to place the same side arm around the client's waist and place your other hand at the other side of the client's waist. You have now encircled the client and are holding him at his center of gravity.

3. "On the count of three, push down with your arms, lean forward, stand up." Remember to count to three. It allows you both to know when to start the motion and work as a team. Hold the client closely. The more assistance needed, the closer you hold the client. On the count of three, rock your weight to your back foot (Figure 14.7b ■).

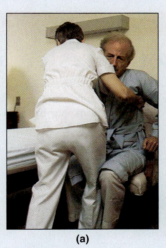 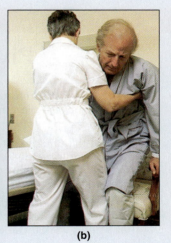

(a)   (b)

FIGURE 14.7 ■

SAMPLE CHARTING:	7/19/04 2:00 P.M.
	Assisted client to his feet. Using a walker, he walked on the patio and saw his beloved flowers. Tomorrow he says he will walk twice around the patio.
	Rosario Stone H/HHA

Help him only when necessary, but remain in good position to guard him as he stands. You may choose to use a gait belt or transfer belt for additional support.

Keep your directions short. Memorize the following sequence. Then you need not stop and remember what to say to clients each time you help them. You should be able to concentrate on how the client is following your directions, not on trying to remember them yourself.

PROCEDURE 42

Helping a Client to Sit

RATIONALE: Some clients require assistance to sit down safely. Providing this assistance contributes to their independence and sense of well-being.

Your body mechanics and positioning are the same as in helping the client to stand. Just reverse the directions.

1. Be sure that the wheels on the bed or chair are locked.
2. Remind the client to feel the bed or chair with the back of his legs.
3. Direct the client to reach back for the arms of the chair or the bed.

4. You support and direct the activity as he sits down.

SAMPLE CHARTING: 8/15/05   5:00 P.M.
Assisted client to sit down in his favorite chair near the window, where he will remain for about an hour until his wife returns home. Phone and water left near him on the table. Walker within reach.
James Monahan H/HHA

PROCEDURE 43

Pivot Transfer from Bed to Chair

RATIONALE: Pivot transfer provides a safe manner in which to move a client from one place to another.

1. Prepare the equipment. Place the wheelchair at a 45° angle to the bed. Place the chair so that the client will move toward his stronger side.
2. If you are transferring the client to a wheelchair, lock the wheels of the chair. If the bed has wheels, lock these wheels, too.
3. Wash your hands.

4. Tell the client what you are going to do.
5. Bring the client to a sitting position with his legs over the edge of the bed (Figure 14.8a ■).
6. Place slippers or shoes on his feet.
7. Explain the procedure to the client:
   a. He will come to a standing position.
   b. He will then reach for the arm of the chair, pivot, and sit (Figure 14.8b ■).
   c. You will remain in good support position and guide him.

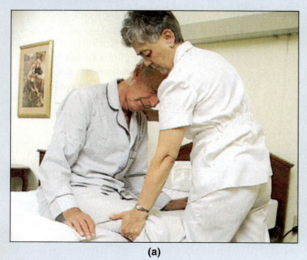 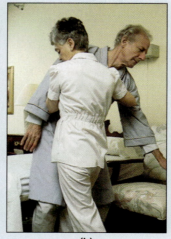 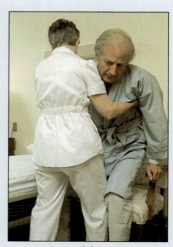

(a)   (b)   (c)

FIGURE 14.8 ■

d. You will keep your foot near the client's foot for extra support (Figure 14.8c ■).

e. You will use good body mechanics to support him and prevent injury to yourself.

8. When you are sure that the client understands the procedure, perform the transfer.

9. Secure the client in the chair. Make him comfortable. Leave him in a safe place.

10. Wash your hands.

11. Chart any observations you may have made during this procedure.

> **SAMPLE CHARTING:**   5/7/04   2:00 P.M.
> Client transferred to wheelchair and back to bed an hour later without incident. Remains unable to put weight on left leg.
> Selma Walker H/HHA

PROCEDURE 44

Transfer from Chair to Bed

> **RATIONALE:** Pivot transfer provides a safe manner in which to move a client from one place to another.

Your body mechanics and positioning are the same as in helping the client into the chair. Just reverse the directions.

1. Wash your hands.

2. Prepare the bed.

3. Place the chair at a 45° angle to the bed so the client moves toward his stronger side.

4. If you are transferring the client from a wheelchair, lock the wheels of the chair. If the bed has wheels, lock these, too.

5. Stand in a good position using a firm base of support and proper body mechanics.

6. Direct the client to come to a standing position.

7. Direct the client to reach for the bed and pivot. Help and guide him.

8. Make the client comfortable. Reposition the side rails.

9. Wash your hands.

10. Chart any observations you may have made during this procedure.

> **SAMPLE CHARTING:**   7/13/05   7:30 P.M.
> Transferred client from chair to his bed following dinner. Remains unable to put weight on right leg. Client left in bed watching television. His daughter-in-law will get him ready for bed in about 2 hours.
> Kate McGuire H/HHA

MINIMAL ASSISTANCE

As the client gains strength and confidence, he will require less assistance. You will use the same basic body positioning but will not hold him. You may remain with him for directions and in case you are needed. When minimal assistance is needed, it is best to stand on the weaker side of the client and support him with a guarding belt. This way, as the client is changing position, you will be available if he falls or loses balance.

Ambulation Activities

Ambulation refers to the action of walking. If the client requires a special gait or must learn a new way to walk, the physical therapist will set up a plan for the client and you to follow. However, the same basic assisting positions can be used for clients with all types of gaits.

ambulate
to walk

■ Use the proper procedure for the client to come to a standing position.

■ Use a guarding belt for extra support.

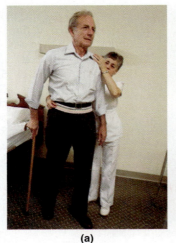
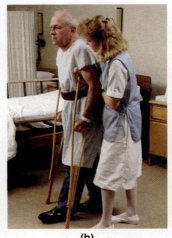
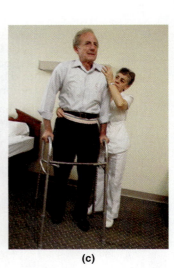

(a)   (b)   (c)

FIGURE 14.9 ■
Clients using assistive
devices for walking:
(a) cane; (b) crutches;
(c) walker.

- Stand on the client's weaker side and a little behind him.
- One hand should be on the guarding belt, the other hand in front of the collarbone on the weaker side.

Assistive Walking Devices

Canes, crutches, and walkers help people support themselves while walking (Figure 14.9 ■). Use of this equipment may be permanent or temporary. A client may use different pieces of equipment at different times. The decision as to which piece of equipment to use will take into consideration the client's needs and abilities. Do not change the equipment or the way in which the client has been instructed to use it. If you have a suggestion or a safety concern, discuss it with your supervisor.

■ GUIDELINES

Using Assistive Walking Devices

- Canes, crutches, and walkers must always have rubber tips on the ends.

- Tips should not be worn, wet, or torn.

- Screws and bolts should be securely in place. If one is lost, replace it. Do not use the device without the proper screws in place.

- Wooden canes and crutches should be smooth, without cracks.

- Metal canes, crutches, and walkers should have no sharp edges and should be straight.

- To go up stairs: Advance the strongest leg to the next step. Bring the cane or crutches and then the weaker leg to the step.

- To go down stairs: Advance the cane or crutches to the lower step, followed by the weaker leg and then the stronger one.

- The hand piece of each device should be level with the hip to allow a slight bend at the elbow when the client is standing.

- All equipment is used after the client has come to a standing position.

- Do not come to a standing position pulling up walkers or canes.

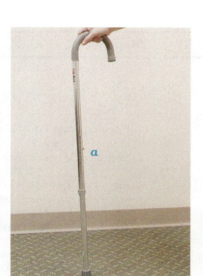
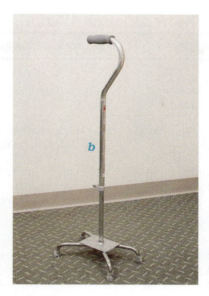

FIGURE 14.10 ■ Two types of canes: (a) single-tipped cane; (b) quad-cane.

Each piece of equipment is prescribed by a physician and fit by a professional nurse or physical therapist to the client's unique needs. This individualized fit decreases the possibility of accidents. If a piece of equipment is borrowed, check it for fit and make sure that it is safe before it is used.

Canes

A client may use either a single-tipped cane, a tripod cane, or a quad-cane (Figure 14.10 ■). A cane is usually used on the stronger side. That way, the client's weight will be balanced between the cane and the involved side. The base of support will change from that of a normal walking gait.

The client walking with the cane will:

1. Place the cane about 12 inches in front on his stronger side (Figure 14.11 ■).
2. Bring the weaker leg forward so that it is even with the cane (Figure 14.12 ■).
3. Bring the stronger leg forward, just ahead of the cane (Figure 14.13 ■).

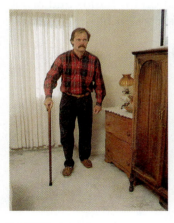
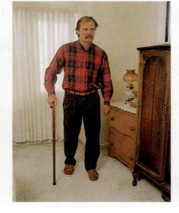
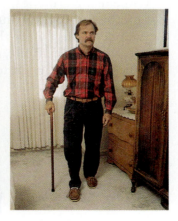

FIGURE 14.11 ■   **FIGURE 14.12** ■   **FIGURE 14.13** ■

Table 14.1: **Crutch Walking**

Gait	Features	Steps
Three-point gait One non-weight-bearing leg		
Swing through (Figure 14.14 ■)	Strong upper arms Some weight bearing	1. Place crutches 8 to 12 inches in front of body. 2. Swing body past crutches.
Swing to crutch	Strong upper arms Some weight bearing	1. Place crutches 8 to 12 inches in front of body while bearing weight on strong leg. 2. Swing body to crutches.
Standard three-point gait (Figure 14.15 ■)	One non-weight-bearing leg Strong upper arms Client can balance well	1. Place crutches 8 to 12 inches in front of body with weaker leg. 2. Bring strong leg forward in front of crutches.
Two-point gait (Figure 14.16 ■)	Weight bearing on both feet Client can balance well	1. Bring right foot and left crutch 8 to 12 inches forward. 2. Bring left foot and right crutch 8 to 12 inches forward.
Four-point gait (Figure 14.17 ■)	Weight bearing on both feet Stable gait, slow	1. Bring right crutch 8 to 12 inches forward. 2. Bring left foot in front of crutch. 3. Bring left crutch in front of left foot. 4. Bring right foot in front of left foot.

Crutches

Crutches assist a client who cannot put complete weight on one or both legs. Crutches are prescribed by a physician and fit by a nurse or physical therapist to the client's unique needs. This individualized fit decreases the possibility of accidents. If the client has a pair of crutches in the house or borrows them, be sure they are checked for fit and they are safe before use. Crutches may be made of wood or aluminum.

While using crutches, the client puts his body weight on his hands and arms, not on the top of the crutch under his arms. Some clients will have to exercise their upper arms before they begin using crutches.

The physical therapist, nurse, or physician will teach the client how to use the crutches and which gait to use (Table 14.1 ■).

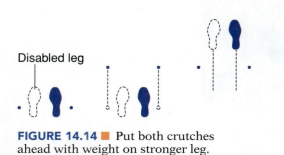

Disabled leg

FIGURE 14.14 ■ Put both crutches ahead with weight on stronger leg.

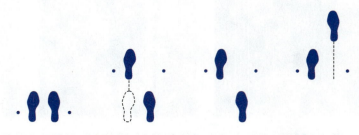

FIGURE 14.15 ■ Advance both crutches and the weak foot. Balance weight on both crutches, then advance the stronger foot.

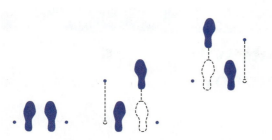

FIGURE 14.16 ■ Advance right foot and left crutch. Then advance left foot and right crutch simultaneously.

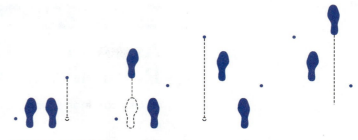

FIGURE 14.17 ■ Put right crutch forward and advance left foot. Then put left crutch forward and advance right foot.

PROCEDURE 45

Going from a Standing Position to a Sitting Position Using Assistive Devices

RATIONALE: Providing assistance while the client uses an assistive device is another step toward independence for the client.

1. Check to see that the chair is secure and safe. Brace it against a wall if possible.

2. The client will walk to the chair.

3. Direct the client to turn his back to the chair and feel it with the back of his legs.

4. Direct the client to let go of the assistive device, reach for the arms of the chair, and slowly lower himself into the chair. (*Note:* The client may need reassurance.)

5. Guide and support him as needed. Remain in front of the client and in good position to assist him.

6. Always use good body mechanics.

SAMPLE CHARTING: 8/17/05   11:30 A.M.
Client able to use his walker and minimal assistance to sit at the table. He enjoys eating with his wife.
Vicki Jones H/HHA

Walker

A walker helps a person who requires support because of greater imbalance or weakness (Figure 14.18 ■). The walker is safe to push down on only when all four legs are on the ground in a level position. If the walker is being moved, the client's feet should be stationary. If the walker is stationary, the client can move his feet. The walker should be picked up and moved, not slid along the ground.

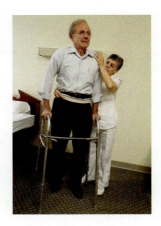

FIGURE 14.18 ■ Using a walker helps support the client when he is walking.

▬ GUIDELINES

As You Help Clients with Rehabilitation Therapy

■ Always apply basic body mechanics.

■ Be sure of your client's abilities before you attempt a procedure. Check each time.

continued

▪ GUIDELINES (*continued*)

As You Help Clients with Rehabilitation Therapy

- ■ Use common sense.
- ■ TCOB.
- ■ Know your own abilities. Do not be ashamed to ask for help or additional instruction with a procedure.
- ■ Communicate through words, gestures, and tone of voice.
- ■ Set an example to the client and the family.
- ■ Use the same procedure each time you assist the client. This will set up a routine with which you will both be familiar.
- ■ Apply what you know from one procedure to help you with another one.
- ■ Clothing should fit well and not block the client's view of the floor. Shoes should be flat with nonskid soles.

SECTION 3

Speech and Language Therapy

OBJECTIVES

What You Will Learn to Do

1. Understand the different ways we can communicate.
2. Understand the meaning of receptive and expressive aphasia.
3. Understand the role of the homemaker/home health aide in working with the speech-language pathologist.
4. Understand what the homemaker/home health aide may do to help a communication-impaired client.

Introduction: Working with a Speech-Language Pathologist

Speech and language therapy is one of the services provided by the home health team. The speech-language pathologist is the professional who evaluates the need for therapy and who plans the therapy program.

Speech and language therapy is given when the client has difficulty communicating. It is important to remember that there is more to communication than just speaking. Communication also means the ability to understand speech, to read, to write, and to gesture (Figure 14.19 ▪).

A client may need speech and language therapy if he has a disorder that affects the parts of the brain, face, lips, tongue, or throat used to form words. Examples of this kind of disorder are Parkinson's disease, cerebral palsy, and cleft palate. A person who has had cancer of the tongue or larynx (voice box) may need therapy after the surgeon has removed the cancer.

APHASIA

Injury to the brain may cause a loss of speech or language abilities, called aphasia. Usually, the injury is from a **cerebrovascular accident (CVA),** often called a stroke. In a cerebrovascular accident, a blood clot, hemorrhage, or vascular spasm in the brain stops oxygen from reaching parts of the brain tissue. When those parts of the brain do not receive oxygen, they stop working. Damage to the brain may also be caused by a blow on the head or by a tumor.

An aphasic person may have difficulty in all areas of communication. It may be hard to speak, understand speech, read, or write. Aphasia may be mild, moderate, or severe. The kind of aphasia is determined by where the brain injury occurs and how much damage is done to the parts of the brain. Aphasia does not mean that the person is unable to make judgments or think. Aphasia only means a person cannot communicate with words.

There are two types of aphasia: expressive and receptive. A client with **expressive aphasia** has difficulty expressing his thoughts and sometimes communicating in writing. Such a client may say things involuntarily. He may have difficulty:

- Naming people and things
- Saying "yes" and "no" at the right time
- Spelling words
- Counting
- Telling time

Everyone has had the experience of having the name of a person or a thing "right on the tip of the tongue." The feeling of knowing what you want to say but not being able to think of the right word is what an expressively aphasic person experiences all day long.

A person with **receptive aphasia** has trouble receiving, or understanding, what he is hearing, seeing, or touching. For example, he can hear words clearly, but they do not have any meaning for him. It is as if he were listening to a foreign language. He might have the same problem when he looks at words. Some aphasic people even have trouble understanding the use of common objects. They might pick up a comb and not know what to do with it.

A person with receptive aphasia may have:

- No interest in watching television or listening to the radio
- No interest in reading the newspaper
- No ability to follow directions
- No ability to answer questions appropriately

The behavior of the aphasic person may seem rude or confusing at times. But think about how *you* might act if you could not say what you wanted to say or if you could not understand what people were saying to you. Always remember that the aphasic person is an intelligent adult. He or she is just as smart as before the brain injury but simply cannot communicate easily. An aphasic person will be most cooperative and least frustrated when you treat him or her as you would any adult.

A client with aphasia:

- Tires easily
- Laughs or cries frequently

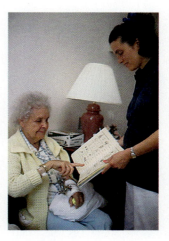

FIGURE 14.19 ■ A client may need to communicate in a nonverbal manner.

cerebrovascular accident (CVA)
blockage of blood vessel within the brain leading to death of brain tissue

expressive aphasia
difficulty communicating in writing and orally

receptive aphasia
inability to understand stimuli due to a deficiency within the brain

- Uses profanity without meaning to
- Repeats the same word over and over

Your Role as a Homemaker/Home Health Aide

Your role in working with the aphasic client is important. You will probably spend more time with the client than any other person on the home health team. You will have a better chance to know the client and to help him adjust to his new schedule of exercises and activities.

The speech-language pathologist will ask you to do two specific tasks. The first will be to help the client practice speech or language activities. These activities are always taught first by the speech-language pathologist. Remember that the aphasic person may have various troubles communicating and with different degrees of severity. For this reason, it is always the job of the speech-language pathologist to determine which activities best fit the needs of a particular client. Never use speech or language activities you practice with one client with another unless so instructed.

If the client has difficulty understanding or using words, you may be taught how to use pictures and printed words to help improve communication. You may be shown how to help your client practice printing or writing. Sometimes, the client may have weakened muscles of the face, lips, or tongue. The speech-language pathologist may teach specific exercises to help improve the strength and coordination of those muscles.

The second task will be to observe and report. It is important to observe how the client makes his needs known and how well he performs the assigned practice tasks. You will want to note how the client makes his feelings known to you. Does he point? Shake his head? Use words? You will also want to keep a record of how often the assigned speech or language tasks are performed.

You will be with the client many more hours during the week than the speech-language pathologist will be. What you report will be useful in planning the therapy program.

Here are some dos and don'ts to keep in mind when you are caring for an aphasic person.

Do

- Get the attention of the client before starting to speak.
- Keep instructions and explanations simple. Speak slowly but naturally. Try to limit your conversation about the client's immediate needs or surroundings.
- Encourage the client to use common expressions, such as "hello," "goodbye," and "I want."
- Encourage the client to be as independent as possible. He is an adult; treat him like one.
- Ask direct questions requiring a simple "yes" or "no" answer. For example, ask "Did you eat lunch?" rather than "What's new?"
- Give the client time to reply.
- Give the client opportunities to hear speech, such as on the radio and television.
- Meals and dressing times are good opportunities to encourage the client's attempts to speak. Let him ask for what he needs. He may say the word

correctly sometimes and forget it at another time. This is usual for the aphasic person.

■ Encourage the client to use whatever speech ability he has. Counting and singing are good activities. Words such as *up-down* or *push-pull* can be used during physical therapy exercises.

■ Show the client understanding, but not pity. Help him verbalize his feeling of frustration ("I know it must be difficult for you.").

■ By your body language, patience, and attitude of acceptance, create an air of relaxation for the client. Avoid directions, such as "Relax."

■ Sometimes, it will be impossible to understand what the client is saying. At such times, tactfully try to change the subject or say, "Let's forget it now and come back to it later. The words will probably come when you're not trying so hard."

You also may encourage the client to learn the words that go with his personal care. When you are helping the client bathe, dress, or eat, say the name of each utensil or body part. For example, say, "Fork, you eat with a fork," or "Arm, I'm washing your arm." Your client may find that he is able to say some of the words with you. If he does, smile and let him know that he has succeeded. If he does not repeat the words, you must not force him. Remember, he wants to talk, and if he could, he would. Talking to him about these activities in the same way each day will help him to relearn what words mean, even if he cannot say them.

Don't

■ Answer for the client if he is capable of speaking for himself. Do include the client in social conversations.

■ Confuse the client with too much idle chatter or too many people speaking at once.

■ Discuss the client's emotional reactions and problems in his presence.

■ Interrupt the client or finish sentences for him. He may require extra time to think of the correct word.

■ Show your concern about the client's speech either through word or facial expression. Do not under any circumstances put the client on display or force him to speak. Such remarks as "Say it for them" upset and embarrass the client.

■ Ridicule or insist that the client give accurate responses, pronounce correctly, or "talk right." (There is nothing the client wants more than to do just that.)

■ Speak to the client as if he were a child, deaf, or retarded. He is not deaf unless a definite hearing loss has been detected. His problem is generally one of understanding the meaning of your words, as though you were speaking a foreign language. Simplify or rephrase your wording without shouting. Treat him like the adult he is.

If you can show the client through your attitude and your work that you understand his problem and that you want to help him, you will often be rewarded by the gratitude of a more relaxed and comfortable client.

One way to have information readily available is a communication board. This has information important to the client such as the day of the week, the name of the caregiver, a picture of his family, names of expected visitors, schedule of care of the day, the weather, and other important information (Figure 14.20 ■).

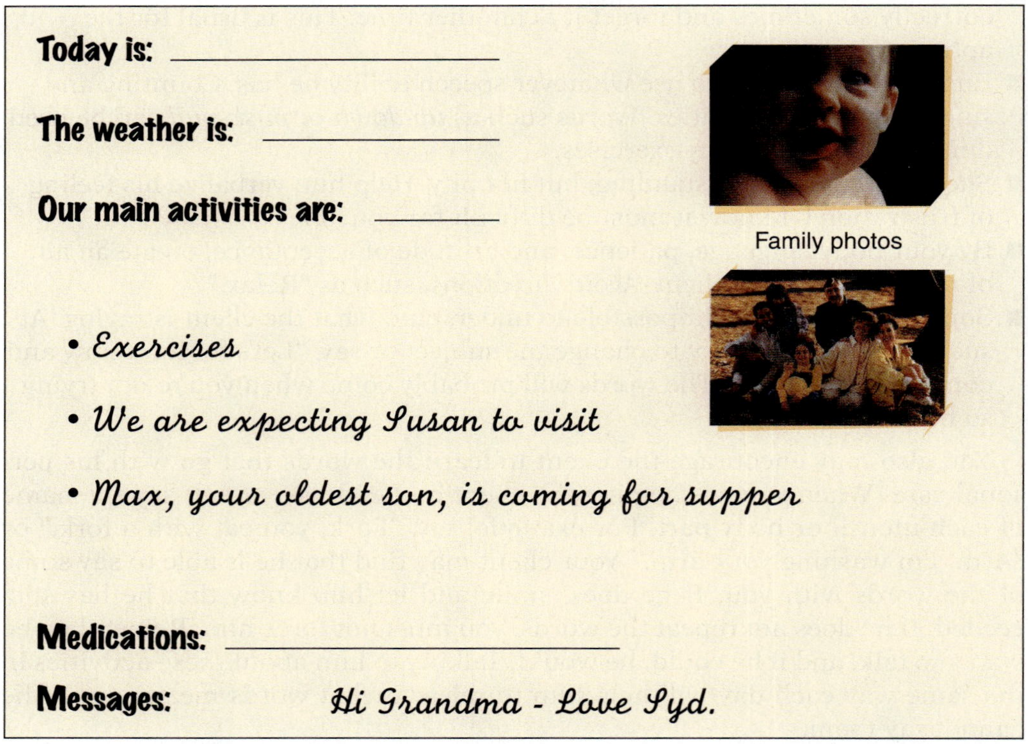

Today is: _____

The weather is: _____

Our main activities are: _____

- *Exercises*

- *We are expecting Susan to visit*

- *Max, your oldest son, is coming for supper*

Family photos

Medications: _____

Messages: *Hi Grandma - Love Syd.*

FIGURE 14.20 ■ Communication board

Dealing with a Hearing Loss

OBJECTIVES

What You Will Learn to Do

1. Identify common causes of hearing loss.
2. Clean a hearing aid earmold.
3. Identify common problems that may prevent a hearing aid from working properly.
4. Identify the best ways to talk to a hearing-impaired person.

Introduction: Hearing and Its Loss

You will likely work with clients with varying degrees of hearing loss. Some are born with a hearing loss. Other people lose their hearing when exposed to loud noise over a long period of time. Head injuries or ear infections can also cause loss of hearing. Many people lose some ability to hear sounds clearly as they age.

Whatever the cause of the hearing loss, it can be a frustrating problem. The person who is hard of hearing may believe that others are mumbling or speaking unclearly. He or she may have to work harder to understand what is being said. If it becomes too frustrating to try to follow a conversation, the hard-of-hearing person may begin to avoid social activities. A **hearing aid** can often be of great help to hard-of-hearing people.

hearing aid
mechanical device used to help a person perceive sounds

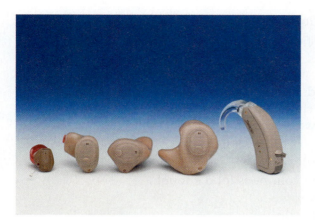

FIGURE 14.21 ■
Hearing aids come in various sizes and shapes.

HEARING AID CARE

The hearing aid **earmold** is custom-made to fit the ear. An earmold that does not fit snugly into the ear will cause a high-pitched whistling noise when the aid is turned on (Figure 14.21 ■).

   The earmold must be kept clean. If earwax or dirt clog the earmold, sound will not pass through. The earmold and aid should be wiped with a dry tissue after each wearing. When not in use, the hearing aid should be kept in a safe place away from extreme heat or cold.

Batteries Make the Hearing Aid Work

   If the hearing aid does not work, the battery may be dead. To insert a new one, match the + on the battery to the + on the hearing aid case. One battery will last about 125 hours, or 10 days. The battery should be removed from the hearing aid whenever the aid is not being worn. This saves the batteries. Store extra batteries in a cool, dry place, such as a dresser drawer.

earmold

an impression of the ear used with a hearing aid

PROCEDURE 46

How to Clean the Hearing Aid Earmold

RATIONALE: Maintaining a hearing aid promotes its good function and client independence.

1. Assemble your equipment:
   Pan of warm water and mild liquid detergent
   Pipe cleaner or toothpick
2. Remove the earmold from the body of the hearing aid.
3. Wash the earmold gently with mild soap and water.
4. Carefully remove any earwax with the pipe cleaner or toothpick.
5. Dry thoroughly. Let it dry overnight, or blow air through the opening to be sure all water has come out of the tubing and earmold.

Remember: Wash only the earmold. Never put the body of the hearing aid in water. Never use alcohol or cleaning fluid on the earmold or the aid. Encourage your client to take the hearing aid off or to protect it during rain and snow to prevent it from getting wet.

SAMPLE CHARTING: 3/3/05   3:00 P.M.
Hearing aid cleaned, as client was complaining of inability to hear well. Earwax removed and mold gently cleaned. Client to keep a record on his calendar so this can be done on a regular basis. Joanne Wan H/HHA

Precautions include the following:

- Keep the hearing aid away from heat sources such as radiators and hair dryers.
- Do not wet the hearing aid.
- Do not drop the hearing aid.
- Do not spray hair spray, perfume, or aftershave lotion on the aid.
- Do not twist the tubing or wires.

If the hearing aid does not work, check to see if:

- The battery is put in correctly and the case is closed tightly.
- The aid is turned on and the volume is loud enough.
- There is wax in the earmold.
- The tubing or wires are twisted.
- The battery is working.

If all of these have been checked and the hearing aid still does not work, it should go to the hearing aid supplier for repair.

HOW TO TALK TO THE HEARING-IMPAIRED CLIENT

- Get his attention before you start speaking.
- Talk face to face whenever possible. Your client will understand more of what you say when he can see your face and expression.
- Keep your hands away from your face so they do not block his view of what you are saying.
- Do not chew food when you are speaking; it will make your words sound unclear.
- Do not exaggerate your words. Speak at a normal rate of speed. You may be asked to speak louder, but do not shout.

The speech-language pathologist may teach you the following exercises to practice with the client. They are often used when the muscles used for speech are weaker. *Never* practice any exercise with a client that was not taught to him by the speech pathologist.

Name _____ Date _____

Do Each Exercise _____

Lips:

1. Open mouth as wide as possible, stretch, close tightly and pucker, hold.
2. Pucker lips, hold, move lips to the left, hold, move lips to the right, hold.
3. Reach out with lower lip, hold. Reach out with the upper lip, hold.
4. Smile with lips closed, frown, repeat.
5. Press lips tightly as if you are saying "mm."
6. Say "ma-me-mi-mo-mu" (as clearly and distinctly as you can).

Tongue:

1. Put the tongue in the outer left corner of the mouth, move to the right and back. Work for speed and rhythm of movement.
2. Extend the tongue straight forward, then pull back vigorously with the whole tongue.
3. Open mouth wide, lift tongue tip up to the roof of the mouth, down. Do not move your jaw; lift your tongue.
4. Say "ta-te-ti-to-tu." Do not move your jaw; lift your tongue.
5. Say "da-de-di-do-du." Do not move your jaw; lift your tongue.
6. Say "la-le-li-lo-lu." Do not move your jaw; lift your tongue.

Throat:

1. Puff up cheeks. Hold air for 5 seconds—then release air as you blow out.
2. Suck in cheeks—then relax.
3. Puff up cheeks with air—move air from one cheek to the other without letting air escape lips. Alternate from one side to the other.
4. Drink liquids whenever possible through a straw.

SECTION 5

Working with an Occupational Therapist

OBJECTIVES

What You Will Learn to Do

1. Discuss your role while working with an occupational therapist.
2. Discuss your role in assisting clients who are relearning daily living skills.
3. Learn techniques to add to your basic knowledge of personal care.
4. Know when and what to report to the OTR.

Introduction: What Is Occupational Therapy?

For most of us, the skills/tasks we perform each day do not require conscious effort or awareness of how we do them. We get out of bed, go to the toilet, bathe, dress, prepare our meals, and feed ourselves. We do not think of the complex movements made by various parts of the body to push; pull; lift; close; zip, hook, and button clothing; or to open or use various objects.

Many clients are unable to perform useful actions with a specific body part. This is called a functional limitation. A client with a **functional limitation** may have to concentrate to hold and lift a spoon to feed himself. Perhaps his grasp is weak. Perhaps he has lost sensation and cannot feel the spoon in his hand. Anyone who needs help with any or all such basic needs as toileting, bathing, dressing, feeding, grooming, or other day-to-day tasks is a candidate for occupational therapy. This training will help him improve his ability to function.

functional limitation
the inability to perform a task due to the deficit of a body part

FUNCTION OF THE OCCUPATIONAL THERAPIST

The occupational therapy program focuses on increasing the functional ability of the client within his familiar environment. The trained person who administers this therapy is a registered **occupational therapist (OTR)**. The client knows what household equipment he has to work with and will learn to adopt new skills in his own home. Being able to learn these skills at home shows the client that he is expected to take an active part in his care. Home is a non-threatening place for relearning basic skills. An OTR can guide and instruct both the client and the homemaker/home health aide in ways to make the transition toward functional independence (Figure 14.22 ■).

General areas in which the OTR works with a homebound client include:

occupational therapist (OTR)
trained person who assists people with performing their daily living tasks

■ *Mobilization.* Teaching the client techniques that he can use to change position; to reach, grasp, or turn while sitting; or to maintain balance during an activity.

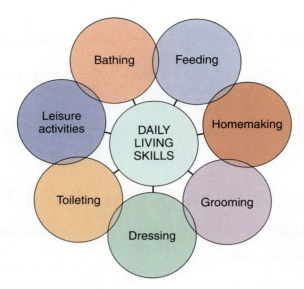

FIGURE 14.22 ■
Helping a client relearn daily living skills will aid him in his recovery and prepare him for independence.

daily living skills (DLS)
those tasks done each day to meet a person's basic needs

- ■ *Daily living skills (DLS).* Tasks we perform each day—toileting, bathing, dressing, feeding, grooming, homemaking, leisure activities.
- ■ *Strength, coordination, and activity tolerance.* The ability to do something without tiring quickly. The client must learn techniques to conserve his energy, perform the skill task to his own satisfaction, and use his physical resources to the fullest.

Your Role As a Homemaker/Home Health Aide

As you begin to assist clients in regaining their independence, your role as teacher, helper, and friend becomes important. Remember:

- ■ Your role in each task will be clearly defined by the OTR.
- ■ If you do not understand what the client is supposed to do and what you are supposed to do, ask the OTR to explain more fully. If it is not clear to you, it will not be clear to the client. It is important for both of you to know what you are expected to do and why you are doing it.
- ■ After each training session with the OTR, you and the client will have an opportunity to practice what has been demonstrated.
- ■ If the client finds it difficult and says, "I can't," assist him with part of the routine to help him start. Example: "You dress your involved arm, and I will help you put on the rest of the shirt."
- ■ If the client shows signs of pain, tiredness, or discomfort during the activity, stop the routine and report your observations to the OTR or the nurse supervisor.
- ■ Observe which parts of each task the client is able and unable to do. Report your observations to the OTR on her next visit.
- ■ Remember, the goal of the client, OTR, and homemaker/home health aide is to help the client become functionally independent, to take care of himself. As he achieves success with each task, your role will change.
- ■ Do not attempt any technique that has not been taught to you and the client by the OTR. A method that was appropriate for a previous client may be wrong for your present client.

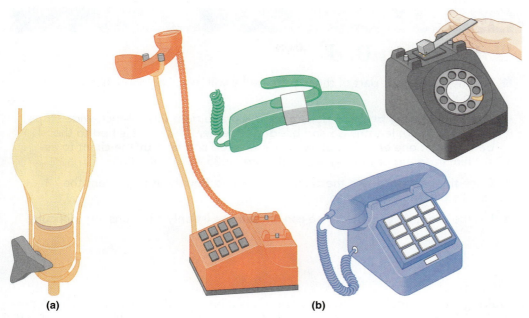

FIGURE 14.23 ■ Using adaptive equipment on everyday devices can help the client return to normalcy. (a) When this piece of adaptive equipment is attached to the lamp switch, the client can turn the switch more easily; (b) Use adaptive equipment on everyday devices such as the telephone.

■ Make the environment a safe and helpful one for your client (Figures 14.23 ■ and 14.24 ■).

■ As the client begins to regain skills, he also may become fearful that he will not be able to manage on his own as well as when you are there. Point out positive changes you have observed.

■ Discuss the outside world, the change of seasons, what is happening in the community, the specials at the grocery store, and who won the ball game. Bring the world into his home so he can begin to relate to it. Help him to realize that his disability does not have to be his whole world and that it no longer requires his total involvement.

■ Observe the client's daily needs such as his glasses, tissues, a glass of water, the newspaper, and the TV. As early in his rehabilitation as possible, make these things accessible to him. Let him begin to assume responsibility for using them without your help.

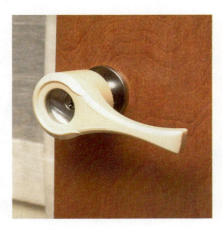

FIGURE 14.24 ■
Door handles are often difficult to turn. Adaptive equipment allows the client greater ease of use.

pulling braid
a device used to assist a
person in moving and/or
sitting up in bed

◆ GUIDELINES

Toileting in Bed

■ Tell the client what part of the procedure he will be doing and what you will do.

■ Provide a **pulling braid.** A pulling braid is made from three 4-inch-wide strips of sheeting torn lengthwise and braided together. This braid is tied to the bedframe at one end. The other end is knotted and held by the client to assist him in sitting or turning in bed (Figure 14.25 ■).

■ Place the bedpan where the client can reach it. Powder it to prevent the client's skin from sticking to it.

■ Let the client do as much as he can himself. Assist only if he runs into difficulty.

Toileting

Taking care of one's own toileting needs is a basic and personal activity. A person who must rely on another person to help with this often suffers a loss of self-esteem or dignity. A person who assumes responsibility for this part of personal care has taken the first step toward functional independence. This is usually the first skill a client wishes to learn. Follow the procedure established by the OTR.

Remember, you may assist the client with toileting, but do not attempt to change the place of toileting until you have been instructed to do so.

Bathing

Bathing stimulates the body. The client who bathes himself stimulates his involved extremities as he touches and rubs them. He becomes aware that the extremity "is there," even if he cannot really "feel" it. He may become aware that the involved extremity moves when he is using other parts of his body. As he bathes, he moves many parts of his body together. He bends, stretches, reaches, grasps, balances, lifts his arms and legs, turns his head, and shifts his eyes.

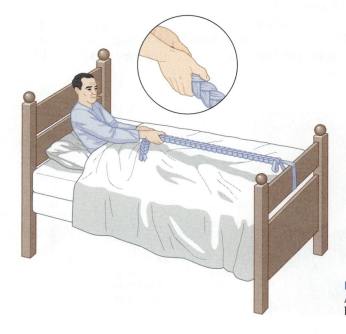

FIGURE 14.25 ■
A client using a pulling braid to sit up in bed.

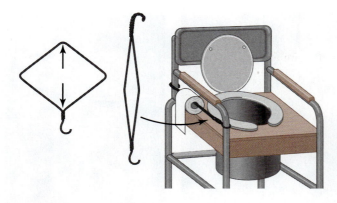

FIGURE 14.26 ■
You can adapt a simple wire coat hanger to make the commode easier for the client to use.

GUIDELINES

Toileting on a Commode

■ Before he begins, explain to the client what he will be doing.

■ Be sure the commode is standing securely.

■ Place the commode in the position in which the client was instructed to use it.

■ Assist the client out of bed as you have been instructed.

■ Fasten the toilet paper to the commode. Tie the roll with a string or make a holder by stretching out a wire coat hanger and threading the roll onto it and hooking it to the frame. If you use a wire hanger, bend the ends and hook them over the front and back of the commode frame. Tape the ends so they do not scratch the client (Figure 14.26 ■).

■ Place the roll on the client's uninvolved side. If he has general weakness, place it on his dominant (most used) side.

■ Provide privacy.

GUIDELINES

Toileting in the Bathroom

■ Place the commode frame over the toilet as instructed or set the elevated toilet seat in place if the client uses such a device (Figure 14.27 ■). If using the commode frame, an 8-by-10-inch sheet of plastic, such as a piece from a garbage or trash bag, can be anchored between the commode seat and frame so it hangs down into the toilet bowl. This will serve as a baffle to prevent urine from splashing out of the toilet bowl. Rinse it off and replace it each time the client uses the toilet.

■ Tell the client what he will do.

■ Allow the client to do as much as he is safely able to do.

■ Assist him with sitting on the toilet as you have been instructed.

■ Provide privacy.

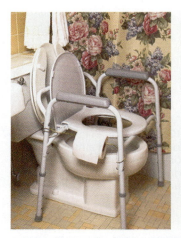
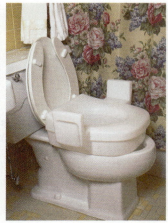
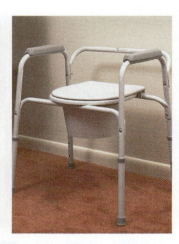

FIGURE 14.27 ■ Various types of adaptive equipment make the commode easier for the client to use.

GUIDELINES

Bathing

■ Do not attempt any technique that has not been taught to you and the client by the OTR. A method that was appropriate for a previous client may be inappropriate for your present client.

■ Provide a safe environment.

■ Assemble everything the client will need for bathing and dressing. Place them where he can reach them (Figure 14.28 ■).

■ Thin washcloths and small face towels may be easier for a weak or arthritic client to handle than thick cloths or large, heavy towels.

■ Stabilize the wet soap by placing it on a dampened sponge, face cloth, paper towel, or rubber suction disk where it is less likely to slide.

■ The client should remove his clothing as he was taught by the OTR.

■ The hemiplegic should wash his involved arm first. He can drape a well-soaped washcloth over the palm of his involved hand, which should be resting palm up on his lap. Then he can lean forward and cradle his uninvolved arm in the hand and slide it back and forth to wash it.

■ Remind your client to rinse off soap and dry each part of his body as he finishes washing it.

■ Place nailbrush, bristles up, in the palm of his involved hand resting on his lap, palm up. Your client can rub his uninvolved fingers across the brush, pushing gently into the palm of the other hand to steady it.

■ The client can also use the nailbrush on the fingers of the involved hand. He may lift the hand into the basin to rinse it, using the other hand for assistance if necessary.

■ If the client is in bed, crank up the bed so that he can see his abdomen and legs. In a regular bed, prop him up with pillows.

■ Place the washcloth and towel over the bed rail where the client can reach them. If he is in a regular bed, use a chair back or the head of the bed.

■ Assist the client with transfers as necessary for safety.

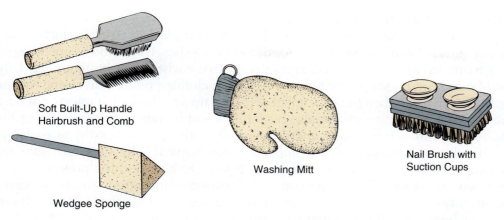

Soft Built-Up Handle Hairbrush and Comb

Wedgee Sponge

Washing Mitt

Nail Brush with Suction Cups

FIGURE 14.28 ■ Adapted equipment assists the client in bathing himself.

- When the client is learning to turn on faucets and run water for himself, make sure he turns on the cold first and then the hot. Run cold water through the faucet last so it will be cool if the client touches it. Certain diseases affect a client's sense of heat and cold, and he cannot judge temperature. Check the water temperature with your hand before the client bathes.

- If your client cannot reach his back, he may use the foam rubber mop or back brush to extend his reach. If not, you should complete this task.

It is particularly important the **hemiplegic** (a person paralyzed on one side of the body), gives this stimulation to involved extremities. Rubbing the affected part with the washcloth or towel may arouse sensory nerves lying close to the skin. The brain, receiving these sensations, may send a message down the motor pathways that could trigger an automatic response in the involved arm.

hemiplegic
one who is paralyzed on one side of his body

When you bathe the client, he does not use his own energy output. His body is not involved with the automatic activity. Therefore, these responses may not be triggered.

The OTR may instruct the client to bathe in bed or when seated on the commode, on a chair in front of a basin in his room, on a chair at the sink or on the toilet seat in the bathroom. As the client regains strength and mobility, the OTR may instruct him in tub bathing or showering using a bench or chair placed in the tub or shower stall. Some states permit the homemaker/home health aide to supervise and assist clients in showers and tubs. Some do not. You will be instructed according to the guidelines in your area.

TUB BATHING AND SHOWERING

By the time the client can bathe in a tub, he should have mastered such skills as balance, hip flexion, and transfers from sitting to standing with minimal assistance. Your role will be to provide a safe environment and provide assistance as the client requires it. Remind the client to transfer to the tub as he has been taught. Be alert for signs of fatigue or weakness.

By the time the client can shower, he will have mastered most skills necessary for this independent activity, but your role is to continue to remain close to provide assistance as needed. Be alert for signs of sudden weakness.

Dressing and Grooming

The client who has been hospitalized or in bed for a long time often starts to feel better about himself when he is dressed in street clothes. He should be encouraged to get dressed for at least part of every day. Even the wheelchair-bound or partially bed-bound person should be assisted to put on clothing other than sleepwear for part of each day. When the dependent person is up and dressed, it affects not only his feelings of self-esteem, but also his family's and friends' perceptions about his health. Let him select clothes and do as much of the actual dressing as possible.

Dressing uses many muscle groups. Dressing himself helps the client improve his coordination, balance, and mobility. Every piece of clothing presents some problem in dressing for the person with functional limitations. However, careful attention to the types of clothing available and the skills needed to put them on may lessen or eliminate many problems.

Clinical ALERT

Use of equipment in the home

Check all equipment for safety before you use it. This includes cleaning equipment, therapeutic aids and eating implements. If you identify an unsafe item and cannot easily fix it, remove it from the client and alert the appropriate people. Be sure and chart this. Do not use unmarked bottles of anything. If you suspect a bottle does not contain what the label indicates, do not use it.

▬ GUIDELINES

Assisting a Client to Dress

- ■ Always dress the weak or most involved extremity first.
- ■ Undress the weak or involved extremity last.
- ■ Help the client select clothing that is roomy and will stretch or give when he puts it on or takes it off. It is easier to put on a garment that opens all the way down the front than one that must be pulled over an involved arm and then pulled over the head.
- ■ Position the client in front of a mirror. The client will see with his own eyes that he has missed a button, his collar is turned in, or his pants are pulled to the side.
- ■ Lay out the pieces of clothing where the client can reach them in the order he will put them on.
- ■ If the OTR has suggested the use of any special tools or adapted equipment for dressing, have them near the client's clothing (Figure 14.29 ■). Always use a shoehorn when putting on the client's shoes. He may use a dressing stick, a buttonhook, or a reacher when he begins to dress himself again.
- ■ Follow the same procedure each time the client dresses and undresses.
- ■ Follow the procedure that the OTR has established for your client.

LAUNDRY AND MEAL PREPARATION

It is important for clients who live alone or are responsible for a family to care for their own basic needs. They should be able to prepare meals, or at least assist in their preparation, and to care for some aspects of housekeeping.

Laundry

Taking care of one's own laundry is a functional activity. Many clients need encouragement to resume this function because they will not do things as neatly and as easily as they once did. Assist the client with handwashing clothes but let the client do as much as possible. Folding, sorting, and stacking clean clothes can be done slowly and should be adapted to the client's individual abilities. Obviously, folding socks and shirts is easier than folding sheets, but stacking sheets is easier than stacking socks. These tasks should be shared as the family sees fit.

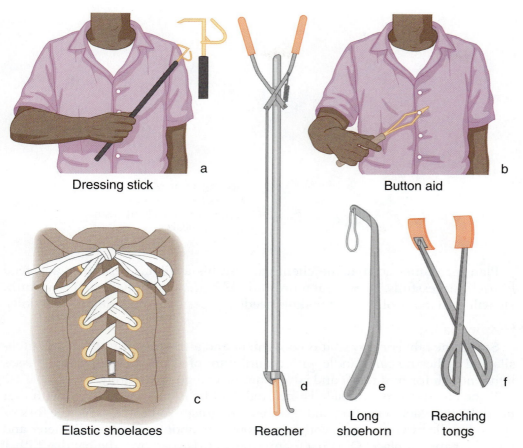

a
Dressing stick

b
Button aid

c
Elastic shoelaces

d
Reacher

e
Long
shoehorn

f
Reaching
tongs

FIGURE 14.29 ■ The client will become more self-sufficient when he learns to dress himself. Adaptive tools may be necessary.

Meal Preparation

If the client must eventually take part in meal preparation, assist him to assume this responsibility slowly. These activities increase his muscular control. Make use of the devices the OTR provides. Be sure the client is instructed by the OTR as to their proper use before he uses them. Supervise the client the first few times he attempts tasks in the kitchen. Praise him and offer support where needed. Point out his successes.

Include the client in all phases of meal planning and preparation. Use a cutting board with two stainless steel nails projecting from it to hold vegetables, fruits, or meats when paring, scraping, and cutting. Supervise as the client begins to place the food onto the nails, and help if he has difficulty turning it or removing it from the spikes.

Use small containers that are easy to handle. Do not fill containers all the way to the top. Use plastic containers instead of glass ones, if available. Let the client assist with the cleanup after the meal—clean off the table, clean dishes, or dry utensils placed in his lap (Figure 14.30 ■).

Feeding

The client who has difficulty feeding himself, drops utensils, spills food, or chokes and drools when swallowing often feels discouraged. He may refuse to feed himself or to eat as much as he should. He becomes dependent and loses his sense of self-esteem.

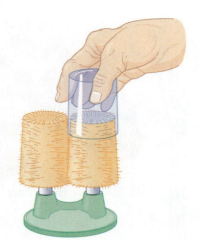

FIGURE 14.30 ■
A glass brush with suction cups can help a client clean up after meals.

Plan mealtimes so that the client can use his available resources and feed himself successfully. He will eat more and feel better emotionally and physically. He will gain many of the motor skills needed to perform other daily living skills.

Helping a Client at Mealtime

Set up the table or tray so it is convenient and attractive. Give the client utensils and dishes he can handle with a minimum of effort. Use cups and glasses light enough for him to lift and silverware he can grasp securely.

If the client's dominant side is involved, and he is still trying to eat with that hand, he may lack sensation and the ability to grasp. You can enlarge the fork or spoon handle by wrapping it with paper towels to about an inch in diameter and tape the paper in place. Or slip a foam rubber curler pad over the handle. Either will enlarge the gripping surface so the client can hold and lift it more easily. The paper towel is temporary and cannot be washed, but the curler can be removed, washed, squeezed dry, and reused on any utensil. Enlarging the handle also makes it easier to use the nondominant hand. If a client has never used his left or right hand to feed himself, he may need the enlarged handle when he first tries.

A rigid plastic cup may be easier and safer for the client to handle than a breakable glass. If the cup has a large hand opening, it will enable the client to put his fingers or hand around the cup for security (Figure 14.31 ■).

A food guard is a plastic ring that slips over the edge of a plate and creates a bumper for the client to push food against when eating. As food is pushed

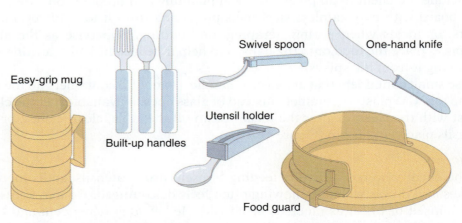

Easy-grip mug

Built-up handles

Swivel spoon

One-hand knife

Utensil holder

Food guard

FIGURE 14.31 ■ Utensils and dishes that are easy to handle will help the client at mealtime.

against an elevated surface, it piles up and spills onto the client's fork or spoon and enables him to get enough on the utensil to feed himself. Plates, bowls, forks, knives, and spoons with specially built-up handles make it easier for the client to grasp and hold onto them while eating.

If a client's grasp is too weak to hold a fork or spoon without dropping it, a feeding cuff may help. It fits over the client's hand. The spoon or fork slips into the pocket and allows the client to lift the utensil without having to grasp it tightly. Cups and glasses with handles open at the bottom can "clip" onto the client's hand, reducing his need to hold tightly while lifting the cup.

Some clients have visual problems. They may be totally or partially blind. Objects placed to the far right or far left may not be visible to them. These clients may need a reminder to "look to your left (right)" when they are eating.

Other clients may have sensory deficits that affect eating. If they lack sensation and the facial muscles are weak on one side, these clients will have difficulty eating. They cannot swallow easily, and they tend to "pocket" food between their cheeks and teeth on the involved side of their face. This can cause them to gag and choke as food builds up. You may have to remind this person to move his tongue to that side of the mouth to dislodge the food.

Place a shaving mirror in front of your client and encourage him to glance at it several times during a meal. This will enable him to use his eyes to make him aware of what occurs when he eats. He may begin to automatically wipe his mouth or to search with his tongue to dislodge stored food or food that remains on his lips.

LEISURE ACTIVITIES

If you can incorporate pleasurable activities into your client's daily routine, you will contribute to his recovery. Ask the client and his family what activities were pleasurable before the illness. Although you could try to introduce new activities, it is always better to start with familiar ones. Look for signs that the client enjoys or at least acknowledges these activities. The client who used to crochet or knit or sew may wish to relearn these skills. The OTR will instruct the client in doing these things again in spite of the disability and you can reinforce the teaching. Use aids to help clients reach objects safely (Figure 14.32 ■).

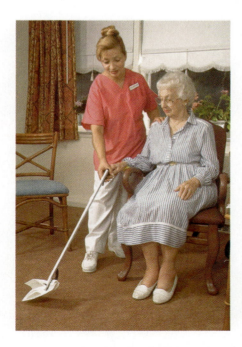

FIGURE 14.32 ■
These tongs are helpful when the client needs to reach an item that is too far away.

Perhaps a client has a perceptual deficit and does not "see" things as they really are. He may not be able to follow the printed lines in a newspaper or read a book because his eyes cannot see the last few words on every line. The OTR works with this client to help him improve his reading ability.

If pleasurable pastimes are used as therapy tools, you may be asked to follow through with the program. Of course, you will be told exactly how to help in any activity of this kind.

On your own, if you have time to play a simple card game with a client, read aloud to him, or turn on the record player for him, it will take his mind off his physical problems and bring him pleasure. Plants and birds both indoors and outdoors provide diversion. Pets provide companionship, love, and stimulation to those who enjoy them. Any extra activity that expands the area of interest for a client is both pleasurable and beneficial. Any activity that stimulates activity and interaction is useful.

CHAPTER REVIEW

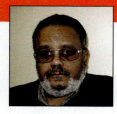

Case Study

Review the case study that appears on the first page of the chapter. Answer two sets of questions about the case study contained in the Explore and Apply sections below.

EXPLORE

1. You have been assigned to assist Mr. Robinson with his exercises and to monitor his medications. When you arrive, three times each week, at the agreed-upon time, he often is not ready, does not want to exercise, or says he has already completed his exercises for the day. He is most reluctant to discuss his medication schedule. What suggestions would you offer to the client so you can complete your assignment? How would you work with your supervisor?

2. How would you work with the neighbors to assist Mr. Robinson when you are not there?

APPLY

1. Identify observations associated with safety that you would complete and report to your supervisor. What would you document?

2. Mr. Robinson has asked that you assist him with his exercises in a way neither safe nor consistent with the way you were trained. When you state that you are uncomfortable with this, he answers, "I always do them this way." What do you do? What do you report? What do you document?

Certification Exam Review Questions

Choose the best answer for each question or statement.

1. **You visit a client three times week and help her with exercises for her shoulder. You notice that the client does not make time for the exercises.**

    a. *You tell her to do them herself, as you are not a policeman.*

    b. *You call your supervisor and report this change in attitude and ask for guidance.*

    c. *You chart the problem and hand it in at the end of the week with your time card.*

    d. *You call the physical therapist and leave a message that you will not help the client anymore.*

2. **An exercise routine should be done**

    a. *at different times of the day so you do not become bored.*

    b. *the exact same way each time or it won't do any good.*

    c. *by the same person each day.*

    d. *at the time of day when the client feels strongest.*

3. **Some clients change their procedure**

    a. *because they like to customize things for themselves.*

    b. *and should be allowed to do this.*

    c. *and insist that everyone uses their way even if it is unsafe.*

    d. *but you are not supposed to use the new procedures if they are unsafe or you are not familiar with them.*

4. **Clients who have speech disabilities should be**

    a. *corrected each time they make a mistake.*

    b. *talked to in a loud voice to attract their attention.*

    c. *ignored unless they say words correctly.*

    d. *allowed to communicate at their own speed and their own way.*

5. **Clients with hearing disabilities should**

    a. *be ignored; eventually they will learn to read lips.*

    b. *never wear hearing aides in the house.*

    c. *tell people they are disabled so that accommodations can be made for them.*

    d. *stay by themselves so they don't bother other people.*

CHAPTER 15

Measuring and Recording Client Vital Signs

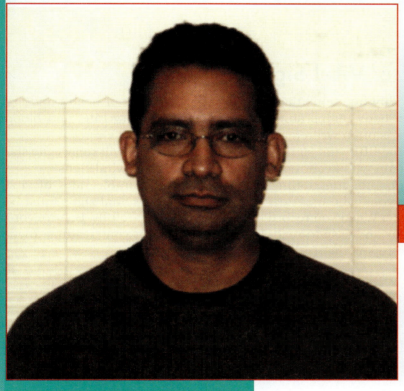

CASE STUDY

Mr. Alvarez, a postman, lives with his wife in a house in which they raised their four children. Mr. Alvarez has recently been diagnosed with hypertension and has been given a diet, a series of exercises, and medication. His wife works hard to cook tasty meals that adhere to the diet, but Mr. Alvarez is not fond of them. He does not do his exercises, saying that he walks all day carrying mail and that is exercise enough. He does take the medication but says he feels different when he takes the pills and, since he didn't feel badly before his physical exam, he doesn't understand why he should take them.

Keep the case study in mind as you read the chapter. After you have read the chapter, answer the Explore and Apply questions at the end of the chapter that relate to the case study.

Vital Signs

OBJECTIVES

What You Will Learn to Do

1. Explain the term *vital signs*.
2. State the average adult normal rates for vital signs.
3. Explain when vital signs are measured.

Introduction: Vital Signs

vital signs

temperature, pulse, respiration, and blood pressure

Vital signs are bodily functions that reflect the body's state of health and are easily measurable: body temperature, pulse rate, respiratory rate, and blood pressure. The term is often written as TPR&BP (Figure 15.1 ■).

In some cases, the fifth vital sign is pain. This means you will report the status of the client's pain when you report and record the other vital signs.

When the body is not functioning normally, the measurable rates of vital signs change. Everyone who measures and records client's vital signs must be careful and accurate. When you record the reading, write carefully. Be sure your handwriting is clear and easy to read. If you are unsure of your reading, mention this when you report the reading to your supervisor.

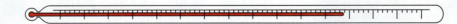

Temperature (T)
The balance between heat
produced by the body and
heat lost by the body

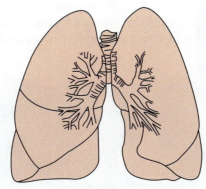

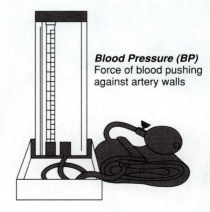

Blood Pressure (BP)
Force of blood pushing
against artery walls

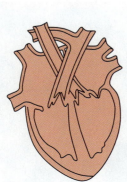

Pulse (P)
The rate at which
the heart is beating

Respiration (R)
Process of inhaling
and exhaling

FIGURE 15.1 ■ Temperature and blood pressure give a picture of the body's status.

WHEN ARE VITAL SIGNS CHECKED?

Your supervisor will tell you when and how often to check your client's vital signs. This decision will be based on the client's present condition, his past history, and his prognosis. Vital signs are not checked in the home as often as they are in the hospital because home-care clients often are in a more stable condition.

You should check the vital signs if you observe any change in your client or after a fall. When you call your supervisor to report the change or the fall, report these vital signs. This information will assist her in making a decision over the telephone. Be sure to record all signs when you take them. If you don't, you will forget.

AVERAGE NORMAL ADULT RATES

- Temperature: 98.6°F or 37°C
- Pulse: 60 to 80 regular beats per minute
- Respiration: 16 to 20 regular breaths per minute
- Blood pressure:

    Infants: 50/40 to 80/58 mm of mercury

    Under 18 years old: below 120/80 mm of mercury

    18 to 50 years and above: below 140/90 mm of mercury
- Pain: none

These rates are given to you as a guide. A person can have a reading that varies from these figures and be healthy. But if you took thousands and thousands of TPR&BPs, you would have these rates as average readings. On an individual basis, it is more correct to compare several of your client's readings than to compare his with the average rates.

REPORTING VITAL SIGNS

When you are assigned to take a client's vital signs, your supervisor will tell you when you should call her with the readings. In the home, you may often take vital signs without reporting them each time. It is most important, however, for you to know when to report your findings. Ask for guidance. If you are in doubt, report. It is far better to report an unnecessary reading than not to report one that is necessary.

TELLING A CLIENT HIS VITAL SIGNS

There was a time when hospitals and doctors did not share information with clients. This time has largely passed. Especially in a person's home, you usually will be expected to share the vital sign readings with your client. Please do so promptly. If you do not, the client may think you are hiding something from him. Remember, it is his body you are caring for and he has the right to know how it is working. If a client does not wish to know his vital signs, do not force the information upon him. You will also work in homes where, for one reason or another, the client will not be told. Your supervisor will tell you how to handle this situation. Remember, you must abide by the wishes of the family and the physician's decision, even if you do not agree with them!

SECTION 2

Measuring Temperature

OBJECTIVES

What You Will Learn to Do

1. Read a thermometer accurately.
2. Become familiar with the proper way to handle a mercury thermometer.
3. Demonstrate the procedure for measuring oral temperatures.
4. Demonstrate the procedure for measuring rectal temperatures.
5. Demonstrate the procedure for measuring axillary temperatures.

Clinical ALERT

Cleaning Thermometers
Wash all thermometers with warm soapy water before use. If you think a thermometer was used to take a rectal temperature, do not use it for an oral temperature, no matter how you wash it. Digital thermometers must also be cleaned after each use and after they have stayed in a drawer for awhile.

temperature
measurement of the amount of heat in the body at a given time. Normal body temperature is 98.6°F (37°C)

Introduction: Body Temperature

Body temperature is a measurement of the amount of heat in the body. The balance between heat produced and heat lost is the body temperature. The normal adult body temperature is 98.6°F or 37°C. There is a normal range in which a person's body temperature may vary and still be considered normal (Figures 15.2 ■ and 15.3 ■).

NORMAL RANGES OF BODY TEMPERATURE

- Oral: 97.6 to 99°F (36.4 to 37.2°C)
- Rectal: 98.6 to 100°F (37.0 to 37.8°C)
- Axillary: 96.6 to 98°C (35.9 to 36.7°C)

For recording the client's **temperature**, three symbols are used:

1. ° degrees
2. F Fahrenheit
3. C Centigrade or Celsius

You will record the client's temperatures according to the method used by your agency.

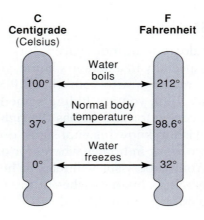

FIGURE 15.2 ■
The two major scales used for measuring temperature.

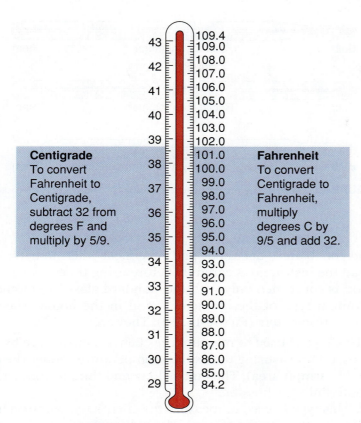

Centigrade		Fahrenheit
To convert Fahrenheit to Centigrade, subtract 32 from degrees F and multiply by 5/9.		To convert Centigrade to Fahrenheit, multiply degrees C by 9/5 and add 32.

FIGURE 15.3 ■ Temperature conversion.

Fahrenheit temperature can be written in two ways:

98.6°F or 98°F

If you are using a centigrade (Celsius) thermometer, the temperature would be written

37.3°C or 37°C

Write an *R* with the temperature reading if a rectal temperature was taken. Write an *A* beside the temperature reading if an axillary temperature was taken.

The body temperature is measured with an instrument called a **thermometer**. This is a delicate, hollow, glass tube with a liquid sealed inside that is sensitive to temperature. The liquid expands when the temperature rises and contracts when the temperature goes down. Even if the temperature rises only slightly, the liquid will expand and travel up the tube, indicating the change. The outside of the glass thermometer is marked with lines, or calibrations, and numbers. These markings make it possible to measure exactly the change in the mercury. By knowing the change, you will know the body temperature.

TYPES OF THERMOMETERS

There are several different types of thermometers. They are:

■ Glass
■ Battery-operated electronic digital readout (Figure 15.4 ■)
■ Chemically treated paper

thermometer
instrument used for measuring temperature

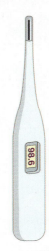

FIGURE 15.4 ■ Battery-operated electronic digital thermometer.

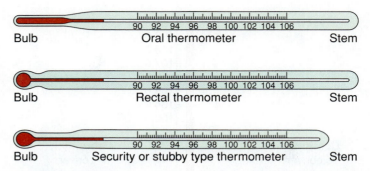

FIGURE 15.5 ■ Use the correct thermometer for the correct purpose.

Each kind of battery-operated and chemical thermometer is slightly different. Read the instructions carefully before using them.

This section is concerned only with the standard glass thermometer. This is the most common type of thermometer found in the home. There are three types of glass thermometers (Figure 15.5 ■). They are:

1. *Oral.* This type is used to measure the client's temperature by mouth and is also used in measuring the axillary temperature (under the client's arm, in his armpit area). The bulb is long and thin, to contact as much of the mouth lining as possible.

2. *Rectal.* This type is used to measure the client's temperature by inserting the thermometer into the rectum. The bulb is small and round. This type of bulb prevents the thermometer from injuring the rectum.

3. *Security.* This type has a strong construction. It is used for taking an infant's rectal temperature. Many agencies use the security or stubby type with a red knob at the stem for rectal temperatures and the one with a green knob at the stem for oral temperatures.

GUIDELINES

Safety Considerations While Using Thermometers

■ Do not expect a client to talk with a thermometer in his mouth.

■ Glass thermometers break and shatter easily. Handle them with care. Be especially careful to avoid breaking a thermometer while it is in a client's mouth or rectum.

■ Keep each thermometer in a case. Do not leave any loose in a pocket, drawer, or dresser.

■ Never clean a glass thermometer with hot water. The liquid will expand so much that the thermometer will explode.

■ If the client thinks that he may be about to sneeze, he should remove the thermometer.

MERCURY

Mercury, the silver metal that, until recently, has been used in thermometers and blood pressure cuffs, is now known to be a poison when it is inhaled, ingested, or comes in contact with skin. If it remains in the thermometer or blood pressure cuff, it poses no danger, but if either instrument breaks, the incident and the area must be treated as a hazardous waste spill.

It is strongly advised not to use a thermometer that contains mercury. If you should find one in a home, notify your supervisor. Many towns have programs that help people trade their mercury thermometer for one with a nontoxic liquid. Encourage your client to buy another type of thermometer if this program is not available.

■ Do not discard a mercury thermometer in the trash. Ask your supervisor the proper way to discard it. One suggestion is to wrap it in paper towels, seal it in a double bagged plastic bag, and call the local heath department for assistance with disposal.

■ If a mercury thermometer should break in the house, open the windows immediately to decrease the amount of vapor that is inhaled. Do not touch the mercury! Do not use a vacuum cleaner to clean the spill. Sweep it onto cardboard, put the mercury, the glass, and the cardboard into a double bagged plastic bag and call the local health department for assistance with disposal. Be sure to document the incident, what you did, and the people who were notified.

PROCEDURE 47

Shaking Down a Glass Thermometer

RATIONALE: The material inside the thermometer must be in the correct place for the temperature reading to be accurate and for the thermometer to be ready for the next use.

1. Assemble your equipment:
   Thermometer in a container
2. Wash your hands.
3. Before using the thermometer, check to make sure that it is not cracked and that the bulb is not chipped.
4. Hold the thermometer firmly between your fingers and your thumb at the stem end farthest from the bulb. The bulb is the end inserted into the client's body.
5. Stand clear of any hard surfaces such as counters and tables to avoid striking and breaking the thermometer while you shake it. For practice, you might stand with your arm over a

pillow or mattress in case you accidentally drop the thermometer.

6. When you are sure that you have a good hold on the thermometer, shake your hand loosely from the wrist. Do it as if you were shaking water from your fingers.
7. Snap your wrist again and again. This will shake down the liquid to the lowest possible point—below the numbers and lines (calibrations).
8. Always do this before and after using a thermometer.

SAMPLE CHARTING: 12/16/05   5:00 P.M.
Thermometer shaken down.
Cecilia Downs H/HHA

Reading a Fahrenheit Thermometer

RATIONALE: Reading a thermometer correctly is an important part of client care.

1. Using your thumb and first two fingers, hold the thermometer at the stem.

2. Hold the thermometer at eye level. Turn the thermometer back and forth between your fingers until you can clearly see the column of liquid.

3. Notice the scale or calibrations. Each long line stands for 1 degree.

4. There are four short lines between each of the long lines. Each short line stands for two-tenths (0.2) of a degree.

5. Between the long lines that represent 98° and 99°, look for a longer line with an arrow directly beneath it. This special line points out normal body temperature.

6. Look at the end of the liquid. Notice the line or number where the liquid ends. If it is one of the short lines, notice the previous longer line toward the silver tip that goes into the client's mouth. The temperature reading is the degree marked by that long line plus two-, four-, six-, or eight-tenths of a degree. If the liquid ends on the fourth short line after the 97 line, the temperature is 97.8°F (Figure 15.6 ■). If the liquid ends between two lines, use the line closer to the silver tip.

7. Write down the client's temperature right away, using the figure you read on the thermometer. Some agencies will write 97.8°F. Others will write 97.8F. Follow the method used by your agency. Always indicate if the reading is oral, rectal, or axillary.

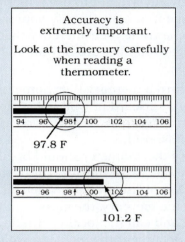

Accuracy is extremely important.

Look at the mercury carefully when reading a thermometer.

97.8 F

101.2 F

FIGURE 15.6 ■

SAMPLE CHARTING: 12/16/05   8:00 P.M.
T 99.4 O.
Cecilia Downs H/HHA

Reading a Centigrade (Celsius) Thermometer

RATIONALE: Reading a thermometer correctly is an important part of client care.

1. Using your thumb and first two fingers, hold the thermometer at the stem.

2. Hold it at eye level. Turn the thermometer back and forth between your fingers until you can clearly see the column of liquid.

3. Notice the scale or calibration. Each long line shows 1 degree.

4. There are nine short lines between each number. These short lines are one-, two-, three-, four-, five-, six-, seven-, eight-, and nine-tenths of a degree. If the liquid ended after the 36° and on the third short line, the temperature would read 36.3°C. If the liquid ended after the long line 37° and on the eighth short line, the temperature would read 37.8°C. If the liquid ends after line 37° on the fifth short line, the temperature would be 37.5°C (Figure 15.7 ■).

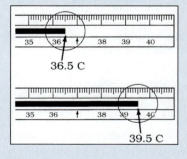

36.5 C

39.5 C

FIGURE 15.7 ■

5. Write down the client's temperature right away. Some agencies write 37°C. Others will write 37.5C. Follow the method used by your agency. Always indicate if the reading is oral, rectal, or axillary.

SAMPLE CHARTING: 11/29/04   12:00 P.M.
T- 37 rectal
Sally Bowles H/HHA

PROCEDURE 50

Cleaning a Thermometer

RATIONALE: Proper cleaning of a thermometer is an important part of infection control in the home.

1. Assemble your equipment:
   Thermometer
   Tissue and/or cotton balls
   Soap
   Disposable gloves
   Cool running water

2. Wash your hands and put on gloves. Wipe the thermometer off from the stem to the bulb. Throw away the tissue (Figure 15.8 ■).

3. Soap a tissue.

4. Holding the thermometer, rotate the soapy tissue around the thermometer from the stem to the bulb.

5. Holding the thermometer under cool running water, repeat the process.

6. Discard the tissue.

7. Dry the thermometer with a dry tissue. Discard the tissue.

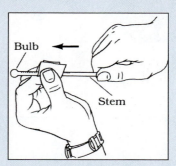

FIGURE 15.8 ■

8. Put the thermometer into a case, bulb first.

9. Dispose of gloves and wash your hands.

SAMPLE CHARTING: 11/29/04   1:00 P.M.
Thermometer cleaned and left in shaken down position in case.
Sally Bowles H/HHA

PROCEDURE 51

Measuring an Oral Temperature

RATIONALE: Taking a client's temperature correctly is an important part of client care.

1. Assemble your equipment:
   Clean oral thermometer in a case
   Tissue or paper towel
   Gloves
   Pad
   Pencil
   Watch

2. Wash your hands.

3. Tell the client that you are going to take his temperature orally.

4. Ask the client if he has recently had hot or cold liquids or if he has smoked. If the answer is yes, wait 10 minutes before taking his temperature.

5. The client should be in bed or sitting in a chair. Do not take a temperature while the client is walking.

6. Take the thermometer out of the container and inspect it for cracks or chips. Do not use it if you see any.

7. Shake the liquid down until it is below the calibrations.

8. Run the thermometer under cool water. This will make the thermometer more pleasant in the client's mouth.

9. Ask the client to lift up his tongue. Place the bulb end of the thermometer under his tongue. Ask him to keep his lips gently around the thermometer without biting it (Figure 15.9 ■). (If the client cannot close his mouth, take the temperature by another method.)

10. Leave the thermometer in place for 8 minutes. (The latest research shows that oral temperature is more accurate when the thermometer remains in the mouth for 8 minutes. However, if it is the policy of your agency to let the thermometer stay only 3 to 4 minutes, follow the policy of your agency.)

11. Stay with your client if you think that he cannot keep his mouth closed. (Wear gloves.)

12. Wash your hands and put on gloves. Take the thermometer out of the client's mouth. Hold

continued

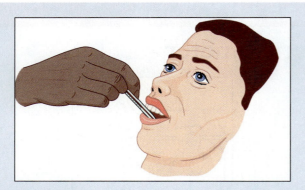

FIGURE 15.9 ■

the stem end and wipe the thermometer with a tissue from the stem toward the bulb.

13. Read the thermometer.
14. Record the temperature and your observations concerning the client during this procedure.
15. Shake down the liquid.
16. Clean the thermometer.
17. Make the client comfortable.
18. Remove gloves and wash your hands.

SAMPLE CHARTING: 7/14/05   11:30 A.M.
T 99.8 orally
Jan Mann H/HHA

Measuring a Rectal Temperature

Always use a rectal thermometer for taking rectal temperatures. Under the following conditions, you would automatically take a rectal temperature:

■ When the client is an infant or a child who cannot safely use an oral thermometer
■ When the client is having warm or cold applications on his face or neck
■ When the client cannot keep his mouth closed around the thermometer
■ When the client finds it hard to breathe through his nose
■ When the client's mouth is dry or inflamed
■ When the client is restless, delirious, unconscious, or confused
■ When the client is receiving oxygen by cannula, catheter, or face mask
■ When the client has had major surgery in the areas of his face or neck
■ When the client's face is partially paralyzed, as from a stroke

PROCEDURE 52

Measuring a Rectal Temperature

RATIONALE: Taking a client's temperature correctly is an important part of client care.

1. Assemble your equipment:
   Rectal thermometer in a case
   Tissue or paper towel
   Lubricating jelly
   Disposable gloves
   Pad
   Pencil
   Watch
   Gloves
2. Wash your hands.
3. Ask visitors to leave the room, if appropriate.
4. Tell the client you are going to measure his temperature rectally.

5. Lower the backrest on the bed.
6. Take the thermometer out of its container. Hold the stem.
7. Inspect the thermometer for cracks or chips. Do not use if you see any. Put on gloves.
8. Shake down the liquid until it is below the calibrations.
9. Put a small amount of lubricating jelly on a piece of tissue. Lubricate the bulb of the thermometer with the jelly. This makes the insertion easier and also makes it more comfortable for the client.
10. Ask the client to turn on his side. If he is unable to turn, position him on his side. Turn back the top covers just enough so that you can see the client's buttocks. Avoid overexposing him.

11. With one hand, raise the upper buttock until you see the anus. With the other hand, gently insert the bulb 1 inch through the anus into the rectum (Figure 15.10 ■).

12. If the client is an infant, remove the diaper. Lay the baby on his back. Raise his legs with one hand. With the other hand, insert the thermometer ½ inch into the rectum. Always hold the thermometer while it is in the child's rectum.

13. Hold the thermometer in place for 3 minutes. Do not leave a client with a rectal thermometer in the rectum, no matter what his condition.

14. Remove the thermometer from the client's rectum. Holding the stem end of the thermometer, wipe it with a tissue from stem to bulb to remove particles of feces.

15. Read the thermometer. Remove gloves and wash hands.

16. Record the temperature and your observations concerning the client during this procedure. (Note that this is a rectal temperature by writing *R* next to the reading.)

17. Make the client comfortable.

18. Put on gloves. Clean the thermometer.

19. Shake the liquid down until it is below the calibrations.

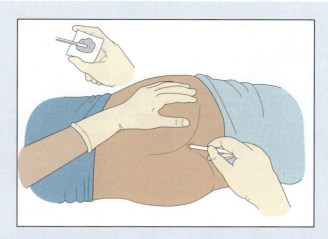

FIGURE 15.10 ■

20. Replace the thermometer in its container.

21. Remove gloves and wash your hands.

SAMPLE CHARTING:	11/30/04 10:30 P.M.
	T 101.4 rectally
	Daughter will call the doctor
	immediately and wait for him
	to call back.
	Judy Elliot H/HHA

PROCEDURE 53

Measuring an Axillary Temperature

RATIONALE: Taking a client's temperature correctly is an important part of client care.

1. Assemble your equipment:
   Oral thermometer in a container
   Tissue or paper towel
   Pad
   Pencil
   Watch

2. Wash your hands.

3. Ask visitors to leave the room, if appropriate.

4. Tell the client that you are going to take his temperature by placing a thermometer under his arm.

5. Remove the thermometer from its case and shake down the liquid so that it is below the calibrations.

6. Inspect the thermometer for cracks or chips. Do not use it if you see any.

7. Remove the client's arm from the sleeve. If the axillary region is moist with perspiration, pat it dry with a towel.

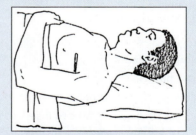

FIGURE 15.11 ■

8. Place the bulb of the oral thermometer in the center of the armpit in an upright position.

9. Put the client's arm across his chest or abdomen (Figure 15.11 ■).

10. If the client is unconscious or too weak to help, you will have to hold the arm in place.

11. Leave the thermometer in place 10 minutes. Stay with the client.

continued

12. Remove the thermometer. Wipe it off with a tissue from the stem to the bulb.

13. Read the thermometer.

14. Record the temperature and your observations concerning the client during this procedure. (Note that this is an axillary temperature by placing an *A* next to the reading.)

15. Shake the liquid down until it is below the calibrations.

16. Clean the thermometer.

17. Replace the thermometer in its case.

18. Make the client comfortable.

19. Wash your hands.

SAMPLE CHARTING: 9/15/05   3:00 P.M.
T 100.6 axillary
Wilma Flint H/HHA

USING A PLASTIC SHEATH OVER A THERMOMETER

A plastic thermometer cover, or sheath, may be used to protect the thermometer from the client's secretions and to aid in thermometer cleanup and reading. Use of a sheath does not mean that you do not have to wash the thermometer after each use; it only makes the washing easier. Be sure to read the directions for each type of sheath, as they differ slightly from manufacturer to manufacturer. Also, remember that sheaths for rectal and oral thermometers are different and should not be used interchangeably.

PROCEDURE 54

Using a Thermometer Sheath

RATIONALE: Using protective equipment correctly is an important part of infection control in the home.

1. Assemble your equipment:
   Thermometer
   Thermometer sheath
   Trash bag
   Tissues
   Disposable gloves

2. Wash your hands.

3. Shake down the thermometer.

4. Hold the sheath so that you can insert the thermometer into the plastic between the paper covering (Figure 15.12 ■).

5. Withdraw the thermometer, now covered with the clear plastic sheath. Be sure the sheath covers the entire thermometer and does not hang off the end (Figure 15.13 ■).

6. Take the client's temperature using the standard procedure. (Lubricating the rectal thermometer may be unnecessary as rectal sheaths usually come prelubricated. Wear gloves.)

7. Put on gloves. Remove the thermometer from the client.
   a. Method A: Remove the sheath with a tissue and discard it in the trash (Figure 15.14 ■).

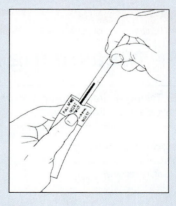

FIGURE 15.12 ■

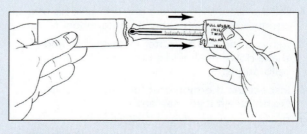

FIGURE 15.13 ■

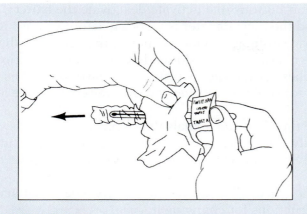

FIGURE 15.14 ■

b. Method B: Insert the sheath back into the package outer sleeve. Remove the

thermometer, leaving the contaminated sheath in the sleeve. Discard it in the trash.

8. Read the thermometer and record the temperature.

9. Wash and store the thermometer according to the standard procedure.

10. Remove gloves and wash your hands.

SAMPLE CHARTING: 10/12/05   4:30 P.M.
Thermometer sheath used
to take client's rectal temperature.
Tina Small H/HHA

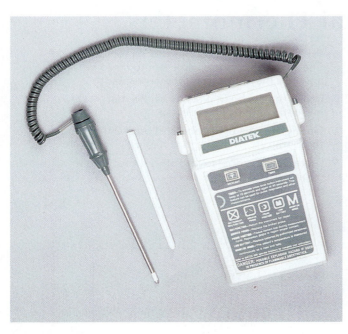

FIGURE 15.15 ■ An electronic thermometer and probe cover.

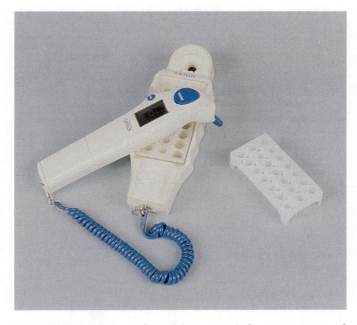

FIGURE 15.16 ■ An infrared (tympanic) thermometer used to measure the tympanic membrane temperature.

DIGITAL OR ELECTRONIC THERMOMETERS

There are several types of **digital thermometers**. It is important that you receive instructions on how to use the model that you have. These may not be used in any other place on the body. Others may be used interchangeably as oral, rectal, or auxiliary thermometers, depending on the probe attached. It is recommended, however, that once a thermometer has been used as a rectal thermometer, it not be used on any other part of the body. (Figure 15.15 ■ and 15.16 ■). Some thermometers are made specifically for use in the ear. These **aural** or tympanic thermometers measure temperature from the blood vessels on the tympanic membrane of the ear.

digital thermometer
thermometer with a temperature readout

aural
tympanic; pertaining to the ear

■ All thermometers have on/off buttons that activate/deactivate the battery. Be sure the battery is good and the thermometer is working before you use it.

■ All digital thermometers have number readouts. That is, they give you the exact temperature they are measuring. You do not have to read calibrations.

■ All thermometers have probes. Electronic thermometers have red probes for rectal use and blue probes for oral use. A cover is used over every probe and is changed after each use.

■ Be sure you know how the thermometer signals that it has measured the client's temperature. Usually, the whole process takes about 10–15 seconds.

■ Observe the same safety precautions with a digital thermometer as you would with a glass one.

■ If the battery is not working, check the instructions for the type of battery needed and follow the instructions for changing it.

■ You may or may not wear gloves for this procedure.

PROCEDURE 55

Measuring an Oral Temperature Using an Electronic or Digital Thermometer

RATIONALE: Using a thermometer correctly helps produce an accurate measure of a client's temperature.

1. Assemble your equipment:
   Electronic thermometer
   Correct sheath
   Trash bag

2. Wash your hands.

3. Tell the client you are going to take his temperature orally.

4. Insert the electronic probe firmly into the probe cover (Figure 15.17 ■).

5. Ask the client to wet his lips and pick up his tongue.

6. Place the probe under the client's tongue on one side of his mouth. Ask him to close his lips. You may have to hold the probe.

7. Leave the probe in place until the thermometer signals it is finished.

8. Gently remove the probe and read the temperature on the digital display.

9. Discard the probe cover without touching it (Figure 15.18 ■).

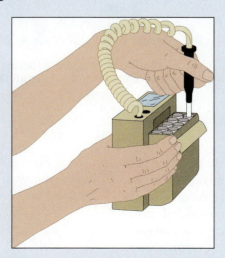

FIGURE 15.17 ■ Insert the electronic probe into the probe cover.

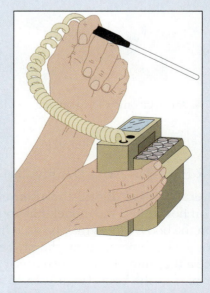

FIGURE 15.18 ■ After reading the temperature on the digital display, discard the probe cover.

10. Return the probe to its holder (Figure 15.19 ■).
11. Return the unit to its holder or charging station.
12. Wash your hands.

SAMPLE CHARTING: 11/01/05   2:00 P.M.
T 98.9 O
Shirley Fine H/HHA

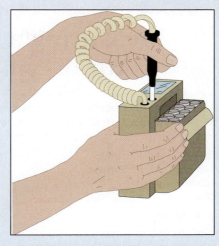

FIGURE 15.19 ■ Return the probe to its holder.

PROCEDURE 56

Measuring a Rectal Temperature Using an Electronic or Digital Thermometer

RATIONALE: Using a thermometer correctly helps produce an accurate measure of a client's temperature.

1. Assemble your equipment:
   Electronic thermometer
   Correct sheath
   Tissues or wet washcloth
   Trash bag
   Gloves
2. Wash your hands.
3. Put on gloves.
4. Ask visitors to leave the room, if appropriate.
5. Tell the client you are going to take his temperature rectally.
6. Insert the electronic probe firmly into the probe cover.
7. Position the client on his left side. Turn back the covers just enough to expose the client's buttocks. Do not overexpose him.
8. Put a small amount of lubricating jelly on the probe cover.

9. With one hand, raise the upper buttock until you see the anus. With the other hand, gently insert the probe into the rectum.
10. Hold the probe in place until the thermometer signals it is finished.
11. Remove the probe and read the temperature on the display.
12. Discard the probe without touching it.
13. Wipe the anal area clean of the lubricant and any fecal matter.
14. Position the client comfortably.
15. Return the unit to its holder or charging station.
16. Remove the gloves and wash your hands.

SAMPLE CHARTING: 9/12/05   4:00 P.M.
T 100 R
Sam Rich H/HHA

Measuring a Temperature Using an Aural/Tympanic Thermometer

RATIONALE: Using a thermometer correctly helps produce an accurate measure of a client's temperature.

1. Assemble your equipment:
   Aural/tympanic thermometer
   Probe cover or sheath
   Trash can

2. Wash your hands.

3. Tell the client you are going to take his temperature using his ear. It will not hurt.

4. Insert the cone-shaped probe into the probe cover.

5. Position the client's head so that it is directly in front of you.

6. For adults, gently pull the outer ear up and back to open the ear canal (Figure 15.20 ■). For children, gently pull the ear straight back (Figure 15.21 ■).

7. Gently insert the probe into the ear canal. You may have to use a gently rocking motion to help the probe slip into the canal and seal the ear canal.

8. Hold the thermometer in place until it signals it is finished.

9. Gently remove the probe and read the digital display.

10. Eject the probe into the trash.

11. Position the client in a safe, comfortable position.

12. Return the thermometer to its holder or charging station.

13. Wash your hands.

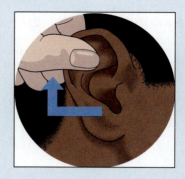

FIGURE 15.20 ■ For adults and children over the age of one year, grasp the outer ear and pull up and back.

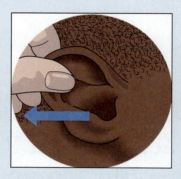

FIGURE 15.21 ■ For Infants under 12 months, pull the outer ear straight back.

SAMPLE CHARTING: 4/30/05   7:00 A.M.
T 97.8 T
Richard Sweet H/HHA

SECTION 3

Measuring a Pulse

OBJECTIVES

What You Will Learn to Do

1. Count the pulse.

2. Report the rate and rhythm of the pulse accurately.

Introduction: The Pulse

Each time the heart beats, it pumps blood into the arteries. This causes the arteries to expand. Between heartbeats, the arteries contract and return to their normal size. The heart pumps the blood in a steady rhythm. The rhythmic expansion

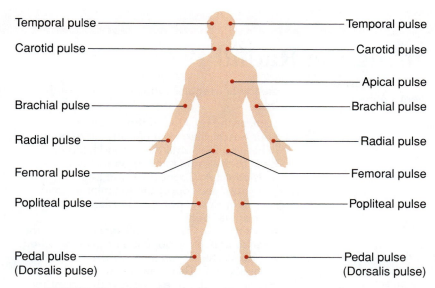

Temporal pulse —————————————— Temporal pulse

Carotid pulse ———————————————— Carotid pulse

——————————————— Apical pulse

Brachial pulse ———————————————— Brachial pulse

Radial pulse ———————————————— Radial pulse

Femoral pulse ——————————————— Femoral pulse

Popliteal pulse ——————————————— Popliteal pulse

Pedal pulse ——————————————— Pedal pulse
(Dorsalis pulse)   (Dorsalis pulse)

FIGURE 15.22 ■ Pulses can be felt at many places on the body.

and contraction of the arteries, which can be measured to show how fast the heart is beating, is called the **pulse.** Measuring the pulse is one method of observing how the circulatory system is functioning.

The pulse measures how fast the heart is beating. At certain places on the body, the pulse can easily be felt under your fingers (Figure 15.22 ■). One of the easiest places to feel the pulse is at the wrist. This is called a radial pulse because you are feeling the radial artery (Figure 15.23 ■). When taking the pulse, you must be able to report accurately the following:

- *Rate:* number of pulse beats per minute
- *Rhythm:* regularity of the pulse beats, that is, whether the length of time between the beats is steady and regular
- *Force:* strength of the beat (weak or bounding)

pulse
rhythmic expansion and contractions of the arteries caused by the beating of the heart

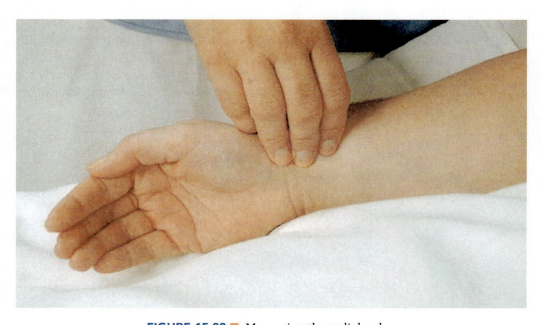

FIGURE 15.23 ■ Measuring the radial pulse.

PROCEDURE 58

Measuring the Radial Pulse

RATIONALE: Correctly measuring a client's pulse is an important part of care.

1. Assemble your equipment:
   Watch with a second hand
   Pad
   Pencil

2. Wash your hands.

3. Tell the client that you are going to take his pulse.

4. If the client is standing, ask him to sit down. Or have him lying in a comfortable position in bed for 5 minutes before you measure the pulse.

5. The client's hand and arm should be well supported and resting comfortably.

6. Find the pulse by placing the tips of your middle three fingers on the palm side of the client's wrist, in line with his thumb directly next to the bone. Press lightly until you feel the beat. (If you press too hard, you may stop the flow of blood and then you will not feel a pulse. Never use your thumb. Your thumb has its own pulse, and you would count it instead of the client's.) When you have found the pulse, notice the rhythm. Note if the beat is

steady or irregular. Notice the force of the beat.

7. Look at the position of the second hand on your watch. Start counting the pulse beats (what you feel) until the second hand comes back to the same number on the clock.
   a. Method A: Count the pulse beats for 1 full minute and report the full-minute count. This is always done if the client has an irregular beat.
   b. Method B: Count for 30 seconds, until the second hand is opposite its position when you started. Then multiply the number of beats by 2. This answer is the number you record. For example, if the count for 30 seconds is 35, the count for 60 seconds is 70 beats.

8. Record the pulse rate, rhythm, and force immediately.

9. Make the client comfortable.

10. Wash your hands.

SAMPLE CHARTING: 7/1/05   7:00 A.M.
Pulse 68 regular
Dina Green H/HHA

apical
refers to the apex of the heart

stethoscope
instrument that allows one to listen to various sounds in the human body

You will use a stethoscope to listen to the **apical** pulse. The apical pulse is the pulse measured at the apex of the heart. The **stethoscope** is an instrument that makes it possible to listen to various sounds in a client's body. The stethoscope is a tube with one end that picks up sound when it is placed against a part of the body. This end is either bell-shaped and called a **bell**, or it is round and flat and is called a **diaphragm** (Figure 15.24 ■).

The apical-radial deficit is the difference between the pulse count at the apex of the heart and the radial artery. This is one way to see if the circulatory system is working properly.

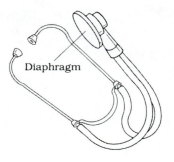
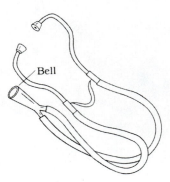

Diaphragm   Bell

FIGURE 15.24 ■ The stethoscope.

Measuring the Apical Pulse

> **RATIONALE:** Correctly measuring a client's pulse is an important part of care.

1. Assemble your equipment:
   Stethoscope
   Antiseptic swabs
   Watch with a second hand
   Pad
   Pencil

2. Wash your hands.

3. Ask visitors to leave the room, if appropriate.

4. Explain to the client that you are going to take his apical pulse.

5. Clean the earpieces of the stethoscope with antiseptic solution. Put the earpieces facing forward in your ears.

6. Uncover the left side of the client's chest. Avoid overexposing the client.

7. Locate the apex of the client's heart by placing the bell or diaphragm of the stethoscope under the client's left breast. Be sure this is the place you hear the heart beating the loudest (Figure 15.25 ■).

8. Count the heart sounds for a full minute.

9. Write the full-minute count on the note paper. Also record the rhythm and the quality of the

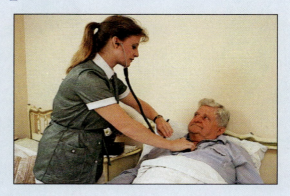

FIGURE 15.25 ■

sounds and your observations concerning the client during this procedure.

10. Cover the client and make him comfortable.

11. Clean the earpieces of the stethoscope. Return the equipment to its proper place.

12. Wash your hands.

> **SAMPLE CHARTING:** 5/17/04   7:00 A.M.
> Apical pulse 60 irregular
> Evelyn Tate H/HHA

Measuring the Apical-Radial Deficit

> **RATIONALE:** Correctly measuring a client's pulse is an important part of care.

1. Assemble your equipment:
   Stethoscope
   Antiseptic swabs
   Watch with a second hand
   Pad
   Pencil

2. Wash your hands.

3. Ask visitors to leave the room, if appropriate.

4. Explain to the client that you are going to take his pulse both apically and radially.

5. There are two methods of taking the apical pulse deficit.

   a. Method A: Two people do this procedure together at the same time. One counts the radial pulse and the other counts the apical pulse for 1 full minute (Figure 15.26 ■). The difference between the two pulses is known as the apical-radial deficit.

   b. Method B: The homemaker/home health aide first takes the apical pulse, then the radial pulse. The difference between the two pulses is known as the apical-radial deficit. Because the readings are not taken at the same time, method B is not considered as accurate as method A.

6. Count the apical pulse and the radial pulse for a full minute, and record both figures.

continued

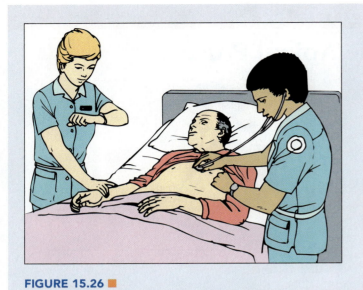

FIGURE 15.26 ■

7. Record the figure for the pulse deficit and your observations concerning the client during this procedure.

8. Make the client comfortable.

9. Clean the equipment and return it to its proper place.

10. Wash your hands.

SAMPLE CHARTING: 8/13/05   10:00 A.M.
Apical pulse 65
Radial pulse is 60
Apical radial deficit is 5
Thelma Green H/HHA and
Sue Johnson RN

SECTION 4

Measuring Respirations

OBJECTIVES

What You Will Learn to Do

1. Count a client's respirations accurately.

2. Determine if the client's breathing is labored or noisy.

Introduction: Measuring Respirations

The human body must have a steady supply of air. When you breathe in, air is drawn into the lungs. The waste products from this process are removed from the body as you exhale.

Respiration is the process of inhaling and exhaling. One respiration includes breathing in once and breathing out once. When a person breathes in, his chest expands. When he breathes out, his chest contracts. When you count respirations, you watch a person's chest rise and fall as he breathes. Or you feel his chest rise and fall with your hand. Either way, you should count respirations without the client knowing it. If he thinks his breathing is being counted, he will not breathe naturally. What you want to count is his natural breathing. Besides counting respirations, you will be noticing whether the client seems to breathe easily or seems to be working hard to breathe. When a person is working hard to breathe, it is called **labored** respiration. You must also notice whether his breathing is noisy.

Normally, adults breathe 16 to 20 times a minute. Children breathe more rapidly. The elderly breathe more slowly. Exercise, digestion, emotional stress, disease conditions, some drugs, stimulants, heat, and cold can all affect the number of times a person breathes per minute.

respiration
process of breathing; inhaling and exhaling air

labored
difficult

ABNORMAL RESPIRATION

While you are counting the client's respirations, it is important to observe and make note of anything about his breathing that appears to be abnormal. Different types of abnormal respiration that you should be familiar with are:

- *Stertorous Respiration.* The client makes abnormal noises such as snoring sounds when he breathes.
- *Abdominal respiration.* The client mostly uses his abdominal muscles to breathe.
- *Shallow respiration.* The client breathes using only the upper part of the lungs.
- *Irregular respiration.* The depth of breathing changes and the chest rise and fall rate is not steady.
- ***Cheyne-Stokes respiration***. At first, the breathing is slow and shallow; then the respiration becomes faster and deeper until it reaches a kind of peak; then the respiration slows down and becomes shallow again. The breathing may then stop completely for 10 seconds and then begin the pattern again. This type of respiration may be caused by certain cerebral (brain), cardiac (heart), or pulmonary (chest) diseases or conditions. It frequently occurs before death.

Cheyne-Stokes respiration
a type of noisy breathing alternating with periods of no breathing; usually precedes death

PROCEDURE 61

Measuring Respirations

RATIONALE: Correctly measuring a client's respirations is an important part of a client's care.

1. Assemble your equipment:
   Watch with a second hand
   Pad
   Pencil

2. Wash your hands.

3. Ask visitors to leave the room, if appropriate.

4. Hold the client's wrist just as if you were taking his pulse. This way he will not know you are watching his breathing. Count the client's respirations, without his knowing it, immediately after counting his pulse rate (Figure 15.27 ■).

5. If the client is a child who has been crying or is restless, wait until he is quiet before counting respirations. If a child is asleep, count his respirations before he wakes up. Always count a child's pulse and respirations before you measure his temperature. (Most children become upset when you measure their temperatures.)

6. One rise and one fall of the client's chest count as one respiration.

7. If you cannot clearly see the chest rise and fall, fold the client's arms across his chest. Then you can feel his breathing as you hold his wrist.

8. Check the position of the second hand on the watch. Count "one" when you see the client's chest rising as he breathes in. The next time

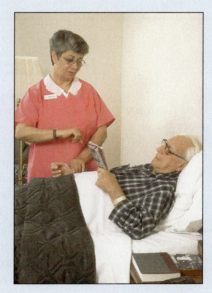

FIGURE 15.27 ■

his chest rises, count "two." Keep doing this for a full minute. Report the number of respirations you count.

9. You may be permitted to count for 30 seconds. Count the respirations for 30 seconds and then multiply the number you counted by 2. For example, if you count 8 respirations in

continued

30 seconds (a half-minute), your number for a full minute is 16.

10. If the client's breathing rhythm is irregular, always count for a full minute. Observe the depth of the breathing while counting the respirations.

11. Immediately write down the number you counted.

12. Note whether the respirations were noisy or labored and your observations concerning the client during this procedure.

13. Make the client comfortable.

14. Wash your hands.

> **SAMPLE CHARTING:** 9/1/05   7:30 A.M.
> Respirations 20 regular
> Gloria Gross H/HHA

SECTION 5

Measuring Blood Pressure

OBJECTIVES

What You Will Learn to Do

1. Explain systolic pressure.
2. Explain diastolic pressure.
3. Demonstrate the use of aneroid and mercury types of blood pressure equipment accurately and efficiently.
4. Measure a client's blood pressure accurately.

Introduction: Blood Pressure

blood pressure
force of blood on the inner walls of blood vessels as it flows through them

Blood pressure is the force of the blood pushing against the walls of the blood vessels. When you take a client's blood pressure, you are measuring the force of the blood flowing through the arteries.

There is always a certain amount of pressure in the arteries. This is because the heart, by pumping, is constantly forcing blood to circulate. The amount of pressure in the arteries depends on two things: the rate of heartbeat, and how easily the blood flows through the blood vessels.

systolic pressure
force with which blood is pumped when the heart contracts

diastolic pressure
the pressure in the blood vessels measured when the heart is relaxed

The heart contracts as it pumps the blood into the arteries. When the heart is contracting, the pressure is highest. This pressure is called the **systolic pressure**. As the heart relaxes between each contraction, the pressure decreases. When the heart is most relaxed, the pressure is lowest. This pressure is called the **diastolic pressure**. When you take a client's blood pressure, you are measuring these two pressures.

In young, healthy adults less than 40 years old, the normal blood pressure range is below 140 millimeters (mm) mercury (Hg) systolic pressure and below 90 millimeters (mm) mercury (Hg) diastolic pressure. These figures are written:

140/90 or 140 = systolic
90 = diastolic

In adults more than 40 years old, 160/90 or less is considered normal.

hypertension
high blood pressure

hypotension
low blood pressure

When a person's blood pressure is higher than the normal range for his or her age and condition, it is referred to as high blood pressure or **hypertension**. When a client's blood pressure is lower than the normal range for his age and condition, it is referred to as low blood pressure or **hypotension**. One reading

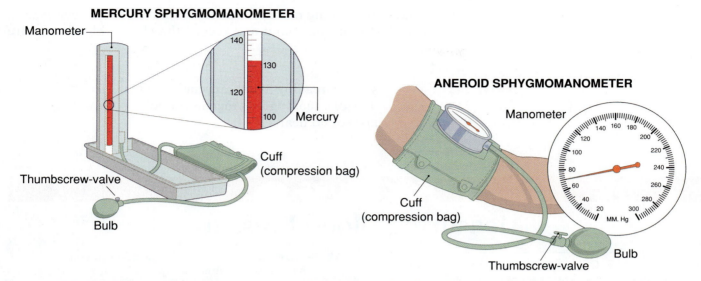

FIGURE 15.28 ■ Sphygmomanometers may look different, but they all measure blood pressure accurately.

of high blood pressure does not mean that a person has hypertension. This diagnosis can only be made by a physician after a complete medical evaluation.

INSTRUMENTS FOR MEASURING BLOOD PRESSURE

When you take a client's blood pressure, you will use an instrument called a **sphygmomanometer**. Sphygmomanometer is a combination of three Greek words:

1. *Sphygmo,* meaning pulse
2. *Mano,* meaning pressure
3. *Meter,* meaning measure

This instrument, however, is usually called simply the **blood pressure cuff**. The four main parts of this instrument are the manometer, valve, cuff, and bulb (Figure 15.28 ■).

Two kinds of instruments are used for taking blood pressure. One is the **mercury** type. The other is called the **aneroid** (dial) type. Both kinds have an inflatable cloth-covered rubber bag or cuff. The cuff is wrapped around the client's arm. Both kinds also have a rubber bulb for pumping air into the cuff. The procedure for measuring blood pressure is the same, except for reading the measurement. When you use the mercury type, you watch the level of a column of mercury or liquid on a measuring scale. When you use the dial or aneroid type, you watch a pointer on a dial.

When you take a client's blood pressure, you do two things at the same time. You listen to the brachial pulse as it sounds in the brachial artery in the client's arm. You also watch an indicator (either a column of mercury or a dial) in order to take a reading.

You use a stethoscope to listen to the brachial pulse. It is important to note the first tapping sound you hear and the last sound you hear. Sometimes, you will hear a tapping sound, then silence, then a tapping sound again. The true reading is the first sound you hear. Often, the first sound is missed through improper technique, and only the second sound is heard and recorded. By following the procedure in this book carefully, you will not miss the first sound and will record an accurate and truthful blood pressure.

sphygmomanometer
apparatus for measuring blood pressure of which there are two types, mercury or aneroid; blood pressure cuff

blood pressure cuff
another term for sphygmomanometer

mercury
one type of sphygmomanometer

aneroid
one type of sphygmomanometer

If you should hear the tapping noise all the way to the "O" on your indicator, try to listen for a change in the sound and record the client's blood pressure reading as follows:

142/72/0

142	systolic reading—first tapping sound heard
72	diastolic reading—change in sound
0	last sound heard

PROCEDURE 62

Measuring Blood Pressure

RATIONALE: Correctly measuring a client's blood pressure is an important part of client care.

This procedure is based on the article "Hypertension—What Can Go Wrong When You Measure Blood Pressure," *American Journal of Nursing* 8, no. 5 (1980): 942–945.

1. Assemble your equipment:
   Sphygmomanometer (blood pressure cuff)
   Stethoscope
   Antiseptic pad to clean earpieces of stethoscope
   Pad
   Pencil

2. Wash your hands.

3. Tell the client that you are going to take his blood pressure.

4. Wipe the earpieces of the stethoscope with the antiseptic pad.

5. Have the client resting quietly. He should be either lying down or sitting in a chair.

6. If you are using the mercury apparatus, the measuring scale should be level with your eyes.

7. The client's arm should be bare up to the shoulder or the client's sleeve should be well above the elbow.

8. The client's arm from the elbow down should be resting fully extended on the bed, the arm of the chair, or your hip, well supported, with the palm upward.

9. Unroll the cuff and loosen the valve on the bulb. Then squeeze the compression bag to deflate it completely.

10. Wrap the cuff snugly and smoothly around the client's arm above the elbow. Do not wrap it so tightly that the client is uncomfortable from the pressure.

11. Leave the area clear where you will place the bell or diaphragm of the stethoscope.

12. Be sure the manometer is in position so you can read the numbers easily.

13. With your fingertips, find the client's brachial pulse at the inner side of the arm above the elbow. Hold the bell or diaphragm there and inflate the cuff until the pulse disappears. Note the reading on the indicator. Quickly deflate the cuff. This is the approximation of the client's systolic reading and is called the palpated systolic pressure (Figure 15.29 ■).

14. Put the earpieces of the stethoscope into your ears and place the bell or diaphragm of the stethoscope on the brachial pulse. Hold it snugly but not too tightly. Do not let the stethoscope touch the blood pressure cuff.

15. Tighten the thumbscrew of the valve to close it. Turn it clockwise. Be careful not to turn it too tightly. If you do, you will have trouble opening it.

16. Hold the stethoscope in place. Inflate the cuff until the dial points to 30 mm above the palpated systolic pressure.

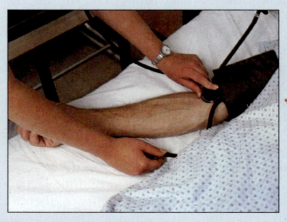

FIGURE 15.29 ■ Part of taking a client's blood pressure is listening to his brachial pulse.

17. Open the valve counterclockwise. This allows the air to escape. Let it out slowly until the sound of the pulse comes back. A few seconds must go by without sounds. If you do hear pulse sounds immediately, you must stop the procedure. Then completely deflate the cuff. Wait a few seconds. Then inflate the cuff to a much higher calibration above 200. Again, loosen the thumbscrew to let the air out. Listen for a repeated pulse sound. At the same time, watch the indicator.

18. Note the calibration that the pointer passes as you hear the first sound. This point indicates the systolic pressure (or the top number).

19. Continue releasing the air from the cuff. When the sounds change to a softer and faster thud or disappear, note the calibration. This is the diastolic pressure (or bottom number).

20. Deflate the cuff completely. Remove it from the client's arm.

21. Record your reading on the client's chart.

22. After using the blood pressure cuff, roll it up over the manometer and replace it in the case.

23. Wipe the earpieces of the stethoscope again with an antiseptic swab. Put the stethoscope back in its proper place.

24. Wash your hands.

25. Record the blood pressure and your observations concerning the client during this procedure.

SAMPLE CHARTING: 2/18/05   4:00 P.M.
Blood pressure 144/88
Sydney Jones H/HHA

Pain Management

OBJECTIVES	
What You Will Learn to Do	1. Identify signs of a client in pain.
	2. Demonstrate reporting pain on the "1/10" scale.
	3. Assist the client with pain medication.

Introduction: Pain Management

Every person has the right to be free of pain. That means that we as health professionals have the responsibility to identify, record, and report the presence of pain and take steps to remove the pain. Everyone experiences pain daily and responds differently to it. Response to pain is an intricate and personal experience. It is the result of personal experiences, health status, and cultural norms. Other influencing factors could be age, family dynamics, and time of day.

Do not compare one client with another. Some people accept pain as normal, some think it is a punishment, and some think it indicates they are getting better. Be objective and nonjudgmental when the client discusses his personal experience.

Clients in pain are unable to participate in rehabilitation, interact with others, or maintain a feeling of control or well-being.

ACUTE AND CHRONIC PAIN

Acute pain is usually short in duration. It has a beginning and an end. An example is pain after an operation. The pain starts after the surgery and is gone when healing is completed.

Chronic pain is always present. The condition that causes this pain is usually chronic, also. An example would be arthritis pain. This pain can be relieved and may even disappear for a time, but will return.

MEDICATION

Each health professional and each client has a different point of view about pain medication. It is important for you to know your point of view of pain and pain medication. Be nonjudgmental as the client and family discuss the situation in the house. Discuss the situation and the plan with your supervisor. If you are not comfortable with the plan, discuss this with your supervisor.

- Be consistent. Follow the plan. Do not change the plan without discussing it with your supervisor or having the client discuss it with the physician.
- Plan your care around administration of medication so that the client will be most comfortable. Discuss this with the client and together you will determine the best schedule for care and medication.
- Observe your client's reaction to the medication. If the reaction is not what is expected, report it to your supervisor immediately!
- If the client is not taking the medication as ordered, report this to your supervisor immediately!

FAMILY DYNAMICS

The ways in which people within a family interact affect their tolerance of and reaction to pain. Some families shun people in pain, some families cater to people in pain, some people see acceptance of pain as "manly"; and some people see acceptance of pain as part of life and do nothing about it. It is important to try to understand how the family treats a person in pain. This will help you and your supervisor determine the best plan of care for the client in his family unit.

MEASURING PAIN

The reporting of pain is strongly subjective. Each of us has his own definition of what is mild pain, bearable pain, and horrible pain. A scale used within the health care industry to quantify pain goes from 1 to 10, with 10 being the worst pain imaginable. (Children use faces instead of numbers.) When asking the client if he is in pain, ask him to rate the pain on this scale. Then report that number. Be sure to record the time of day and the number. It may also be important to record what the client was doing. Having this record will let you compare one day with the next and notice any changes.

It is also important to note other changes in the client that indicate the status of his pain:

breathing pattern	facial expression
skin: dry, clammy, or sweaty	tone of voice
body position	

Your Role as a Homemaker/Home Health Aide

The support and reinforcement you give the client are your most important activities. Your careful observation and the reporting of this to your supervisor will help the plan remain current. Encourage the client to discuss his reaction to pain. Encourage him to continue to try medication and other methods such as relaxation to relieve the pain. Continually observe the client and the environment to be sure it is safe. Some clients try "alternative methods" for pain control. They buy machines, eat unusual foods, or practice rituals. Discuss these with your supervisor, and the two of you can determine if they are harmful or not.

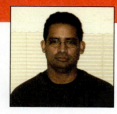

Case Study

Review the case study that appears on the first page of the chapter. Answer two sets of questions about the case study contained in the Explore and Apply sections below.

EXPLORE

1. You visit the Alvarez home twice a week to monitor Mr. Alvarez's blood pressure and assist his wife with maintaining the prescribed diet. Each time, you see markedly different readings for the blood pressure even though you take it the same way. What questions would you ask the client to help you understand the variations? Would you document this conversation?

2. Mrs. Alvarez says the physician's readings are different from yours. What do you reply?

APPLY

1. Mr. Alvarez shows you a new medication he bought through the mail and says he is going to try it along with his usual prescribed medication. What is your response?

2. On your visit to the Alvarez home, Mr. Alvarez refuses to let you take his blood pressure. He says he is afraid he will lose his job because of the high readings you have been recording. How do you respond? What do you do when you leave the house?

Certification Exam Review Questions

Choose the best answer for each question or statement.

1. **Vital signs are**
   a. *all the temperature readings for a month.*
   b. *blood pressure readings for the year.*
   c. *respirations after exercise.*
   d. *considered temperature, blood pressure, and respirations.*

2. **A client asks you what his vital signs are. You reply:**
   a. *"I can only report them to my supervisor."*
   b. *"You will not understand them, so don't worry."*
   c. *"Your temperature is 98 degrees orally; your blood pressure is 122/60, and your respirations are 22. Do you have any questions?"*
   d. *"I only take them because it makes your daughter happy. They don't mean much anyway."*

3. **You are used to using a digital thermometer that measures a client's temperature from his ear. Your client, however, only has a glass oral thermometer. You,**
   a. *ask him to buy a digital thermometer.*
   b. *use the glass thermometer.*
   c. *borrow a digital thermometer from your last client.*
   d. *ask your supervisor if his daughter can take his temperature so you do not have to use the glass thermometer.*

4. **You have taken three clients' blood pressures today, and each of them have been significantly different from the previous ones.**
   a. *You attribute this difference to the holiday season and their excitement.*
   b. *You note the differences and take your blood pressure cuff to be checked by your office.*
   c. *You leave your blood pressure cuff in the car overnight and go back and check the client's blood pressure the next day.*
   d. *You don't do anything about it.*

5. **A glass thermometer slips out of your hands and breaks in the bathroom.**
   a. *You close the bathroom door and call your office for instructions.*
   b. *You sweep up the glass and the mercury. Put it in a plastic bag and mark it "Hazardous material."*
   c. *You clean up the material and flush it down the toilet.*
   d. *You sweep up the material and throw away the material and the broom.*

CHAPTER 16

Intake and Output

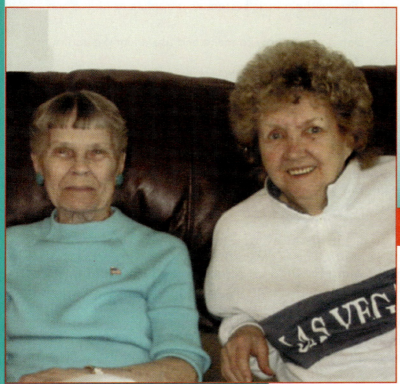

CASE STUDY

Mrs. Oates, an elderly widow, lives with her older sister, Ms. Davis, in the family home on a large piece of land. Living in this rural area has been a family tradition, and both Mrs. Oates and her sister will not discuss leaving the house or hiring help to maintain it. Several nieces and nephews live in the city about 50 miles away and visit infrequently. Mrs. Oates is receiving chemotherapy for cancer and seems to be tolerating it well. She is grateful to the Red Cross person who drives her to the city every week for the treatment. Ms. Davis, although she is older, appears able to cook the meals and do the laundry. A local church member does the shopping weekly and brings it to the sisters. The sisters enjoy listening to the radio, watching television, and talking to their dog, Lucky.

Keep the case study in mind as you read the chapter. After you have read the chapter, answer the Explore and Apply questions at the end of the chapter that relate to the case study.

SECTION 1

Fluid Balance

OBJECTIVES

What You Will Learn to Do

1. Explain fluid balance and imbalance.
2. List the factors that affect intake and output.
3. List the reasons for keeping accurate records of intake and output.
4. Discuss the metric system as it applies to intake and output.
5. Demonstrate how to make and use an intake and output record.

Introduction: Fluid Balance

fluid intake
liquid taken into the body

fluid output
liquid excreted by
the body

fluid balance
the relationship of intake
fluid with excreted fluid
output

edema
abnormal swelling of
a part of the body
caused by fluid collecting
in that area

dehydration
condition in which the
body has less than normal
amount of fluid

Water is essential to human life. Next to oxygen, water is the most important nutrient the body requires. A person can lose half his body protein and almost half his weight and still live, but losing only one-fifth of his body fluid will result in death.

Through eating and drinking, the average healthy adult will take in about 3½ quarts of fluid every 24 hours. This is called **fluid intake**. The average adult also will eliminate about 3½ quarts of fluid every 24 hours. This is **fluid output**. The human body has several ways of keeping the amount of fluid it eliminates balanced with the amount of fluid it takes in. This balance is what allows the body to continue to function in a healthy state. When this balance is disturbed, the body is said to be in a state of **fluid imbalance** (Figure 16.1 ■). In some medical conditions fluid may be held by the body tissues. This causes swelling and is called **edema**. In other conditions much fluid can be lost, and this is called **dehydration**. Fluids can be discharged from the body through:

- The kidneys in the form of urine
- The skin in the form of perspiration
- The lungs during breathing
- The intestinal tract

REASONS FOR KEEPING RECORDS OF FLUID BALANCE

When a person is healthy, the fluid balancing system works by itself; however, when a person is ill or disabled, this system often does not function to its maximum. Accurate records of an individual's intake and output indicate how his fluid balancing system is functioning. Many factors can affect the fluid balance system:

- Medication
- Emotional stress
- Exercise
- Nourishment
- Weather
- General health

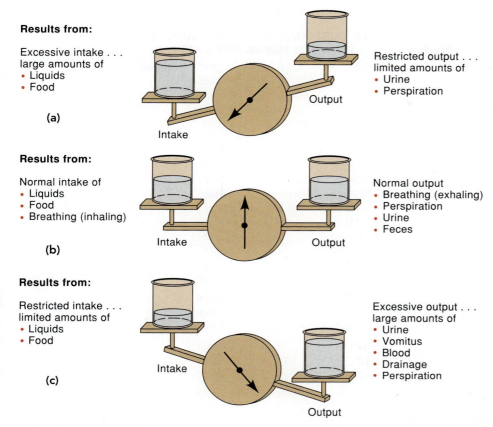

Results from:

Excessive intake . . .
large amounts of
• Liquids
• Food

(a)

Intake

Output

Restricted output . . .
limited amounts of
• Urine
• Perspiration

Results from:

Normal intake of
• Liquids
• Food
• Breathing (inhaling)

(b)

Intake

Output

Normal output
• Breathing (exhaling)
• Perspiration
• Urine
• Feces

Results from:

Restricted intake . . .
limited amounts of
• Liquids
• Food

(c)

Intake

Output

Excessive output . . .
large amounts of
• Urine
• Vomitus
• Blood
• Drainage
• Perspiration

FIGURE 16.1 ■ (a) Intake exceeds output; (b) Intake equals output; (c) Intake is less than output.

THE METRIC SYSTEM OF MEASUREMENT

You probably have already noticed that many quantities used in the health-care field are measured in cubic centimeters. Because this method of measurement is used more and more, you should understand what it means (Figure 16.2 ■).

The term *cc* is an abbreviation for **cubic centimeter**, a unit of measurement in the metric system. The **metric system** of measurement is used in many countries of the world. In the United States, we normally use one system for measuring liquids (ounces, pints, quarts, and gallons) and a different system for measuring lengths (inches, feet, yards, and miles). Scientists, engineers, and many health-care personnel use the metric system for measuring liquid, length, and weight. The basic unit of measurement is the meter, which is a little longer than the yard. A centimeter (one one-hundredth [$\frac{1}{100}$] of a meter) is about four-tenths ($\frac{4}{10}$) of an inch long.

A cubic centimeter can be thought of as a square block with each edge of the block 1 centimeter long. If we filled this block with water, we would have a cubic centimeter (1 cc) of water. The list in Figure 16.2 includes liquid amounts with which you are probably familiar. It also gives about the same amounts in cubic centimeters.

MAKING AN INTAKE AND OUTPUT SHEET

The amounts of **intake** and **output** (I&O) are written on a special sheet of paper. It is called the intake and output sheet and is usually kept near the client's bed. Some agencies have special forms for this purpose; some do not.

cubic centimeter
a unit of measure used in the metric system

metric system
a method of measuring temperature, length, and volume of fluid which is based on the decimal system

intake
all substances ingested by the body, sometimes refers only to fluid consumed

output
material discharged from the body, may refer only to fluids

U.S. CUSTOMARY LIQUID MEASURE WITH EQUIVALENT METRIC MEASUREMENTS

cc	=	cubic centimeter
ml	=	milliliter
oz	=	ounce
1 cc	=	1 ml
1/4 teaspoon	=	1 cc
1 teaspoon	=	4 cc
30 cc	=	1 oz
60 cc	=	2 oz
90 cc	=	3 oz
120 cc	=	4 oz
150 cc	=	5 oz
180 cc	=	6 oz
210 cc	=	7 oz
240 cc	=	8 oz
270 cc	=	9 oz
300 cc	=	10 oz
500 cc	=	1 pint
1,000 cc	=	1 quart
4,000 cc	=	1 gallon
pt	=	pint
qt	=	quart
gal	=	gallon

FIGURE 16.2 ■ Liquid measurements must be recorded and reported on the same measurement scale.

The illustration will give you a guide as to how to make up an I&O sheet in the client's home (Figure 16.3 ■). The intake and output sheet is divided into two parts, intake on the left and output on the right. After measuring intake and output, you will record the amount in the proper column. You will also indicate the time and what was drunk or expelled. The amounts in each column are totaled every 24 hours.

Starting an Intake and Output Record

A 24-hour intake record is started with the first fluids the client drinks in the morning. The first urinary output of the morning, however, is considered a part of the previous day's I&O because the fluid that formed the urine was consumed within the previous 24 hours. Therefore, the first urine recorded on the output sheet will actually be the second urination of the day.

Responsibility for Keeping an I&O Record

The responsibility for keeping an accurate I&O record is a shared one. A family member must be taught to keep the record when you are not in the home. It is most important that all people who write on the sheet use the same procedure; otherwise, the total will not be accurate. If you are asked to keep additional information, such as the amount of solid food the client eats, your supervisor will show you how to do it.

Usually, the supervisor of your client's case will teach the family members how to keep a simple I&O record. You will, of course, have to answer any questions they may have and reinforce the teaching. Be sure to report to your supervisor any difficulty the family may have with keeping the records.

Client name _____			Date _____		
INTAKE			OUTPUT		
Time		Amt.	Time		Amt.
Total			Total		

FIGURE 16.3 ■ Intake and output sheet.

SECTION 2

Fluid Intake

OBJECTIVES

What You Will Learn to Do

1. List the fluids considered as intake.
2. Measure fluids accurately.
3. Demonstrate that you can accurately measure and record intake.

Introduction: Fluid Intake

Although solid foods also contain liquid, most fluids in the body are taken in when a person drinks liquids. A client's intake includes all liquids (Figure 16.4 ■).

HOW MUCH DOES EACH SERVING CONTAINER HOLD?

A container or measuring cup is used to measure intake and output. It is marked or **calibrated** with a row of short lines and numbers. These show the amount of liquid in both cubic centimeters and ounces. You can use a regular measuring cup. Another calibrated container may be a baby bottle. Be sure that you use one container to measure intake and a different one for output.

calibration
graduations on a measuring instrument

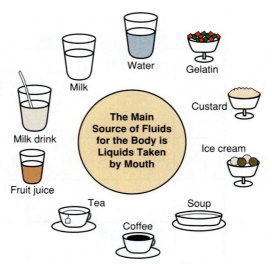

The Main Source of Fluids for the Body is Liquids Taken by Mouth

Water
Gelatin
Custard
Milk
Ice cream
Milk drink
Soup
Fruit juice
Tea
Coffee

FIGURE 16.4 ■
Fluid intake includes many things. Record all of them.

To record accurately the exact amounts of fluids taken by the client, you will have to measure the amount of liquid contained in each serving container, bowl, glass, and cup the client uses. It is helpful to make a list of how much each one contains. Then you can refer to it rather than measuring the liquid each time you fill the container.

PROCEDURE 63

Measuring the Capacity of Serving Containers

RATIONALE: Knowing the capacity of serving containers aids accurate planning for client intake.

1. Assemble your equipment:
   Complete set of dishes, bowls, cups, and glasses used by the client
   Measuring cup
   Water
   Pen
   Paper
2. Fill the first container with water.
3. Pour this water into the measuring cup.

4. Look at the level of the water and determine the amount in cc (cubic centimeters).
5. Write this information on the paper. For example, a carton of milk equals 240 cc.
6. Repeat these steps for each dish, glass, bowl, or cup used by the client.

SAMPLE CHARTING: 9/9/05   8:30 A.M.
Seven serving containers measured. Capacity indicated on list on refrigerator.
Elaine Coors H/HHA

MEASURING FLUID INTAKE

Tell the client that his intake is being measured. Encourage him to help you as much as he can by asking him to keep track of how much liquid he drinks. Record the fluid intake as soon as the client has consumed the fluids. Do not wait. You will forget. Think about fluid intake every time you remove a tray, glass, or cup.

When measuring fluid intake, you will have to note the difference between the amount the client drinks and the amount he leaves in the serving container.

It is a good idea to list the intake and output in the same unit of measurement. If you keep the output in cc, record the intake in cc, too. If you keep the output in ounces, also record the intake in ounces.

PROCEDURE 64

Determining the Amounts Consumed

RATIONALE: Correctly measuring and recording intake assists in determining the client's ability to process fluid.

1. Assemble your equipment:
   Measuring cup
   Pen
   Paper
   Leftover liquids in serving containers
2. Pour the leftover liquid into the measuring cup.
3. Look at the level and determine the amount in cc.
4. From your list, determine the amount in the full serving container.

5. Subtract the leftover amount from the full container amount. This figure is the amount the client actually drank.
6. Immediately report this amount on the intake side of the intake and output sheet.

SAMPLE CHARTING:	9/9/05 8:30 A.M.–2:30 P.M.
9:00 A.M.	4 oz orange juice
	6 oz decaffeinated tea
	2 oz milk
11:00 A.M.	8 oz chicken soup
2:00 P.M.	6 oz water
2:30 P.M.	4 oz water
	Elaine Coors H/HHA

SECTION 3

Fluid Output

| **OBJECTIVES**
What You Will Learn to Do	1. List the fluids considered output.
	2. Demonstrate the technique for measuring and recording output.

Introduction: Measuring Fluid Output

Fluid output is the sum total of liquids that come out of the body. Most fluid is discharged from the body as urine. Other terms for this bodily function are "void" or "pass water." Output also includes **emesis (vomitus)**, drainage from a wound, loss of blood, and excessive perspiration. Every time your client uses the urinal, emesis basin, or bedpan, the urine and other fluids must be measured.

You should tell a client his output is being measured and ask him to cooperate. All clients who are measuring their output must urinate in a bedpan, urinal, or container. Ask the client not to place toilet paper in this container. Provide a

emesis
vomitus

vomitus
material that is vomited; emesis

plastic bag for this purpose. Then dispose of the tissue into the toilet. If at all possible, ask your client not to move his bowels while urinating.

DOCUMENTING FLUID OUTPUT

It is important to notice all qualities about the urine when you measure it. If the urine should change, this is also important and should be reported immediately. Some medications can change the color of urine. Some foods can change the odor of urine. Discuss this with your supervisor so you know what to expect and what is "usual" for a client.

- Color
- Odor
- With particles or clear
- Amount

PROCEDURE 65

Measuring Urinary Output

RATIONALE: Measuring urinary output is one way to assist in assessing the body's ability to maintain fluid balance.

1. Assemble your equipment:
   Bedpan and cover or urinal or container for urine
   Disposable gloves
   Measuring container
   Pad
   Pencil

2. Wash your hands and put on gloves.

3. Pour the urine from the bedpan or urinal into the measuring container.

4. Place the container on a flat surface for accuracy in measurement.

5. At eye level, carefully look at the container to see the number reached by the level of urine. Remember it.

6. Rinse and return the measuring container to its proper place. (Pour the urine and the rinse water into the toilet.)

7. Rinse and return the urinal or bedpan to its proper place. (Pour the rinse water into the toilet.)

8. Remove gloves and dispose of them. Wash your hands.

9. Record the amount of urine in cc and the character of the urine on the output side of the I&O sheet.

SAMPLE CHARTING: 8/5/05 8:30 P.M.
230 cc yellow urine voided without difficulty.
Walter George H/HHA

MEASURING OUTPUT FROM AN INDWELLING CATHETER

catheter
a tube used to remove body fluids from a cavity

Sometimes, a client has a **catheter** (tube) inserted into his urinary bladder by the doctor or nurse. This catheter drains all the client's urine into a plastic urine container, which hangs below the level of the urinary bladder (Figure 16.5 ■ and Figure 16.6 ■). You will empty this container, measure the urine for amount, and record the amount. This will always be done whenever it is full and always before the end of your working shift. The measurement is not taken from the soft, expandable, plastic urine container. A hard plastic container is always used, as it is more accurate.

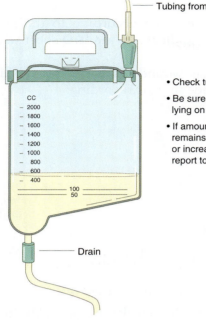

Tubing from the client

CC
— 2000
— 1800
— 1600
— 1400
— 1200
— 1000
— 800
— 600
— 400
—————100
—————50

• Check tubing for obstructions.
• Be sure client is not lying on tubing.
• If amount of urine remains the same or increases rapidly, report to nurse.

Drain

FIGURE 16.5 ■ A plastic urine collection container should be hung on the bed frame below the level of the bladder.

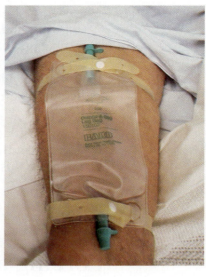

FIGURE 16.6 ■ Leg drainage bag for ambulatory patient.

PROCEDURE 66

Emptying a Urinary Collection Bag from an Indwelling Catheter

RATIONALE: Periodically emptying a collection bag is an important step in determining the patency of the catheter and in preventing infection.

1. Assemble your equipment:
   Measuring container
   Paper towels
   Pad
   Pencil
2. Wash your hands.
3. Protect the floor with paper towels.
4. Open the drain at the bottom of the plastic urine container and let the urine run into the measuring cup. Then close the drain. Be sure the urine does not touch the floor. Be sure the tubing from the catheter bag does not touch the floor.

5. Place the measuring container on a flat surface for accuracy in measurement.
6. At eye level, carefully look at the container to see the level of urine. Remember it.
7. Rinse the measuring container and put it in its proper place. (Put the urine and rinse water into the toilet.)
8. Wash your hands.
9. Record the time, amount in cc, and anything unusual concerning the urine on the output side of the I&O sheet.

SAMPLE CHARTING: 7/4/05   7:30 A.M.
Collection bag emptied of 500 cc yellow urine. No blood or sediment noted.
Ruth Jacobs H/HHA

Fluid Output from the Incontinent Client

If the client is **incontinent** (cannot control bowels and/or urine), record this on the output side of the I&O sheet each time the bed is wet. Even though the urine cannot be measured, it will be obvious that the client's kidneys are functioning.

incontinence
the inability to control one's bowel movements or urination

Measuring Fluids Other than Urine

Vomitus and diarrhea are also measured according to the procedure for measuring urinary output. Be sure to indicate on the I&O sheet what fluid you are recording.

If a client bleeds a great deal, has wound discharge, or perspires heavily, indicate this on the I&O sheet. Include in your recording:

- What was wet
- How wet (damp, dripping, etc.)
- The size of the wet area
- The time this occurred

SECTION 4

Forcing and Restricting Fluids

OBJECTIVES

What You Will Learn to Do

1. Explain the terms *force fluids* and *restrict fluids*.

2. Demonstrate the homemaker/home health aide's role when a client is on restricted fluids.

3. Demonstrate the homemaker/home health aide's role when a client is to force fluids.

Introduction: Balancing Fluid Intake

force fluids
extra fluids taken in according to a doctor's orders

Clients who need fluids added to their normal intake are told to **force fluids**. Fluids should never be forced or restricted without discussing this with your supervisor first. FF is the abbreviation for force fluids. A client who is to force fluids often needs encouragement to drink. Be sure you know how much fluid the client is to have within a 24-hour period. Some ways you can assist the client to drink the amount of fluids are:

- Show enthusiasm and be cheerful
- Provide different kinds of liquids that the client prefers, as permitted
- Offer liquids without being asked
- Offer hot and cold drinks
- Offer liquids in divided amounts; for example, 800 cc every 8 hours means the client ought to drink 100 cc an hour

Record the amount taken in by the client in cc and on the intake side of the I&O. Report to your supervisor if the client is unable to drink the amount required.

Some clients must restrict their fluid intake. This means that fluids must be limited to a certain amount. Follow orders and measure accurately. Your calm and reassuring attitude can make a big difference in how the client feels and reacts.

- Record the amount of intake on the intake side of the I&O sheet.
- Frequent oral hygiene is often necessary.
- Discuss with your supervisor the client's reaction to this restriction.
- If the restriction is severe, the client may be permitted to suck on ice chips or candy. Check with your supervisor before you start any of these practices.

Straining Urine

OBJECTIVES		
What You Will Learn to Do	1.	Explain why urine may be strained.
	2.	Demonstrate the correct procedure for straining and labeling the urine.

Introduction: Straining Urine

You may be asked to strain urine after you have measured it or you may be instructed to only strain it. In either case, you will collect the urine in the same manner as if you were to measure it. Be sure the client knows he is to save all his urine and has a container available. The toilet tissue should not be dropped into the container with the urine but disposed of in a plastic bag. The client should not move his bowels at the same time or the specimen is useless.

PROCEDURE 67

Straining Urine

RATIONALE: Collecting the sediment in urine is important in noting calculi (stones).

1. Assemble your equipment.
   Disposable paper strainers or gauze that fits into the container
   Specimen container with label
   Urine specimen
   Disposable gloves

2. Wash your hands.

3. Put on gloves.

4. Pour the urine through the strainer into a calibrated container (Figure 16.7 ■).

5. Put the strainer with any particles into the specimen container. Do not remove any particles.

6. Record the amount of urine measured, if appropriate. Record the date and time of the collection.

7. Discard the urine.

8. Clean the containers.

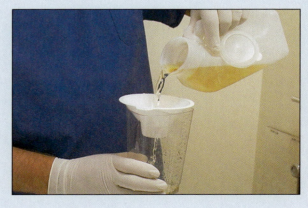

FIGURE 16.7 ■

9. Put the specimen in the appropriate place until it can be sent/taken to the laboratory.

10. Remove gloves and wash hands.

SAMPLE CHARTING:	2/7/05 7:30 A.M.
	300 cc pink-tinged urine strained. Sediment saved in specimen jar for nurse.
	Irene Beatty H/HHA

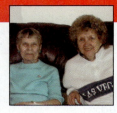

Case Study

Review the case study that appears on the first page of the chapter. Answer two sets of questions about the case study contained in the Explore and Apply sections below.

EXPLORE

1. You visit each morning to assist the sisters with personal care, make general observations, and help organize their day. You notice that Mrs. Oates' urine is dark in color and has a strong odor. When you question her, she says she does not have time to drink fluids. Why should Mrs. Oates increase her fluid intake? How will Mrs. Oates know she has increased her fluid intake sufficiently? What types of fluids would you encourage her to drink?

2. One morning, you meet Mrs. Oates's nephew. He questions you about his aunts' status. You share with him your concern about the small amount of fluids his aunt drinks. He asks how he can help. What do you tell him?

APPLY

1. While Mrs. Oates is having chemotherapy, you have the opportunity to assist Ms. Davis with her bath and talk with her. How would you display concern for this client and also enlist her help in increasing her sister's fluid intake?

2. How would you set up a documentation system for the sisters so that they could readily see what they drink and you could review it each morning when you arrive?

Certification Exam Review Questions

Choose the best answer for each question or statement.

1. **Maintaining fluid balance is important. Therefore you should**

    a. *set up an intake and output chart for every client.*

    b. *observe intake and output for each client and report to your supervisor if you notice something unusual for that client.*

    c. *insist that all clients drink water with their meals.*

    d. *carry water with you and drink it while you work.*

2. **In order to maintain an accurate intake and output record,**

    a. *instruct your client and his family that you will measure all urine.*

    b. *allow your client to drink only from a glass that you have measured.*

    c. *teach a member of the family or your client to measure intake and output when you are not in the house.*

    d. *let the family estimate intake and output when you are not in the house.*

3. **If your client has an indwelling catheter, forcing fluids will**

    a. *not be your responsibility and should not be initiated unless the client has been told to do so by his physician.*

    b. *only result in you having to empty the bag more often.*

    c. *help the client maintain the patency of the catheter and help decrease the risk of infection.*

    d. *help the client if it is done during the day but not at night.*

4. **Once the intake and output sheets are completed,**

    a. *they should be attached to the documentation and turned in to the office.*

    b. *they should be sent to the physician's office.*

    c. *they should be left in the home.*

    d. *you will be told what to do with them.*

5. **If a client voids in the toilet and does not measure his urine,**

    a. *forget about it and start keeping track of the urine next time he voids.*

    b. *indicate on the sheet that a specimen was not counted.*

    c. *call the supervisor so she can insert a catheter.*

    d. *keep the client in bed and do not let him use the toilet again.*

CHAPTER 17

Specimen Collection

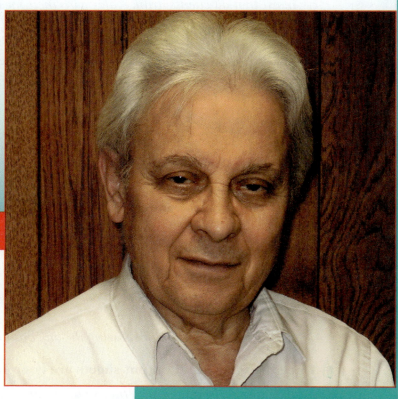

CASE STUDY

Mr. Hogan lives with his wife and son, Ronald, in a large house. Ronald suffered a diving accident when he was 15 and has been mentally challenged since then. Although he can care for himself when reminded, he cannot live independently. The Hogans have a housekeeper who has been with them for many years. She does the cooking and the cleaning. Now that Mr. Hogan is becoming more and more forgetful, the housekeeper and Mrs. Hogan share the work and the care of Mr. Hogan and Ronald.

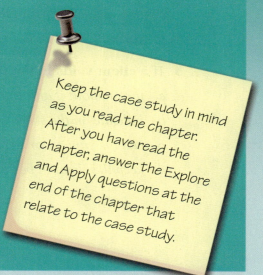

Keep the case study in mind as you read the chapter. After you have read the chapter, answer the Explore and Apply questions at the end of the chapter that relate to the case study.

Specimen Collection

OBJECTIVES	1. Explain the term *specimens*.
What You Will Learn to Do	2. Collect specimens correctly.

Introduction: Specimen Collection

As one of its natural functions, the human body regularly rids itself of various waste materials. Most of the wastes are discharged in the form of urine and feces. The body also discharges waste in sputum, which is coughed up from the lungs.

When bodily wastes are tested in the laboratory, changes in the body function can be detected. The doctor uses this information to decide on an appropriate treatment for the client. **Specimens** are samples of bodily products that are collected and sent to the laboratory for examination.

When you are collecting a specimen, you must be accurate in following the procedure and labeling the specimen. You have to collect the specimen at exactly the right time. The name of the client, his address, the date, and the time of specimen collection should be printed on the label in clear letters. This label must be attached securely to the specimen container. All laboratories throw away unlabeled specimens. If this happens, another one will have to be collected, resulting in extra time and cost for the client.

Many specimens must be stored in the home for a short period before they are taken to the laboratory. It is your responsibility to be sure of the correct storage procedure for a specimen.

Urine specimens must be free of fecal matter. They must also be free of menstrual blood. If your client is menstruating, a vaginal tampon must be in place while the urine specimen is collected. Before you suggest this, however, discuss it with your supervisor.

specimen
samples of bodily products that are collected and sent to a laboratory for examination

OBTAINING A SPECIMEN

Few of us can urinate on demand, but if we know we will be expected to give a urine specimen, we will cooperate. Tell your client that a specimen will be needed some time before you actually try to collect it.

Some clients are embarrassed by the procedures involved in obtaining certain types of specimens. Your client will be calm and cooperative if you show understanding and assist him when necessary. If your client understands the procedure, he should obtain the specimen himself.

Human waste material has many names. Street language uses one set of terms. Many cultures use other sets of terms. Many people do not know the correct English words for human waste material. It is usually a good idea to try to use the words that the client and his family use (this is especially true of children). If these words are offensive to you, discuss this situation with your supervisor.

NEED FOR ACCURACY

Be sure you follow all the "rights" listed here:

- *The right client:* from whom the specimen is to be collected.
- *The right specimen:* as ordered by the doctor.
- *The right time:* when the specimen should be collected.
- *The right amount:* amount needed for the laboratory to test.
- *The right container:* the correct cup for each specimen.
- *The right label:* filled out properly and neatly.
- *The right method:* procedure by which you collect the specimen.
- *The right asepsis:* washing your hands before and after collecting the specimen. Use disposable gloves.
- *The right attitude:* how you approach and speak to the client.

ASEPSIS IN SPECIMEN COLLECTION

As you learned from Chapter 8 on infection control, asepsis means "free of disease-causing organisms." When collecting specimens, it is important to use good medical aseptic technique to prevent contamination. Wash your hands carefully before and after collecting each specimen. Handwashing before you collect the specimen prevents contamination of the specimen by anything that may be on your hands. Handwashing after you collect the specimen prevents microorganisms from the specimen from remaining on your hands.

SECTION 2

Collecting Urine for a Specimen

OBJECTIVES

What You Will Learn to Do

1. Define a routine urine specimen.
2. Demonstrate the correct procedure for collecting a routine urine specimen.
3. Demonstrate the correct procedure for collecting a urine specimen from a client who has a Foley catheter.
4. Demonstrate the correct procedure for collecting a urine specimen from an infant.
5. Define a clean-catch urine specimen.
6. Demonstrate the correct procedure for collecting a clean-catch urine specimen.
7. Demonstrate the correct procedure for collecting a 24-hour urine specimen.

Introduction: Urine Collection

ROUTINE URINE SPECIMEN

This is a single sample of urine taken from the client as he voids the usual way. No special precautions are taken. At times, you will be told to take a specimen of the first urine of the day, but if you are not given time instructions, this specimen may be taken when convenient. Be sure that the client's perineal area or penis is clean before obtaining the specimen.

PROCEDURE 68

Collecting a Routine Urine Specimen

RATIONALE: A properly collected specimen allows a laboratory to evaluate the chemical structure of the urine and evaluate for possible further testing.

1. Assemble your equipment:
   Bedpan or urinal
   Disposable gloves
   Measuring container for measuring output
   Urine specimen container and lid
   Paper or plastic bag for toilet tissue
   Label
   Wet washcloth
   Towel

2. Prepare the label. Write clearly the client's name and address, the date, and the time. Also write what type of specimen this is—Routine Urine.

3. Wash your hands and put on gloves.

4. Ask visitors to leave the room, if appropriate.

5. Tell the client a urine specimen is needed. Explain the procedure to him. If he is able to collect the specimen himself, he should do so.

6. If the client is able, he can urinate directly into the container. If he is not, ask him to urinate into the bedpan or urinal. Remind the client to put toilet tissue not into the bedpan but into a paper bag or a plastic bag. You will discard the tissue in the toilet. Remove gloves and wash hands.

7. Offer the client a washcloth and towel to wash his hands.

8. Make the client comfortable.

9. Put on gloves and take the bedpan or urinal into the bathroom.

10. If the client is on I&O, pour the urine into a clean measuring container and note the urine amount on the I&O sheet.

11. Pour the urine into the specimen container. Fill it ¾ full.

12. Put the lid on the container. Wipe off the outside of the container. Secure the label to the container.

13. Pour the urine remaining in the bedpan, urinal, or measuring container into the toilet.

14. Clean and rinse the bedpan, urinal, or measuring container and return to their proper place.

15. Remove gloves and wash your hands.

16. Make a notation on the client's chart that you collected the specimen, the time, and anything you observed about the client during this procedure.

17. Store the specimen in the correct place before it is taken to the laboratory.

SAMPLE CHARTING: 1/29/05   4:15 P.M. Routine urine specimen obtained and placed in the refrigerator so client's daughter can take it to the lab tonight. Urine appeared yellow and clear.
MaryJo Heaton H/HHA

COLLECTING A URINE SPECIMEN FROM A CLIENT WITH A FOLEY CATHETER

A urine specimen from a client with a Foley catheter in place takes time to collect. Be sure the client has had fluid to drink before you attempt this. Tell the client what you will be doing because he will be unable to see the procedure or take an active part in it. It is imperative that the specimen be labeled properly. Include the fact that the specimen was obtained from a catheter.

MIDSTREAM CLEAN-CATCH URINE SPECIMEN

A special method is used to collect a client's urine when the specimen must be totally free from contamination. This special type of specimen is called a midstream clean-catch urine specimen. **Clean-catch** refers to the fact that the urine is not contaminated by anything outside the client's body. The procedure requires careful washing of the genital area. Midstream means catching the urine specimen between the time the client begins to void and time he stops.

clean-catch
urine specimen, following the careful cleansing of the urinary meatus and surrounding area, directly by the client into a sterile container

PROCEDURE 69

Obtaining a Urine Specimen from a Client with a Foley Catheter

RATIONALE: A properly obtained urine sample allows a laboratory to evaluate the chemical structure of the urine and evaluate for possible further testing.

1. Assemble your equipment:
   Specimen container and lid
   Measuring container
   Label
   Disposable gloves
   Padding to protect the bed
   Protective cap for drainage tubing or sterile gauze pads

2. Prepare the label. Write clearly the client's name and address, the date, and the time. Write the type of specimen and how it was obtained.

3. Wash your hands.

4. Explain the procedure to the client.

5. Put on gloves.

6. Clamp indwelling urinary catheter below the port by folding plastic tubing in half and applying a metal/plastic clamp.

7. Wait no more than 15 minutes for a small amount of urine to collect in the tubing above the port.

8. Insert a sterile syringe gently into the port (after swabbing with alcohol) taking care not to poke the needle through the tubing.

9. Withdraw approximately 10 cc of urine.

10. Insert the urine into a sterile specimen cup. Take care not to touch the rim or inside cover of the cap (prevents contamination of the specimen).

11. Unclamp the tubing and straighten it out. Be sure that the urine is now freely flowing.

12. Apply the correct lab label to the specimen cup and bag according to policy.

13. Report the results of the procedure to your supervisor.

14. Remove gloves and wash your hands.

15. Make a notation on the client's chart that you collected the specimen, the time, and anything observed about the client during this procedure.

16. Store the specimen in the correct place before it is taken to the laboratory.

SAMPLE CHARTING: 3/3/05   3:30 P.M.
Routine urine specimen obtained via catheter and placed in the refrigerator so client's daughter can take it to the lab tonight. Urine yellow and clear.
Denise Kelly H/HHA

All the equipment and supplies necessary for this specimen are usually found in a special kit the laboratory sends to the client. If you are unable to get such a kit, sterilize a jar. Wash the genital area with a nonirritating sterile cleansing solution and sterile gauze. Be sure all soap is off the area before collecting the specimen.

PROCEDURE 70

Collecting a Midstream Clean-Catch Urine Specimen

RATIONALE: A properly collected sample allows a laboratory to evaluate urine free from bacteria.

1. Assemble your equipment:
   Clean-catch kit or sterilized jar
   Sterile cleansing solution

   Sterile gauze
   Disposable gloves
   Bedpan or urinal if the client is unable to go to the bathroom
   Wet washcloth
   Towel
   Waste bag

2. Prepare the label if it is outside the kit. If not, wait until the end of the procedure. Write clearly the client's name and address, the date, and the time. Write the type of specimen and how it was obtained.

3. Wash your hands.

4. Ask visitors to leave the room, if appropriate. You may want to explain this procedure to a family member.

5. Tell the client you need a midstream clean-catch urine specimen.

6. Explain the procedure. If the client is able, he may collect the specimen himself.

7. If the client is not able to collect the specimen, assist him with the procedure.

8. Open the disposable kit.

9. Put on the gloves. Remove the towelettes and the urine specimen container. Do not put your hand inside the container or lid.

10. For female clients:
    a. Separate the folds of the labia and wipe with one towelette from the front to the back along one labia. Throw away the towelette. The labia must be separated during cleansing and collection of the specimen.
    b. Wipe the opposite labia with the second towelette. Throw it away.
    c. Wipe down the middle using the third towelette. Throw it away.

11. For male clients:
    a. If the male is not circumcised, pull the foreskin of the penis back before cleansing the penis. Hold it back during urination.
    b. Use a circular motion to clean the head of the penis. Use all three towelettes. Throw each one away after you use it.

12. Ask the client to start urinating into the bedpan or the toilet. Then ask him to stop. Place the sterile urine container under the stream of urine and ask the client to start urinating again. Fill the container ½ to ¾ full. The remaining urine may be discarded.

13. If the client is on I&O, all the urine must first be voided into a sterile measuring container and measured, then put into the sterile specimen container provided. Be sure to note on the I&O sheet the amount of urine sent as a specimen.

14. Cover the urine container with the proper lid. Be sure not to touch the inside of the lid or the container. Wipe off the outside of the container.

15. Take off your gloves.

16. Wash your hands.

17. Make the client comfortable. Offer the client a wet washcloth and towel to wash his hands.

18. Clean all the equipment and replace it.

19. Wash your hands.

20. Make a notation on the client's chart that you collected the specimen, the time, and anything observed about the client during this procedure.

21. Store the specimen in the correct place before it is taken to the laboratory.

SAMPLE CHARTING: 5/5/05   6:30 P.M.
Clean-catch urine obtained and taken to the lab by daughter.
Wilma Ruck H/HHA

24-HOUR URINE SPECIMEN

A 24-hour urine specimen is a collection of all urine voided by a client over a 24-hour period. All urine is collected for 24 hours, usually from 7 A.M. on the first day to 7 A.M. the following day (Figure 17.1 ■).

When you obtain a 24-hour urine specimen, it is necessary to ask the client to void and discard this voided urine at 7 A.M. This is done because this urine has been in the bladder an unknown length of time. The test should begin with the bladder empty. For the next 24 hours, save all the urine voided by the client. On the following day at 7 A.M., ask the client to void and add this specimen to the previous collection. This way, the doctor can be sure that all of the urine for the test came into the urinary bladder during the 24 hours of the test period.

The client and his family must understand the importance of collecting *all* urine voided within the 24 hours. If one urination is accidentally thrown away, the test is not accurate and must be repeated.

It is your responsibility to be sure of the correct placement of the 24-hour urine collection bottle. Some specimens must be kept on ice and others not. Ask!

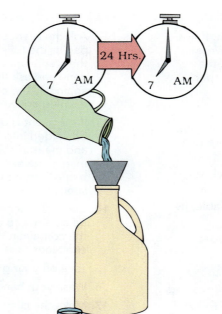

FIGURE 17.1 ■
Write down the 24 hours in which you are collecting the urine.

COLLECTING URINE FROM AN INFANT

It is often difficult to collect urine from an infant because he cannot cooperate and void when we ask him. Therefore, it is important to gather the specimen in the correct manner the first time so that the procedure need not be repeated. The procedure may appear uncomfortable to the child, but it does not hurt him. Reassure the child's parent or guardian that you are not hurting the child and that the information the doctor will have after the laboratory examination of the urine will help in the child's care. Be kind, efficient, and thoughtful of both child and parents.

PROCEDURE 71

Collecting a 24-Hour Urine Specimen

RATIONALE: A properly collected sample allows a laboratory to evaluate the chemical structure of the urine and evaluate for possible further testing.

1. Assemble your equipment:
   Large container, usually a 1-gallon bottle (the laboratory usually supplies this)
   Bedpan or urinal
   Disposable gloves
   Funnel, if the neck of the bottle is small
   Measuring container used for measuring output if the client is on I&O
   Label for the container
   Wet washcloth
   Towel

2. Fill out the label. Clearly write the client's name and address, the date, and the time the collection started.

3. Wash your hands and put on gloves.

4. Ask visitors to leave the room, if appropriate.

5. Tell the client that a 24-hour specimen is needed. Explain the procedure to him and his family. Discuss the placement and care of the gallon container of urine.

6. You may be instructed to refrigerate the urine. If so, one way is to keep it in a bucket of ice. This ice must be changed as it melts. It may, of course, be kept in the refrigerator if that is acceptable to the client and his family.

7. During the collection of the specimen, ask the client to use the bedpan or urinal each time he voids. Remind him not to throw toilet tissue into the bedpan or urinal and to try to urinate without moving his bowels at the same time. Provide a waste bag for the toilet tissue and then discard the tissue promptly in the toilet.

8. If the client is on I&O, measure all urine each time the client urinates and write it on the I&O sheet.

9. When the collection starts, have the client urinate. *Throw away this first urine.* This is to be sure that the bladder is completely empty as the collection starts. If this urine is discarded at 7 A.M., the collection will continue until 7 A.M. the following morning.

10. For the next 24 hours, save all the client's urine. At the end of the collection, write the time the collection stopped on the label. Store the bottle in the proper place until it is sent to the laboratory.

11. Offer the client a washcloth and towel to wash his hands each time he voids.

12. Be sure to clean all equipment *after each urination*. Note in your charting that the collection was done and your observations about the client during this procedure.

SAMPLE CHARTING: 5/9/04   7:00 A.M. 24-hour urine specimen started. Client and her daughter aware of how to collect urine throughout the day and night. Client's daughter will take completed specimen to the laboratory tomorrow morning following the 7:00 A.M. specimen. Joanne Deal H/HHA

PROCEDURE 72

Collecting a Urine Specimen from an Infant

RATIONALE: A properly collected sample allows a laboratory to evaluate the chemical structure of the urine and evaluate for possible further testing.

1. Assemble your equipment:
   Urine specimen bottle or container
   Plastic disposable infant urine collector
   Gloves

2. Prepare a label. Write the client's name and address, the date, and the type of specimen. Fill in the time when the actual specimen is obtained.

3. Wash your hands.

4. Ask visitors to leave, except the parent or guardian of the child.

5. Explain to the child and his parent that you want to collect a urine specimen. A toddler who is not yet toilet-trained often can understand language and is more likely to cooperate if he knows what is expected of him. Use language the child understands and is familiar with.

6. Put on gloves and take off the child's diaper.

7. Clean the genital area. Be sure it is dry or the collector bag will not stick.

8. Remove the outside piece that surrounds the opening of the plastic urine collector. Be sure the skin is not folded under the sticky part as you apply it. Place the opening of the bag around the male penis or the female meatus (Figure 17.2 ■). Do not cover the rectum. The specimen is useless if it is contaminated with fecal matter.

9. Put the child's diaper on as usual.

10. Check every half-hour to see if the infant has voided. You cannot feel the diaper. You must look inside the diaper.

11. When the infant has voided, remove the urine collector gently. Do not spill the urine. Pour the urine into a specimen container.

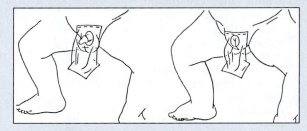

FIGURE 17.2 ■

continued

12. Wash off any excess sticky material on the genitalia. Make the baby comfortable.

13. Remove gloves and wash your hands.

14. Make a notation on the client's chart that you collected the specimen, the time, and anything you observed about the client during the procedure.

15. Store the specimen in the correct place before it is taken to the laboratory.

SAMPLE CHARTING: 11/1/04   11:00 A.M. Collection bag placed on infant. Urine collected within 30 minutes. Placed in specimen cup. Mother to take to laboratory this afternoon. Specimen to be held in refrigerator until then. Urine appeared yellow. Thelma Lowe H/HHA

SECTION 3

Collection of a Stool Specimen

OBJECTIVES

What You Will Learn to Do

1. Define stool specimen.

2. Demonstrate the correct procedure for collecting a stool specimen.

---

stool

solid waste material discharged from the body through the rectum and anus. Other names include "feces," "excreta," "excrement," "B.M.," and "fecal matter"

Introduction: Stool Specimen

"The solid waste from a person's body has many names—"**stools**," "feces," "fecal matter," "excreta," "excrement," "B.M.," and "bowel movement." They all mean the same thing. The doctor sometimes requires a sample of the client's feces to assist him in diagnosing the client's illness or in monitoring the client's progress. A feces sample is a stool specimen. Certain tests must be performed only on a warm stool. You will be told whether the specimen is to be warm or cold.

PROCEDURE 73

Collecting a Stool Specimen

RATIONALE: To determine if blood, parasites, or foreign bodies are present in the stool.

1. Assemble your equipment:
   Bedpan
   Stool container
   Disposable gloves
   Label
   Wooden tongue depressor
   Plastic bag for warm specimen if used by your agency
   Washcloth
   Towel

2. Fill in the label with the client's name and address, the date, and the type of specimen.

   Fill in the time when the actual specimen is obtained.

3. Wash your hands and put on gloves.

4. Ask visitors to leave the room, if appropriate.

5. Tell the client that a stool specimen is needed. Explain that he is to call you whenever he can move his bowels.

6. Have the client move his bowels in the bedpan. If the client is unable to use the bedpan, place several layers of toilet tissue in the bottom of the toilet and have the client move his bowels on the paper (Figure 17.3 ■). This way you will be able to take a specimen easily.

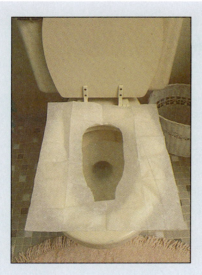

FIGURE 17.3 ■

7. Ask the client not to urinate into the bedpan and not to put toilet tissue into the bedpan. Provide him with a plastic or paper bag to dispose of the tissue temporarily. Then discard the tissue in the toilet.

8. After the client has had a bowel movement, take the bedpan into the bathroom.

9. Remove gloves and wash your hands.

10. Offer the client a washcloth and towel for his hands.

11. Make the client comfortable.

12. Put on gloves. Using the wooden tongue depressor, take 1 to 2 tablespoons of stool from the bedpan and place it into the stool specimen container (Figure 17.4 ■).

13. Cover the container. Do not touch the inside of the container or the top of it.

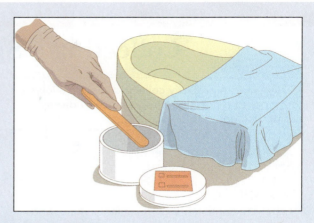

FIGURE 17.4 ■

14. Wrap the depressor in a piece of toilet tissue and discard it into a plastic or paper bag.

15. Empty the remaining feces into the toilet.

16. Clean the bedpan and return it to its proper place.

17. Remove gloves and wash your hands.

18. Make a notation on the client's chart that you collected the specimen, the time, and anything you observed about the client during this procedure.

19. Store the specimen in the correct place before it is taken to the laboratory.

SAMPLE CHARTING:	9/9/04 12:00 P.M.
	Soft, brown stool collected. Son took it to the laboratory within half an hour.
	Carol Baker H/HHA

SECTION 4

Collection of Sputum

OBJECTIVES

What You Will Learn to Do

1. Define *sputum*.

2. Demonstrate the correct procedure for collecting a sputum specimen.

Introduction: Sputum Collection

Sputum is a substance collected from a client's lungs. It contains saliva, mucous, and sometimes blood or pus. It is usually clear in color but can be gray, yellow, green, or red. The best time to collect a sputum specimen is in the morning, right after the client awakens.

PROCEDURE 74

Collecting a Sputum Specimen

RATIONALE: A properly collected sample allows a laboratory to determine the presence of disease-causing bacteria or blood.

1. Assemble your equipment:
   Sputum container with lid
   Tissues
   Disposable gloves

2. Label the container with the client's name and address, the date, and the type of specimen. Fill in the time when the actual specimen is obtained.

3. Wash your hands and put on gloves.

4. Ask visitors to leave the room, if appropriate.

5. Tell the client a sputum specimen is needed.

6. If the client has eaten recently, have him rinse out his mouth. If he wants oral hygiene at this time, help him as necessary.

7. Give him the sputum container. Ask him to take three consecutive deep breaths. On the third breath, ask him to exhale deeply and cough. He should be able to bring up sputum from within the lungs. Explain to him that saliva is not adequate for this test.

8. Have the client spit the sputum directly into the specimen container.

9. Cover the container immediately. Be careful not to touch the inside of either the container or the cover.

10. Offer the client oral hygiene.

11. Make the client comfortable.

12. Remove gloves and wash your hands.

13. Make a notation on the client's chart that you collected the specimen, the time, and anything you observed about the client during this procedure.

14. Store the specimen in the correct place before it is taken to the laboratory.

SAMPLE CHARTING: 8/8/04   3:00 P.M.
Specimen collected. Appears yellow. Niece took it to the lab.
 Pamela Gott H/HHA

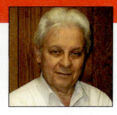

CHAPTER REVIEW

Case Study

Review the case study that appears on the first page of the chapter. Answer two sets of questions about the case study contained in the Explore and Apply sections below.

EXPLORE

1. You visit the Hogans three times weekly to assist with the personal care of both father and son. You are also assigned to report changes in the activity level of either client. You notice that, with Mr. Hogan becoming more forgetful, his wife is keeping him more sedentary because she cannot trust him to safely be away from her. He has developed a cough. You also notice that Ronald is becoming less active because he is staying near his father. How would you explain the effects these changes in activity level seem to have produced?

2. What activities would you suggest to safely increase the client's activity?

APPLY

1. You have been asked to obtain a sputum specimen from Mr. Hogan. Why? What do you say to Mr. Hogan when he asks the reason?

2. You notice that Mrs. Hogan visits the bathroom frequently while you are in the house. You mention your observation and she says, "I don't drink much when you don't come because I am afraid to leave the men alone. So, when I know you are coming, I drink more." How do you respond to her? How do you chart this conversation?

Certification Exam Review Questions

Choose the best answer for each question or statement.

1. **Gathering specimens**
   a. is a job you can delegate to a family member.
   b. includes you taking the specimen to the laboratory.
   c. includes keeping the specimen at the correct temperature until it reaches the laboratory.
   d. is the responsibility of the supervisor, and you do not have to worry about it.

2. **Collecting a regular urine specimen**
   a. can be done at any time of the day.
   b. should always be done in the morning.
   c. should always be done after a shower.
   d. should be done by the client whenever he has a clean jar.

3. **Collecting a mid-stream clean-catch urine specimen**
   a. can never be done by the client alone.
   b. must always be done with your help.
   c. must always be done at the laboratory.
   d. can be done either alone or with your help depending on the capabilities of the client.

4. **When obtaining a urine specimen from an infant, it is**
   a. important to put the collection bag on so that no fecal matter enters.
   b. important to leave it on as long as possible so that as much urine as possible is collected.
   c. important that the area where the collection bag will be placed is wiped with alcohol to clean it.
   d. important that the child be immobile while the collection bag is in place.

5. **Sputum collection**
   a. always means the client has tuberculosis.
   b. is never done if the client is not a smoker.
   c. may be done more than once.
   d. means the client is contagious and should be isolated.

CHAPTER 18

Special Procedures

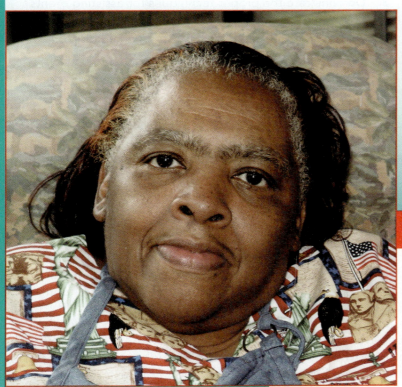

CASE STUDY

Mrs. Collins, a retired nursery nurse, lives in a boarding house. She shares a small kitchen with her neighbor. The refrigerator is small, and periodically food goes missing. The bathroom is shared by three people. Mrs. Collins does not leave her room unless she goes to the doctor or the corner store where she buys her groceries. She spends her days in her chair looking out of the window and watching television. Her family does not live nearby, and she has no friends who visit. Mrs. Collins has some savings, but she is frugal because she does not know how long her money will last. Her two big expenses are her medication and her food. She has recently accepted oxygen, but you are not sure how much she uses it.

Keep the case study in mind as you read the chapter. After you have read the chapter, answer the Explore and Apply questions at the end of the chapter that relate to the case study.

Assisting with Medications

OBJECTIVES

What You Will Learn to Do

1. Discuss the difference between administering medication and assisting with medication.

2. Define the homemaker/home health aide's role in relation to medication.

3. Demonstrate the proper techniques for assisting clients with various types of medication.

4. Discuss methods of medication storage and disposal.

5. Define the homemaker/home health aide's role when oxygen is in the home.

Introduction: Assisting with Medications

medication

substance or preparation used in treating a disease

administer

to give a client medication without his assistance

Medication is prescribed by a physician, dispensed by a pharmacist, and **administered**, or given without client assistance, by a nurse. All these professionals are licensed by the state to perform their duties. These duties are specific. Failure to stay within the state guidelines can result in a legal action ending in a fine, revoking a license to practice the profession, and possibly jail. In addition, these people are paid for their services. As a homemaker/home health aide, you are not licensed to administer medication, nor are you paid to do so. You are, however, expected to assist your clients as they take their own medication. When you *administer* to a client, you take all responsibility that goes along with giving medication. When you *assist* a client, he shares the responsibility. If you ever have a question about a situation with your client, ask your supervisor.

Prescription drugs are prescribed by a physician and cannot be bought without a prescription. Over-the-counter drugs can be bought without a prescription. As a homemaker/home health aide, you will not administer either type of drug and will assist the client with only those drugs about which you have been instructed specifically.

Your Role as a Homemaker/Home Health Aide

As a homemaker/home health aide, you probably will spend more time with the client than any other member of the health-care team. During this time, you often will be assigned to assist the client with his medication. To do this correctly, you will have to have certain information. Without this information, an accident could happen. Accidents involving medication are serious because they can cause the client pain, delay his recovery, and sometimes even cause death.

Your supervisor will find out all information about your client's medication. She then will make a medication plan for the client and review it with the client, the family, and you. Your supervisor will tell you your specific duties about the client's medication. You must be sure you have all the information you need to perform your duties to the best of your ability.

To perform your duties well, you must know the Five Rights of Medication (Figure 18.1 ■).

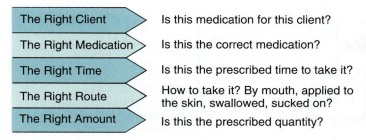

The Right Client	Is this medication for this client?
The Right Medication	Is this the correct medication?
The Right Time	Is this the prescribed time to take it?
The Right Route	How to take it? By mouth, applied to the skin, swallowed, sucked on?
The Right Amount	Is this the prescribed quantity?

FIGURE 18.1 ■ The Five Rights of Medication must be observed every time a client takes medication.

You should also know the side effects of each client's medication, how to store it, and how it reacts with food. If you observe any side effects after your client has taken the medication, report them immediately to your supervisor. Some most common side effects are identified in Figure 18.2 ■. However, any change in behavior, associated with the taking of medication should be noted.

As you spend time in your client's house, you will observe many things. Here are a few of the observations you should report to your supervisor immediately:

■ If your client is not taking the medication exactly as it has been prescribed (Figure 18.3 ■)
■ If your client is taking medication (prescription or over-the-counter) of which your supervisor is unaware
■ If your client does not know why he is taking his drugs
■ If your client has nausea, vomiting, diarrhea, itching, difficulty breathing, a rash, or hives soon after he takes his medication

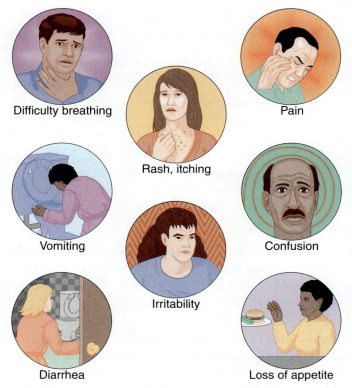

FIGURE 18.2 ■ Changes in usual patterns of behavior may indicate a medication reaction. Report any change you note or are told about immediately to your supervisor.

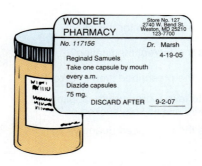

FIGURE 18.3 ■
The label on the medication bottle must be checked every time the client takes the medication.

■ If his orientation, concentration, memory, or mood changes soon after he takes his medication
■ If your client is confusing his medications

PROCEDURE 75

Assisting a Client with Medication

RATIONALE: Correctly assisting with medication is an important part of client care.

1. Assemble your equipment:
   Medication
   Spoon
   Water or juice
   Dressings if medication is applied to the skin
   Tissues or cotton balls
2. Wash your hands.
3. Ask visitors to leave the room, if appropriate.
4. Remind the client it is time for his medication.
5. Check the Five Rights of Medication.
6. Place the medication within reach of the client. Loosen the tops of bottles or tubes.
7. Assist the client as necessary:
   a. *Oral medication.* Hold client's hand, assist him with liquid.

   b. *Ointments.* Assist him as needed with medication and dressing.
   c. *Eyedrops.* Guide his hand and wipe excess liquid or ointment from under eye from nose to outer area.
8. Make the client comfortable.
9. Put the medication in its proper place. Dispose of the used equipment.
10. Wash your hands.
11. Make a notation on the client's chart that he took his medication, the time, and how he took it. Also note your observations of the client during this procedure.

SAMPLE CHARTING: | 12/12/04   10:30 A.M. Brought client his Lopressor. He took 50 mg with a glass of milk.
Rose Davis H/HHA

MEDICATION STORAGE

Each year, many accidents result from improper storage of medication. As you make your first tour of your client's house, observe how he keeps his medication. If it is poorly stored, you will want to correct this. If you cannot discuss the problem with your client directly, discuss it with your supervisor and together make a plan to correct the situation.

■ Clients save medications, but some medications change chemical makeup as they stand. Clients save medication so they can medicate themselves if they have symptoms—yet the same symptoms can be caused by different physical problems. The practice of saving medication is extremely dangerous. Old medication should be disposed of with the client's permission.
■ Many medications have similar names and look alike. Store these separately.

- Do not assist a client with a medication from an unlabeled container.
- Do not change the place your client stores his medication without his permission. People do not always read labels but take medications from the places they expect to find them.
- Keep medication out of reach of children and confused, forgetful clients.
- Keep medication away from extreme heat, cold, or light.
- It is important to dispose of medication in a safe manner that does not promote environmental pollution, such as flushing it down the toilet, or leave the medication so that other people will be tempted to use it or animals will be tempted to eat it. You can put it in with the kitchen trash in a plastic bag and throw the whole bag into an outside garbage container.

ASSISTING A CLIENT WITH OXYGEN THERAPY

Oxygen is considered a medication. All the rules and responsibilities that apply to you while you assist a client with medication apply to you while you assist a client with oxygen (Figure 18.4 ■). Oxygen is prescribed by a physician. It is delivered to the home by a special company. The tank may look like a vacuum cleaner canister or a piece of furniture. It may also look like the tanks in the hospital.

The three main kinds of oxygen storage are:

- *Portable liquid unit.* This small unit is intended to be used for short time-spans, usually outside the house. It is filled from a stationary unit in the house (Figure 18.5a ■).
- *Stationary unit.* Several different types of cylinders are all designed to remain stationary and deliver oxygen over several days. The tubing connected from the cylinder to the client can be adjusted in length to increase client mobility (Figure 18.5b ■).
- *Oxygen concentrator.* This device removes oxygen from the air and delivers it, through tubing, to the client. The tubing length can be adjusted (Figure 18.5c ■).

The company delivering the oxygen is responsible for refilling the tank, servicing the equipment, and teaching the client and his family how to use the equipment. The company should provide a telephone number to call in case of an emergency. If this is not the case, report it to your supervisor.

oxygen
a colorless, odorless gas making up about one-fifth of the air we breathe. It is essential for life.

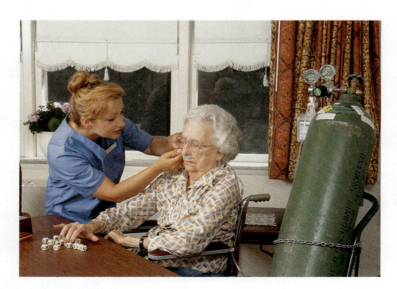

FIGURE 18.4 ■ Assisting a client with oxygen

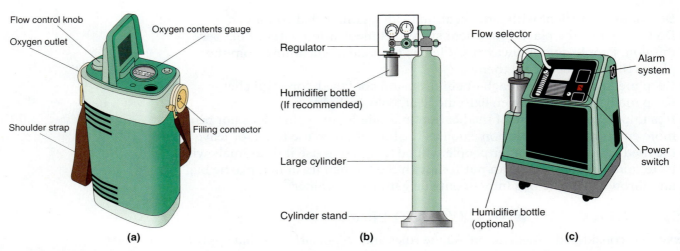

FIGURE 18.5 ■ (a) Portable oxygen unit used to increase client mobility for short periods of time; (b) stationary cylinder is most commonly used for clients confined to their home; (c) oxygen concentrator may be prescribed for prolonged need of oxygen therapy.

Although the oxygen may be dispensed in several ways, all oxygen is dispensed from a tank to the client through a rubber tube connected to a nasal cannula or catheter. Oxygen is extremely drying, so a nebulizer filled with water or medication usually is attached to the tank. The oxygen passes through the water and takes on moisture before it goes to the client (Figure 18.6 ■).

The following are important parts of oxygen delivery systems:

Nasal catheter. This catheter is a piece of tubing longer than a cannula. It is inserted through the client's nostril into the back of his mouth. The nasal catheter is used when the client must have additional oxygen at all times. The nasal catheter is fastened to the client's forehead or cheek with a piece of tape that holds it steady.

Nasal cannulas. Nasal cannulas, or tubes, are used to give oxygen to a client. The cannulas are inserted into the client's nostrils. The plastic cannula is a half-circle length of tubing with two openings in the center. It fits about ½ inch into the client's nostrils. Nasal cannulas are held in place by an elastic band around the client's head and are connected to the source of oxygen by a length of plastic tubing (Figure 18.7 ■).

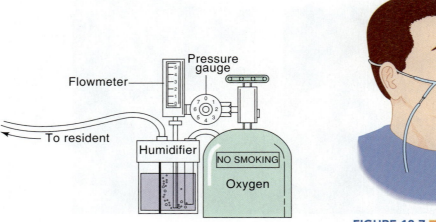

FIGURE 18.6 ■ Oxygen delivery systems may look different, but they have the same parts and function.

FIGURE 18.7 ■ Nasal cannulas move easily, so check their placement frequently.

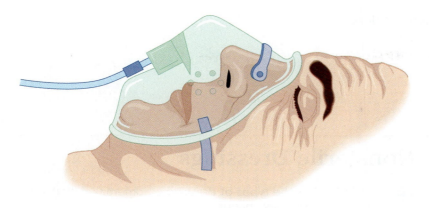

FIGURE 18.8 ■ A client can say little with a face mask in place. Be sure the client can signal for assistance.

Face mask. This is a piece of plastic shaped like a cup that covers the client's nose and mouth and has holes in it. A tube connects the mask to the oxygen tank, and a piece of elastic holds the mask securely to the client's face. This mask is used when the client requires more oxygen than can be given by cannula or catheter. The mask must be removed for the client to eat. A client can say a few words with the mask in place but usually removes it to speak (Figure 18.8 ■).

HOMEMAKER/HOME HEALTH CARE AIDE RESPONSIBILITIES

■ Put up a "No Smoking" sign in the room where the client uses the oxygen. *Enforce this rule without exception!*

■ Report to your supervisor if the client uses the oxygen other than as prescribed.

■ Use cotton bedclothes to decrease static electricity.

■ Do not use electric shavers or hair dryers while the oxygen is running. Keep electric plugs out of walls while the oxygen is running. If an electric plug is pulled from an outlet while the oxygen is running, a spark could cause an explosion. Use a three-pronged plug, if possible.

■ Do not use candles or open flames in the room.

■ Avoid combing a client's hair while he is receiving oxygen. A spark of electricity from his hair could set off an explosion.

■ Ask for careful instructions as to which valve turns the oxygen on and off.

■ Do not change the setting on any oxygen equipment. The setting has been chosen by the physician. Too much or too little oxygen can cause the client to change his breathing pattern, his heart rate, and his speech pattern. Call your supervisor immediately if you notice any of these signs. *Do not change the oxygen setting.*

Indications of too much oxygen are:

■ Sleepiness or difficulty waking up
■ Headache
■ Difficulty speaking
■ Slow, shallow breathing

Indications of too little oxygen are:

■ Tiredness
■ Blue fingernails and/or lips

- Anxiety, restlessness
- Irritability
- Confusion

Nonsterile Dressings

OBJECTIVES

What You Will Learn to Do

1. List the types of dressing a homemaker/home health aide may change.

2. Demonstrate the correct technique for changing a nonsterile dressing.

Introduction: Nonsterile Dressings

dressing
bandage for an external wound

nonsterile
not subjected to the sterilizing process and therefore possibly having pathogens

Some of your clients will have wounds or areas of their bodies that must be covered by a bandage or **dressing**. Dressings that do not require you to use sterile technique or to apply medication to the wound will often be assigned to your care. These are called **nonsterile**. When applying a dressing, it is important to keep in mind the following:

- Protection of the wound
- Protection of the surrounding tissue

The type of dressing used will address these issues. Sometimes, a dressing will use tape to secure it; sometimes, additional bandage material will be wrapped around the area; and sometimes, an occlusive dressing will be used (Figure 18.9 ■). Do not change the type of dressing unless you have discussed it with your supervisor.

drainage
discharge from a sore, wound, or body part

When you change a dressing, always note the color, odor, amount, and consistency of the **drainage** (discharge) on the old dressing. Also note how big the wound is and the condition of the skin surrounding the wound. Note any change in the wound since you last saw it. If the nurse is scheduled to visit, save the old dressing for her to see. Each dressing is somewhat different, but the following procedure is a general rule for changing all nonsterile dressings.

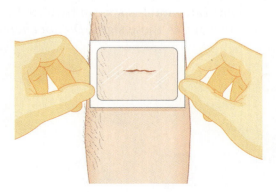

FIGURE 18.9 ■
A dressing that encloses the wound to keep air away from it is called an occlusive dressing.

EXAMPLE OF CHARTING FOLLOWING A DRESSING CHANGE

7/3/05   10 A.M.
Dressing changed on Mrs. C's right thigh. Old dressing has light-red drainage, 25-cent size, no odor. Wound 5-cent size. Surrounding skin had several small, red raised areas. Clean dressing applied. Tape not applied to red areas. Called supervisor to report this.
Mary Jones H/HHA.

PROCEDURE 76

Changing a Nonsterile Dressing

RATIONALE: Correctly dressing a wound prevents infection and contributes to the client's comfort.

1. Assemble your equipment:
   Clean dressing
   Tape
   Cleansing solution
   Disposable gloves
   Paper bag or plastic bag for old dressings
   Medication the client will apply

2. Wash your hands and put on gloves.

3. Ask visitors to leave the room, if appropriate.

4. Tell the client you will change his dressing.

5. Open the paper bag.

6. Open the clean dressings without touching the center of them. Prepare the tape in a convenient place.

7. Position the client so that the wound is exposed.

8. Remove the old dressing. Note the drainage for amount, color, odor, and consistency. Note the size of the wound and the condition of the surrounding skin. Place the soiled dressing in the paper/plastic bag.

9. Cleanse the wound and the skin as you have been instructed. Use circular motions and clean from the clean areas to the dirty. The wound is considered clean and the skin dirty. Discard cleaning materials in the paper/plastic bag.

10. Allow the client to assist you as much as possible.

11. If a medication is to be applied to the wound, assist the client with the application as needed.

12. Apply clean dressings. Hold all dressings by the corners as you apply them. Do not contaminate the center of the bandages. Tape the dressing in place, leaving the edges free. Do not put tape completely around the edges of the bandage (Figure 18.10 ■).

13. Make the client comfortable.

14. Close the bag and discard it in a covered container, preferably outside. If possible, put the paper/plastic bag into another plastic bag to prevent leakage and contamination of the large trash can.

15. Remove gloves and wash your hands.

16. Make a notation on the client's chart that you changed the client's dressing. Also note your observations of the client during this procedure.

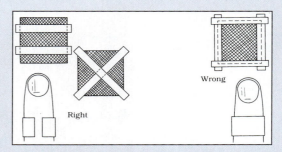

FIGURE 18.10 ■

SAMPLE CHARTING: 8/4/05   8:23 A.M.
Nonsterile dressing applied to abrasion of left leg. Wound is about 50-cent size, slightly red, no drainage, and not painful.
Sally Lind H/HHA

Care of the Indwelling Catheter

OBJECTIVES

What You Will Learn to Do

1. Understand what an indwelling catheter is and when it is used.
2. List your responsibilities as a homemaker/home health aide in caring for an indwelling catheter.
3. Demonstrate the proper technique for giving catheter care.
4. Demonstrate the proper technique of changing the catheter from a straight drainage bag to a leg drainage bag.

Introduction: Indwelling Catheter

catheter

a tube used to remove body fluids from a cavity

The urinary catheter is the most common kind of **catheter** used for taking fluids out of the body. This catheter is made of plastic or rubber and is inserted by a nurse or physician through the client's urethra into his bladder. A catheter may be used when a client is unable to urinate naturally, or it may be used to measure the amount of urine left in the bladder after a client has urinated naturally. It may also be used to help keep an incontinent client dry. An incontinent client is one who cannot control his urine or feces.

Sometimes, a urinary catheter is used for only one withdrawal of urine. Sometimes, it is kept in place in the bladder for days or even weeks. This type of catheter is called an indwelling catheter or Foley catheter (Figure 18.11 ■). This catheter is specially made so that it will stay in the bladder. It has two tubes, one inside the other. The inside tube is connected at one end to a balloon. After the

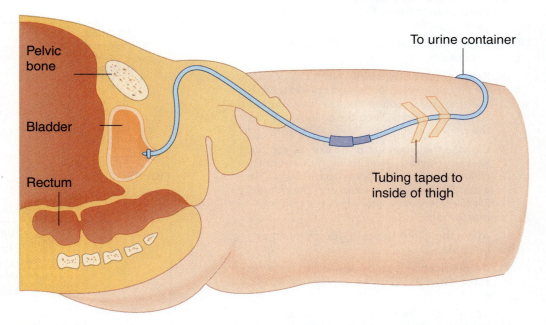

FIGURE 18.11 ■ A catheter is a possible source of irritation and infection. Tend it carefully and according to the plan of care.

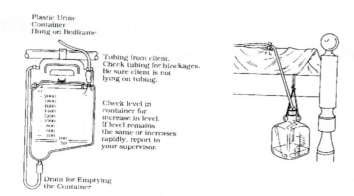

FIGURE 18.12 ■ Check the tubing from the client to the drainage bag frequently to be sure it is free of blockages.

catheter has been inserted, the balloon is filled with water or air so the catheter will not pass out through the urethra. Urine drains out of the bladder through the outer tube. The urine collects into a container. The container is attached to a point lower than the client's urinary bladder. An indwelling catheter is always a closed system, which means it is never opened except when the urine collecting bag is emptied.

Sometimes, in male clients, the catheter is secured to the abdomen. This reduces the pressure on the catheter and provides the straightest route for the urine to drain.

Urinary indwelling catheters drain by **straight drainage** from the client into a bag. This type of drainage gets its name from the fact that the tubing from the bed to the bag must be kept straight and all other tubing must be kept above this. When the tubing is in its proper position, the urine will drain freely into the bag. If the tubing is not in the proper position, the urine could back up into the bladder or the kidneys (Figure 18.12 ■).

straight drainage
method of collecting urine from a Foley catheter into a closed container

GUIDELINES

Indwelling Urinary Catheter

It is normal for urine to change from light yellow to dark yellow, depending on the concentration and the amount of fluid the client has consumed.

■ Check from time to time to make sure the level of urine has increased. If the level stays the same, report this to your supervisor.

■ If the client says he feels that his bladder is full, or that he needs to urinate, report this to your supervisor.

■ If the client is allowed to get out of bed for short periods, the bag goes with him. It must always be held lower than the client's urinary bladder to prevent the urine in the tubing and bag from draining back into the urinary bladder.

■ Check to make sure the catheter and tubing flow freely and without obstruction.

■ Be sure the client is not lying on the catheter or the tubing. This would stop the flow of urine.

■ Be sure the tubing from the bed to the bag is always straight.

continued

GUIDELINES (continued)

Indwelling Urinary Catheter

■ The catheter should be secured at all times to the client's inner thigh or, in the case of male clients, the abdomen. This keeps it from being pulled on or being pulled out of the bladder. Either tape or special straps made for this purpose can be used.

■ Most clients with urinary drainage through a catheter are on intake and output measurement.

■ If urine leaks around a catheter, report this to your supervisor.

■ A male client may have an erection while the catheter is in place. This is a natural occurrence. Assure him there is nothing the matter with him, and maintain a concerned attitude. Discuss this with your supervisor for additional information.

■ Empty the collection bag frequently and from the correct port. Protect the floor from spillage. There are many types of collection bags. If you find one that is new to you, ask your supervisor for assistance.

■ Clean the collection tubing and the bag as instructed by your agency. Some agencies discard collection equipment after a specified amount of time. Some agencies use a cleansing procedure.

■ Keep the client's urinary opening clean. Even though he is not urinating, mucous and perspiration collect in the area.

■ Be sure the tubing is free of fecal matter and mucous.

■ Cover the exposed ends of tubing only with sterile covers.

■ Notify your supervisor if you see sediment or blood in the tubing or collection bag.

PROCEDURE 77

Catheter Care

RATIONALE: Correct catheter care decreases risk of infection and contributes to the client's overall comfort.

Note: This procedure may be incorporated into the morning bath routine. Be sure you use clean water for this procedure.

1. Assemble your equipment:
   Basin of water and mild soap or cleaning solution
   Washcloth or gauze pads
   Paper or plastic bag for waste
   Disposable gloves
2. Wash your hands.
3. Ask visitors to leave the room, if appropriate.
4. Tell the client you are going to give him catheter care.

5. Position the client on his back so the catheter and urinary meatus are exposed. Put on your gloves.
6. Wash the area gently. Do not pull on the catheter, but hold it with one hand while wiping it with the other.
7. Observe the meatus for redness, swelling, or discharge.
8. Wipe away from the meatus. Wipe from the meatus to the anus (Figure 18.13 ■).
9. Wipe one way and not back and forth.
10. Remove your gloves.
11. Dry the area.
12. Apply lotion or powder in small quantities to the thighs. Ask your supervisor if this area should be kept dry or moist.

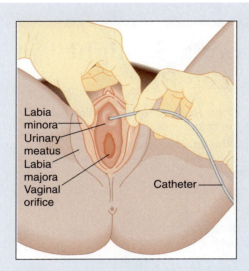

Labia
minora
Urinary
meatus
Labia
majora
Vaginal
orifice

Catheter

FIGURE 18.13 ■ Be sure to keep the entire perineum clean in female clients to prevent irritation and possible infection.

13. Make the client comfortable.

14. Dispose of the dirty water into the toilet. Clean your equipment and put it in its proper place.

15. Wash your hands.

16. Make a notation on the client's chart that you have completed this procedure. Also make a note of your observations of the client during this procedure.

SAMPLE CHARTING:	3/29/04 6:30 A.M. Catheter care given. Meatus slightly red. Client reminded to wipe herself after each bowel movement from front to back. Daughter will also be reminded. Thelma Justt H/HHA

LEG BAG

A leg bag is a small plastic bag worn on the client's leg. This apparatus allows the client to be more active than when using the traditional straight drainage. It cannot be used when the client is lying down, as the drainage is improper in that position (Figure 18.14 ■).

The same rules of asepsis that apply to changing a straight drainage bag apply to putting on a leg bag. Be sure to put the top of the bag at the top, and the bottom at the bottom. Empty the bag immediately after it is removed or when it is full. If the client is on I&O, record the amount of urine collected. Clean the bag as you have been taught by your supervisor.

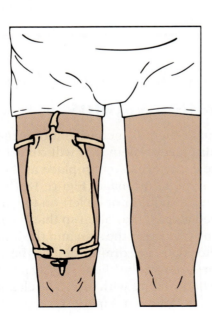

FIGURE 18.14 ■

Using a leg bag increases the client's mobility but it must be emptied frequently.

PROCEDURE 78

Changing a Catheter from a Straight Drainage Bag to a Leg Bag

RATIONALE: Correctly changing to and from a leg bag increase the client's comfort and mobility and decreases risk of infection.

1. Assemble your equipment:
   Leg bag with straps
   Disposable gloves
   Alcohol wipes or antiseptic solution
   Sterile cover for straight drainage tubing
   Sterile 4 × 4 bed protector
2. Wash your hands and put on gloves.
3. Ask visitors to leave the room, if appropriate.
4. Tell the client you are going to put on his leg bag.
5. Expose the end of the catheter and the drainage tubing. Put the bed protector under this area.
6. Disconnect the drainage tubing from the catheter and allow it to drain. Put a sterile cover on the end of the tubing, and place it out of the way but not on the floor. Do not put the catheter on the bed.
7. Wipe the attachment tube of the leg bag with an alcohol swab and insert the tube into the catheter.
8. Secure the leg bag to the client's thigh.
9. Make the client comfortable.
10. Empty the drainage bag. Measure the urine and note it on the chart.
11. Remove gloves and wash your hands.
12. Make a notation on the client's chart that you have completed this procedure. Also note your observations of the client during this procedure.

SAMPLE CHARTING: 5/6/05   2:35 P.M.
Client wore leg bag for 5 hours. Bag contained 250 cc of yellow urine. Client walking well.
Samuel Jones H/HHA

SECTION 4

Care of External Urinary Drainage

OBJECTIVE
What You Will Learn to Do

1. List the reasons a male client may have an external urinary drainage system.

Introduction: Uses of External Urinary Drainage Systems

When a male client is incontinent of urine, the nurse may suggest the use of an external drainage system that will collect the urine and keep the client dry. One end of the catheter is kept in place at the end of the penis and one end is connected to straight drainage (Figure 18.15 ■).

This device should not be left on for more than 24 hours at a time and must be removed at least that often so that the penis may be washed and inspected. If there is any change in the skin and the client complains of pain or discomfort or the catheter does not drain, remove the entire device, discard it, and call your supervisor. Observe the client shortly after you put on the catheter and then frequently when you are with him. The cleaning of the bag and the catheter should be discussed with your supervisor.

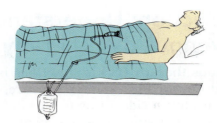

FIGURE 18.15 ■
Check the placement of external drainage frequently and change it at least every 24 hours.

PROCEDURE 79

External Urinary Drainage

RATIONALE: Correctly applying external drainage decreases the risk of infection and skin breakdown and increases the client's general well-being and dignity.

1. Assemble your equipment:
   External urinary system, consisting of a condom, a catheter, and a straight drainage system
   Material to secure condom to penis: tape, strap, or adhesive foam
   Soap
   Water
   Towel
   Disposable gloves
2. Wash your hands.
3. Ask visitors to leave the room, if appropriate.
4. Tell the client you are going to put on an external urinary collection device. Put on gloves.
5. Position the client on his back so that the penis is exposed. Cover the client so he is not exposed.
6. Wash the entire penis and dry thoroughly. Observe the penis for any discharge or redness.

7. Roll the condom onto the entire length of the penis.
8. Secure the condom. Be sure the strap is tight enough to hold the condom in place but not so tight as to hurt the client.
9. Attach the catheter to the condom and to the straight drainage. Secure the collection bag on a bed or chair.
10. Make the client comfortable.
11. Dispose of the dirty water into the toilet. Clean your equipment and put it in its proper place.
12. Remove gloves and wash your hands.
13. Make a notation on the client's chart that you have completed this procedure. Also note your observations of the client during this procedure.

SAMPLE CHARTING: 4/9/04   6:30 P.M.
External drainage in place for the evening. Daughter will check it before she goes to bed. Skin intact, dry, and not red.
Wilma Flint H/HHA

SECTION 5

Intravenous Therapy: Peripheral or Central

OBJECTIVES
What You Will Learn to Do

1. Define the difference between peripheral and central intravenous therapy.
2. List two reasons for intravenous therapy.
3. Discuss the homemaker/home health aide's role in caring for a client receiving intravenous therapy.

Introduction: Understanding Intravenous (IV) Therapy

intravenous therapy (IV)
giving of fluids or medication directly into the vein

continuous infusion
uninterrupted; without a stop

intermittent infusion
alternating; stopping and beginning again

peripheral line
intravenous lines in place in the upper extremities

central venous lines
intravenous lines surgically placed in large veins of the body

Intravenous therapy (IV) is prescribed by a physician and administered by a registered nurse. During this procedure, the nurse inserts a needle into the client's veins to provide a way to give fluids or medication. The medication or fluids are given by single injection, continuous drip slowly from a bottle or bag, or by a pump that regulates the flow of medication or nourishment through a tube secured to the needle (Figure 18.16 ■).

- *Continuous infusion*. Fluid and/or medication is always running. This type of therapy is most often prescribed for a client who has a family member or friend who can assume responsibility for the insertion site and care of the bottles or bags.
- *Intermittent infusion*. Small amounts of fluid or medication are given for short times. Each time a dose is needed, the IV must be started again.

There are three types of intravenous therapy:

- *Peripheral line*. Veins, usually of the upper extremities, are used.
- *Central venous line*. A catheter surgically implanted into one of the large veins is used. This type of catheter is used when the medication is irritating to the blood vessels or must be given frequently or when large amounts of medication must be given. The end of the catheter used for medication administration is visible on the chest area. Catheter care will be carefully discussed with you and the family. Do not touch the catheter until you have received the instructions (Figure 18.17 ■).
- *Peripherally inserted central venous catheter (PICC)*. This is inserted at the bedside by a specially trained nurse or physician. The care of this catheter and the dressing will be discussed with you and the family. Do not remove the dressing unless you have been instructed to do so.

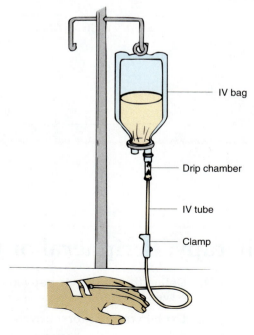

FIGURE 18.16 ■ Clients with IVs do not have to be in bed, but they must be in a relaxed environment.

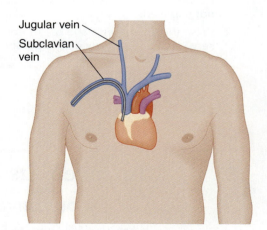

FIGURE 18.17 ■ Central lines should be cared for as prescribed by the physician. Be sure to immediately report to your supervisor any discomfort the client describes.

Your Role as a Homemaker/Home Health Aide

Be observant and supportive. Support the client and the family as they learn to care for the equipment. A client who has a continuous infusion may walk around as long as the bottle of fluid is above the insertion site and does not pull on the tubing. Remind the client not to sit or lean on the tubing.

You will not be responsible for care or dressing changes of the IV site. Central venous lines will be covered by a dressing when they are not in use. Sometimes, a peripheral line will have a cap on it when it is not in use. This cap is usually covered by a dressing. Do not disturb either type of dressing. You will be asked to keep the dressing dry and clean. Check the dressing at least every 8 hours to be sure it is secure. You should also be alert to changes in the site and report them immediately. Report if:

- The client complains of pain in the area.
- The area is red, hot, and/or swollen.
- You notice blood or any drainage from the area.
- The client removes the needle or tubing, or either falls out.
- The tubing has blood in it.
- The level of fluid in the bag or bottle does not decrease.
- The bag or bottle breaks.

Be sure to document when you check the dressing. Write down that you checked the area and the condition of the dressing and the skin.

Example:

> April 11, 2000   2:00 P.M.
> IV site on left arm checked. Client did not complain of discomfort. Skin intact. No drainage noted on dressing, which was secure and dry.
> Mary Cummings, H/HHA

SECTION 6

Cast Care

OBJECTIVES

What You Will Learn to Do

1. List the reasons for plaster casts.
2. Describe the homemaker/home health aide's role in caring for clients with plaster casts.

Introduction: Casts

A client who has broken a bone or sprained or strained a muscle may have a **cast** or splint placed on the body part to immobilize it. The procedure provides support to the injured part and prevents deformity by keeping it in the correct body alignment. Splints and casts are temporary. Permanent support to the bones in the form of pins, plates, and replacement of joints may also be necessary (Figures 18.18 ■ and 18.19 ■).

Plaster casts are, in reality, a form of a bandage. They are used as a support to hold injured bones in alignment while they are healing. Casts are wet when

cast
rigid dressing molded to the body to give support and proper alignment

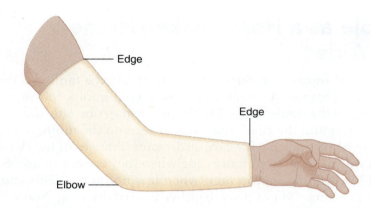

FIGURE 18.18 ■ Report immediately any changes in the casted limb or the cast that you notice or the client reports.

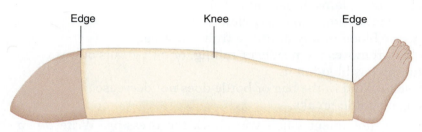

FIGURE 18.19 ■ Check the edges of the cast several times a day. Report immediately any sharp areas to your supervisor.

applied, then allowed to dry. Once they are hardened, the casts should be kept dry. Plastic or fiberglass casts perform the same task but are lighter, cleaner, and easier to use and remove.

While a plaster cast is drying, the client's position must be maintained and the cast left uncovered. It is normal for the cast to feel hot to the touch and to the client as it is drying. Pillows can be placed to support the cast so it will not move while it is still soft.

■ A cast should not restrict circulation to the part.
■ A cast should not cause pain. The pain should be only from the healing bone or muscle.
■ The skin under a cast frequently itches. Do not put anything into the cast. This might cause a scratch and lead to a skin infection.

Your Role as a Homemaker/Home Health Aide

Keep the cast clean and dry. It should be protected while a client is using the bedpan or toilet. Do not wash a plaster cast, as it will crumble.

There are casts that can be wet and allowed to air dry. Check with the client and your supervisor as to how to care for each cast. Just because casts look alike, they are not all cared for in the same way.

Encourage your client to take an active part in his care. Some people feel restricted in a cast and do not use the part as much as they are able. This unnecessary restriction of activity leads to a feeling of uselessness and loss of muscle tone.

Frequent careful checking of the cast and the injured part will help prevent complications. Call your supervisor if you notice any of the following:

- Client complaints of numbness or tingling of toes or fingers
- Discoloration of toes or fingers
- Swelling of the limb at the edge of the cast
- Unusual odors coming from the cast
- Rough or cracked edges of the cast
- Loosely fitting cast
- Discolorations on the cast

A client will often ask you how much movement he will have when the cast is removed. Tell him that you will find an answer for him. Then call your supervisor and discuss what to tell the client. Do not promise the client he will be fine unless that is what the physician has told him. Beware of telling him that everyone who has a broken arm is eventually fine. Everyone heals differently.

SECTION 7

Assisting with Ostomy Care

OBJECTIVES
What You Will Learn to Do

1. Define ostomy.
2. Demonstrate the proper techniques for assisting with ostomy care.

Introduction: The Ostomy

The creation of an ostomy is a surgical procedure. An **ostomy** is a new opening in the abdomen for the release of wastes from the body. The opening is called a **stoma**. This operation is necessary when the colon or urinary system is diseased or injured. Ostomies are created for many reasons—not only because a client has cancer. Sometimes, the surgery is done to permit the colon to heal following an injury. Some ostomies are temporary and others are permanent. The word *ostomy* means "opening into." A **colostomy** is an opening into the colon. An **ileostomy** is an opening into the ileum. A **ureterostomy** is an opening into the ureter. The opening is from the abdominal wall to the affected organ. The part you see, the stoma, will look like a pink rosebud (Figure 18.20 ■).

There are several types of colostomies. The type of colostomy takes its name from the placement of the stoma. It can be in the ascending, descending, or transverse colon. It can have one opening (single barrel) or two openings side by side (double barrel). The surgeon decides which type of colostomy is made.

A person with an ostomy must wear an appliance to collect the matter released through the stoma (Figure 18.21 ■). This collecting bag is held over the stoma by special paste, adhesive, and/or a belt. Some ostomy appliances are permanent. This means that they are reused after they are cleaned and dried. Some bags are disposable and used only once (Figure 18.22 ■).

Having an ostomy is usually a traumatic occurrence. It requires a big change in the way the client excretes either urine or fecal matter. It requires changes in

ostomy
artificially created opening through the abdominal wall that provides a way for the intestinal organs to discharge waste products

stoma
artificially made opening connecting a body passage with the outside

colostomy
surgical procedure that creates an artificial opening through the abdominal wall into a part of the large bowel through which feces can leave the body. Can be temporary or permanent

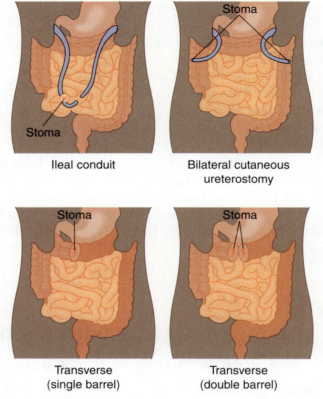

Ileal conduit

Bilateral cutaneous ureterostomy

Transverse (single barrel)

Transverse (double barrel)

FIGURE 18.20 ■ The physician determines the placement and type of ostomy before surgery.

ileostomy
surgical procedure that makes an artificial opening through the abdominal wall into the ileum, through which waste is discharged

ureterostomy
an incision through the abdominal wall into the ureters resulting in drainage to the outside of the body

the daily routine of the client and often of family members. The client's body image changes. Having an ostomy is a life-altering experience.

Everyone reacts differently to this experience. Families react differently to this experience. Some people learn the new routines and return to their previous lifestyles. Some people do not. Be alert to the coping mechanisms of your client and his family. Support them as they learn how to care for the ostomy and become familiar with the appliances.

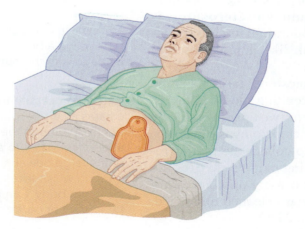

FIGURE 18.21 ■ The choice of a collection device is a personal one.

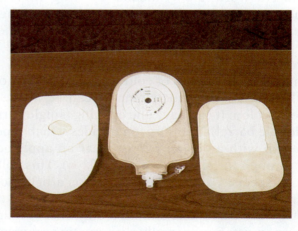

FIGURE 18.22 ■ There are various types of ostomy appliances.

Your Role as a Homemaker/Home Health Aide

When you receive your assignment, your supervisor will tell you the reasons the client had an ostomy. You will be told exactly for how much of the client's care you will be responsible. You will also be told what the client knows about his operation.

Your client's goal is to be as self-sufficient as possible. If the client cannot assume his total care, you will assist the client and his family as they establish a routine that they can maintain when you are no longer in the home.

A client and his family may want to discuss this operation with you. They will ask you questions. Do not lie to them. If they ask you questions that you cannot answer, assure them you will get the answers and call your supervisor. If the client asks you questions about death, recovery, and the future, and you are uncomfortable, discuss this with your supervisor. Frequently, a client or family member will ask you the same question many times. This is a way of confirming that the first answer you gave was the real one. Report this to your supervisor. Your supervisor can then help you plan your care to meet this client's need.

All ostomy care is based on several considerations. They are:

- Aseptic technique (rules of cleanliness)
- Client and family reaction to the procedure
- Client prognosis
- Frequent changing of the collection bag

A collection bag must be changed when it is full or when the adhering seal is broken. Some clients will be well enough to sit in the bathroom on the toilet to do this procedure. Also, many clients will be learning to do this procedure independently, in which case you will assist them less and less.

PROCEDURE 80

Assisting with an Ostomy

RATIONALE: Assisting with ostomy care contributes to the client's independence and overall well-being and decreases risk of skin irritation.

Note: Each client has his own routine for caring for his ostomy. This procedure is a general guide.

1. Assemble your equipment:
   Bedpan
   Disposable bed protector
   Bath blanket
   Clean ostomy belt (ostomy appliance), adjustable
   Toilet tissue
   Basin of water
   Soap or cleanser
   Washcloth
   Disposable gloves
   Towels
   Lubricant or skin cream, as ordered
   Plastic waste bag

2. Wash your hands.

3. Ask any visitors to leave the room, if appropriate.

4. Tell the client that you are going to assist him with changing his ostomy appliance.

5. Cover the client with the bath blanket. Ask the client to hold the top edge of the blanket. Without exposing him, fanfold the top sheet and bedspread to the foot of the bed under the blanket.

6. Place the disposable bed protector under the client's hips. This is to keep the bed from becoming wet or dirty.

7. Place the bedpan within easy reach.

continued

8. Put the wash basin, soap, washcloth, and bath towels near the bed. Put on gloves.

9. Open the belt. Protect it if it is clean and can be used again. If the belt is dirty, remove it. It must be replaced with a clean one.

10. Remove the soiled plastic stoma bag from the belt carefully.

11. Put the soiled plastic bag into the bedpan. Wipe the area around the ostomy with toilet tissue. This is to remove any loose feces. Place the dirty tissue in the plastic bag. Flush the tissues down the toilet later.

12. Wet and soap the washcloth. Wash the entire ostomy area with a gentle circular motion.

13. Dry the area gently with a bath towel.

14. Apply a small amount of lubricant or protective cream (if ordered) around the area of the ostomy. The lubricant is to prevent irritation to the skin around the ostomy. Wipe off all excess lubricant so that the ostomy device will adhere to the skin.

15. If using a wafer, secure it around the stoma. Be sure the size is correct (Figure 18.23 ■).

16. Put a clean adjustable belt, if the client wears one, on the client. Place a clean stoma bag in place through the loop.

17. Remove the disposable bed protector. Change any damp linen.

18. Replace the top sheet and bedspread, and remove the bath blanket.

19. Make the client comfortable.

20. Remove all used equipment. Dispose of waste material into the toilet. Do not throw the plastic collection bag down the toilet but into the plastic liner in the wastebasket.

21. Clean the bedpan and put it in its proper place.

22. Empty the wash basin into the toilet. Wash it thoroughly with soap and water. Rinse and dry it and return it to its proper place.

23. Remove gloves and wash your hands.

24. Make a notation on the client's chart that you have completed this procedure. Also make a note of your observations about the client during this procedure.

SAMPLE CHARTING:	5/29/04 2:20 P.M. Client able to apply ostomy bag with minimal assistance. Bag held all day. Client pleased with his increasing skill. Skin appears intact with no irritation. Client wearing street clothes. Carly Kitt H/HHA

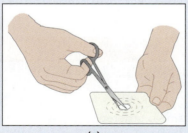

(a)
Cut the hole in the center of the wafer 1/8-inch larger than the stoma.

(b)
Peel the backing from the wafer.

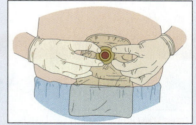

(c)
Place the wafer around the stoma and attach a clean bag.

FIGURE 18.23 ■

irrigate
cleanse or wash with water or fluid

Some clients **irrigate** their colostomy as part of their routine. Irrigating a colostomy is like giving an enema into the ostomy. You may, after you have been instructed, assist the client as he carries out this procedure.

As a homemaker/home health aide, you will be assisting clients and their families in many phases of ostomy care. Clients are often afraid of or disgusted by this procedure. Be patient and understanding. Let the clients and their families express their feelings. Listen. Although most ostomy clients are encouraged to assume their own care, they do so at different paces. Respect the clients' feelings and their individual wishes. Discuss your clients' reactions and your feelings and

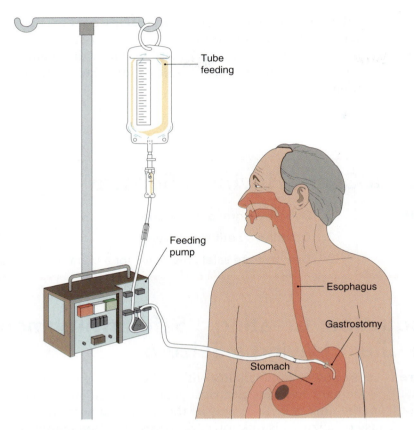

FIGURE 18.24 ■ A pump keeps the tube feeding drain at a predetermined rate.

activities when you see your supervisor. In this way, you will gain a better understanding of your client and yourself.

GASTROSTOMY, DUODENOSTOMY, AND JEJUNOSTOMY

These ostomies are surgical openings directly into various parts of the upper gastrointestinal tract. These incisions are kept open by the presence of a tube or a screw cap. The client will receive part or all of his nourishment through this opening. He may also take his medication through this opening (Figure 18.24 ■).

Your Role as a Homemaker/Home Health Aide

Your role in working with a client who has one of these openings is to assist him in feedings and in the care of the area. You will not be given complete responsibility for the procedure as it is important that a family member be able to assist the client when you are not there.

Cleanliness is an important part of the care. Be sure that the client's or family member's hands are clean before caring for the site and before starting the feeding.

Assist the client in making the feeding or in preparing commercially prepared feeding. Be sure to read directions and to follow them closely. When mixing the solution, date the container with important information such as date and time of mixing and initial use. It is wise to discard any feeding that is more than 24 hours old. Warm the solution to room temperature. Observe the client as to how he tolerates the feeding. Report your observations to your supervisor.

Note the time of the feeding, how long it lasts, and how the client tolerates it. Also note if he complains of any nausea, vomiting, diarrhea, cramps, or sweating after the feeding.

SECTION 8

Assisting a Client Having a Seizure

OBJECTIVES
What You Will Learn to Do

1. Describe a grand mal seizure.
2. Describe a petit mal seizure.
3. Demonstrate safety measures for a client having a seizure.

Introduction: Creating a Safe Environment for a Client Having a Seizure

seizure
convulsions or involuntary muscular contractions and relaxations

A **seizure** is caused by an abnormality within the central nervous system. This abnormality is thought to be an electrical problem in the nerve cells. Seizures can occur from the time of birth or may be the result of a head injury or disease. Often, the cause of seizures is unknown. Seizures are often controlled by medication.

As a homemaker/home health aide, you may be present when a client has a seizure. Therefore, it is important for you to know the warning signals of a seizure and what to do if one occurs.

aura
sensation before an epileptic seizure

A client may know when he is going to have a seizure. He experiences what is called an aura. An **aura** may be a smell or sensation that always occurs before the client has a seizure.

There are two types of seizures. One type is known as grand mal. The other type is a partial-body seizure known as a petit mal.

grand mal seizure
type of epileptic seizure

The **grand mal seizure** may include stiffness of the total body followed by a jerking action of the muscles. Usually, the client becomes unconscious. The client may bite his tongue or become incontinent. These seizures can last for several minutes.

petit mal seizure
type of epileptic seizure

In the **petit mal seizure**, the client may appear to be daydreaming. His eyes may roll back and there may be some quivering of the body muscles. The petit mal seizure usually lasts less than 30 seconds. The client usually has no memory of the seizure. A client who has been diagnosed as having epilepsy or who has seizures due to other diseases often leads a normal, productive life. Other people's ignorance about seizures is his biggest enemy.

Your Role as a Homemaker/Home Health Aide

Your role as a homemaker/home health aide in caring for a client having a seizure is to prevent the client from injuring himself. If you are present at the beginning of a seizure, you may place a padded tongue depressor, padded tongue blade, or a belt in the client's mouth, depending on the policy of your health-care agency. Some health-care agencies prefer that you simply turn the client's head to the side. If the client's jaw is already tight or he has his teeth clenched, *do not try to pry his teeth apart to insert a tongue depressor.* Help the client to lie down on the floor. Loosen his clothing and move any furniture that he might hit as he moves. Place a pillow or something soft under his head. *Turn his head to the side to promote drainage of saliva or vomitus. Never try to move or restrain the client.* Protect the client from people who may stare at him. Protect him from embarrassment.

Comfort the client after the seizure. Clean him of any saliva, urine, or fecal matter. Assist him with mouth care and care of his body after the seizure. After the client is comfortable and safe, chart the client's actions and your actions during this occurrence. Notify your supervisor of the entire incident.

Testing for Glucose (Sugar) and Acetone

OBJECTIVES

What You Will Learn to Do

1. Discuss the reasons for testing a client's blood for sugar and the urine for acetone.

2. Demonstrate the proper techniques for testing blood and urine.

Introduction: Testing Urine for Acetone and Blood for Glucose (Sugar)

Testing urine provides an accurate and easy method of checking how much acetone may be present. These procedures are usually for diabetic clients (see Chapter 19) and may be done with clients who have other disorders. The Acetest or Ketostix reagent strip determines the amount of **acetone** or **ketones** in the urine. The physician will prescribe when the test should be done and what equipment to use.

For each test you will use either a reagent strip or a reagent tablet. A **reagent** is a substance used in a chemical reaction to determine the presence of another substance. The names of these tablets or strips vary greatly according to geographical area and the pharmaceutical company that makes them. Instructions for these tests are on the package of reagent strips or reagent tablets. Be sure to follow the instructions exactly. All tablets and strips used for these tests are poisonous. Always put equipment in a safe place where children cannot reach them. Be sure to wash and dry all equipment between tests and keep bottles tightly closed. Some readings are recorded as percentages and some as "plus" (++, etc.). Be sure you ask how the client reports his readings.

For testing the urine, a small amount of fresh specimen is needed. The word *fresh* is used to refer to urine that has accumulated recently in the client's urinary bladder. The word *fractional* is used to refer to a small portion of the urine voided. To obtain fresh urine, it is necessary to discard the first urine voided because this urine has remained in the bladder for an unknown length of time. One-half hour after discarding the urine, collect a fresh urine specimen for the test. This will be urine recently accumulated in the urinary bladder.

acetone
a chemical found in urine

ketones
chemical compounds sometimes found in urine

reagent
a substance used to measure or detect another substance

The amount of glucose in the blood indicates the amount of medication and food the diabetic person must have. Diabetic clients are taught how to monitor their blood glucose by using one of several testing devices. They are also instructed how to record their findings and how to adjust their medication. The device and the timing of the tests are prescribed by the physician and may be different for each client.

PROCEDURE 81

Testing Blood for Glucose

RATIONALE: Correctly testing blood contributes to the client's general well-being and assists with ongoing monitoring of his medication, diet, and exercise regime.

1. Assemble your equipment:
   One-Touch Profile meter
   Test strips
   Penlet and lancet
   Disposable pipet
   Disposable gloves
   Band-Aid

2. Wash your hands.

3. Explain to the client that you are going to test his blood sugar.

4. Make the client comfortable and wash his hands with soap and water.

5. Put on disposable gloves.

6. Match the code on the test strips to the number on the meter. Check the expiration date on the test strips. Discard them if they have expired. The code number may have to be reset. Follow the manufacturer's instructions.

7. Remove test strip from container. Close the container. Do not touch the white area of the strip.

8. Press Power and insert the strip into the meter (Figure 18.25 ■).

9. Insert the lancet into the Penlet according to the manufacturer's directions.

10. Place the end of the lancet firmly against the side of a fingertip of the client.

11. Press the button on top of the Penlet.

12. Squeeze the finger gently to obtain a large drop of blood.

13. Using a disposable pipet, slowly draw up the drop of blood and apply the sample to the test strip. This method prevents contamination of the client and is preferred in a hospital or nursing-home setting where several patients or residents use the same blood glucose meter. An alternative method for individual use (at home, for example) is to apply the blood sample directly to the strip (Figure 18.26 ■).

14. Wait a short time for the results to appear on the blood glucose meter (Figure 18.27 ■).

15. Apply the Band-Aid to the client's finger.

16. Remove disposable gloves and wash your hands.

17. Record the results. Notify the supervisor if the results are above or below normal.

SAMPLE CHARTING: 11/11/04   12:30 P.M.
Blood sugar tested   95.
Ruth Sapp H/HHA

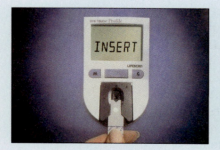

FIGURE 18.25 ■ (Photo courtesy of Johnson & Johnson)

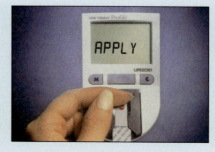

FIGURE 18.26 ■ (Photo courtesy of Johnson & Johnson)

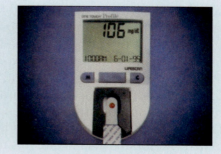

FIGURE 18.27 ■ (Photo courtesy of Johnson & Johnson)

SECTION 10

Deep-Breathing Exercises

OBJECTIVES

What You Will Learn to Do

1. State the reasons for shallow breathing. State your role in assisting clients with deep-breathing exercises.

2. Demonstrate the correct technique for assisting clients with deep-breathing exercises.

Introduction: Deep Breathing

Shallow breathing takes place in the upper lobes of the lungs, which are surrounded by bony areas on all sides. The lungs cannot expand much in the bony enclosure, so they cannot take in much oxygen or exhale much carbon dioxide. People who have had lung disease for a long time have "barrel chests." The chest cavity has taken on this shape in an attempt for the lungs to inhale more oxygen.

Deep breathing helps people inhale more air with less effort than their usual type of breathing. When people breathe deeply, the lower lobes of the lungs push the soft tissue of the abdomen out of the way and expand to take in more air.

People who have lung disease continue to breathe with shallow breaths because of fear and misinformation about how their bodies are built. You can help clients trust deep breathing by explaining how their lungs work.

Your supervisor will do this, too, but it will be your responsibility to answer questions. If you do not know the answer, tell the clients that you will get the information and ask your supervisor.

Your Role as a Homemaker/Home Health Aide

A client who is learning to deep breathe is often frightened. Have patience and be gentle. Praise the client, and point out small successes. Continue to reinforce the reasons why deep breathing is important.

When the client takes a deep breath, his shoulders and chest should *not* move. His abdomen should expand. When he exhales his abdomen should become *flat*. If the client is confused about how to do this, tell him to cough. The squeezing of the abdominal area will make him aware of where the muscular activity should take place.

Coughing is forced expiration. Deep breathing sometimes produces a coughing response. This is true especially if the lungs are congested. Keep a basin, tissue, or specimen container (if ordered) near the client. Collect any mucous he may bring up. Encourage him to spit it out. Note the color, amount, and odor.

Protect the client from visitors and friends when he is coughing. Deep breathing is frequently unpleasant, although it is important. Because it can also make people cough and bring up mucous, plan this exercise between mealtimes. By doing this, you will not cause vomiting or loss of appetite.

The physical therapist will instruct you as to how often to do this exercise. She may also give you special instructions for your client. Remember, all clients are different, and although the exercise may look the same for two people, it may be done for different reasons. The physical therapist will also tell you of any special observations you are to make while you help the client.

Even though you can do these exercises, do not start them until you have been instructed to do so. The aim of teaching clients deep breathing, or "abdominal breathing," as it is also called, is to change their breathing habits permanently.

PROCEDURE 82

Helping a Client with Deep-Breathing Exercises

1. Assemble your equipment:
   Equipment for mouth care following this procedure
   Tissues and basin or specimen container
   Plastic bag for waste

2. Wash your hands.

3. Ask visitors to leave the room, if appropriate.

4. Tell the client you are going to help him with deep-breathing exercises.

5. Direct the client to breathe in deeply through his nose

6. Direct the client to blow out through his mouth with his lips "pursed," as though he were blowing out a match (Figure 18.28 ■).

7. Repeat the steps 10 times.

8. Offer the client mouth care.

9. Dispose of the tissues into a plastic bag.

10. Make the client comfortable.

11. Make a notation on the chart that you have completed this procedure. Also note anything you observed about the client while doing this procedure.

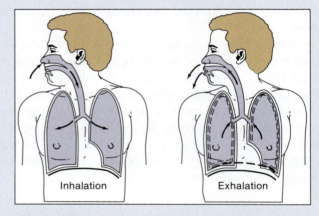

Inhalation   Exhalation

FIGURE 18.28 ■

SECTION 11

Making Normal Saline

OBJECTIVES

What You Will Learn to Do

1. Describe uses of normal saline.

2. Demonstrate the procedure for making normal saline.

Introduction: Making Normal Saline

Normal saline is a solution of salt and water that has many uses. Its chemical makeup is close to the fluids in the body. It is usually used to wash open areas or to clean sore bony prominences or bedsores. It may also be used by a nurse to irrigate a Foley catheter.

PROCEDURE 83

Making Normal Saline

RATIONALE: Making normal saline decreases the need for the client to purchase this and contributes to infection control in the home.

1. Assemble your equipment:
   Large pot
   Sterilized 1-quart jar and lid
   2 teaspoons of salt
   1 quart of water
   Source of heat (stove, sterno, fire)
2. Wash your hands.
3. Measure 1 quart of water into pot. Add 2 teaspoons of salt. Boil covered for 10 minutes (Figure 18.29 ■).

4. Pour into sterilized jar, and replace cover. Allow solution to cool (Figure 18.30 ■).
5. The solution may be used up to 48 hours after preparation.

SAMPLE CHARTING: 7/24/04   12:20 P.M.
A bottle of normal saline made and left in sterile bottle. Client will use it to irrigate his wound.
Joanne White H/HHA

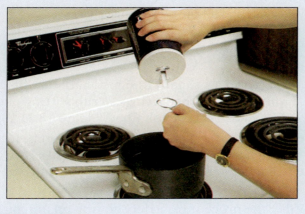

FIGURE 18.29 ■

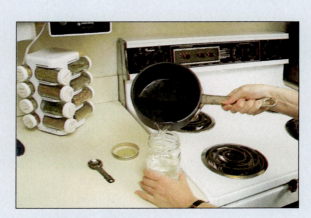

FIGURE 18.30 ■

SECTION 12

Sitz Bath

OBJECTIVES

What You Will Learn to Do

1. List three reasons a client may need a sitz bath.
2. Describe the safety precautions you will take when assisting a client with a sitz bath.
3. Demonstrate what you will report to your supervisor after your client has taken a sitz bath.

Introduction: The Sitz Bath

The term **sitz bath** means "seat bath" or a bath taken while seated. The area bathed is the perineal area. Such a procedure may be ordered to promote healing of the area, to decrease pain following surgery or a procedure, and to increase relaxation of the muscles in the perineal area.

sitz bath
bath in which the client sits in a specially designed chair or tub with his hips and buttocks in water

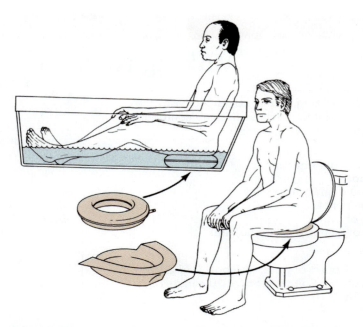

FIGURE 18.31 ■ Provide a safe and private place for the client during a sitz bath. Be sure he can signal for assistance.

The client can take a sitz bath either in a specially designed bath that fits into the toilet or commode or in a bathtub that has had a covered rubber ring placed in it so that the perineal area is suspended off the tub floor (Figure 18.31 ■).

Safety Considerations: Be sure the water is the correct temperature. It should be comfortable to the touch and measure between 95° and 110°F or between 35° and 43°C. Water that is too hot will burn the client, and water that is too cold will cause the muscles to tighten up rather than relax.

Help the client start and finish the procedure. Safely getting on and off the commode or in and out of the tub should be done slowly and at the client's speed. Protect the client from slipping and falling on towels, clothes, or dressings.

Maintain the water temperature by adding warm water when necessary.

Help the client keep track of the time. The usual length of time for a sitz bath is between 10 and 15 minutes. You will be told how long and how often your client should have a sitz bath. Check on your client frequently and tell him how long he has yet to go. Ask your client how he feels and also observe him.

Your Role as a Homemaker/Home Health Aide

Your role is to help the client take his sitz bath as it has been ordered. If you find the client deviates from the order, report that to your supervisor.

You will also be responsible for cleaning the sitz bath or the bathtub following the procedure. Be sure that the bath area is clean and dry and ready for the next time the client must bathe. Assist the client with dressings that he may have to apply and dispose of old soiled dressings in plastic bags in the outside trash.

Following the procedure, after the client is comfortable and the area is clean, you will chart your activities. These are the elements to include:

- The length of time the client remained in the bath
- The client's reaction to the bath
- A description of any drainage from the wounds
- How the client finished the procedure—new dressing, returned to bed, and so on

SECTION 13

Hyperalimentation

OBJECTIVES

What You Will Learn to Do

1. Recognize the reasons that a client would receive hyperalimentation.

2. Discuss the homemaker/home health aide's role as an observer during the feeding.

3. List at least five occurrences when you would call your supervisor.

Introduction: Working with Hyperalimentation

Clients who are severely malnourished and who are unable to eat may receive their nutritional requirements by means of **hyperalimentation**. For long-term administration a catheter is surgically placed in a large vein and the nutrition is administered directly into the blood stream. A physician orders the exact dose of the supplement, which must be mixed by a pharmacy. A pharmacy or company specializing in this service has the responsibility for delivering the correct feeding to the client every 24 hours. The catheter used for the feeding is used for no other purpose. Some bottles or bags must be kept refrigerated. Some must be at room temperature. If the delivery does not arrive on time or you notice that the feedings are stored improperly, call your supervisor. Do not discard any unused feedings. Return them to the pharmacy.

Clients may receive this treatment for a short amount of time or for several years. Some clients receive their feedings in the evening and work during the day. Others receive feedings over a 24-hour period. Clients who receive this treatment must be able to assume responsibility for feedings or have responsible family members who can. This teaching usually takes place in the hospital and will be reinforced in the home by the company that brings the feedings. Be sure you and the client have the emergency telephone numbers to call with questions. The professionals from the supply company will take responsibility for checking the pump and the catheter insertion site. If family members have any questions between visits, they should be encouraged to contact the suppliers via the emergency telephone numbers.

You will not be asked to administer the feedings or change the dressings on the catheter, but you will be responsible for assisting with preparation of the bottles.

hyperalimentation
process of giving nutrients directly into the blood stream

Your Role as a Homemaker/Home Health Aide

You will care for the client's personal needs during administration of the hyper-alimentation and help the family incorporate this into their regular routine. Look for any changes in the client. Report them immediately. If you are to keep a record of intake and output, vital signs, and weights, do so accurately.

- Report any shortness of breath, tingling in arms or feet, weakness, or temperature change.
- Report any irritation or drainage near the catheter site.
- Report any change in the client.
- Help the client maintain a comfortable position during the feeding. The tubes should be straight and not under the client. Help the client identify the place in the house where he prefers the feeding to be administered.

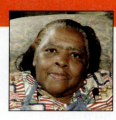

Case Study

Review the case study that appears on the first page of the chapter. Answer two sets of questions about the case study contained in the Explore and Apply sections below.

EXPLORE

1. Mrs. Collins tells you that her neighbor thinks she should go out and sit in the park. She is not sure she will be able to manage her oxygen. She also tells you that one of the reasons she does not leave her house is that she is sometimes incontinent of urine. What do you tell her? What do you do with the information?

2. Mrs. Collins' neighbor has arranged for church members to visit Mrs. Collins and assist her with her bath, her cooking, and with cleaning up her small apartment. What are your responsibilities when you leave the house and you know these ladies are coming to visit?

APPLY

1. You have been asked to check Mrs. Collins' blood sugar twice a day. When you arrive one day, you see that the client and her visitors are eating homebaked cookies. How do you chart your findings from the blood sugar test? Is it important to note that the client is eating cookies?

2. You think someone is using Mrs. Collins' oxygen. What do you do?

Certification Exam Review Questions

Choose the best answer for each question or statement.

1. **You notice that one medication, which your client has taken for a long time, looks different. The pill used to be white and now it is pink and purple.**

   a. *You don't do anything because the client says it is not a problem.*

   b. *You call the pharmacy and ask what the pill is.*

   c. *You call your supervisor and report this and note that the client seems to have a slight rash on his hands.*

   d. *You leave a note for his daughter, who will visit over the weekend.*

2. **Your client has been prescribed oxygen for when he walks around the house. You notice he rarely uses it, and when he does, he seems more sleepy.**

   a. *You advise your client to continue using the oxygen as it has been prescribed.*

   b. *You call your supervisor immediately and report this.*

   c. *You call the oxygen company and report this.*

   d. *You don't do anything.*

3. **When caring for your client, you frequently change his nonsterile dressing and do his catheter care right after his bath. This allows you to keep your gloves on and combine the tasks to save time. You tell your coworkers how you have saved time and are surprised at their reaction.**

   a. *You have created a way for bacteria to be transported from one area of the body to another.*

   b. *The client will be billed for the extra gloves anyway, so your savings does not matter.*

   c. *Since his daughter does not do things the same way, this confuses him.*

   d. *You should not have told anyone because this indicates that you are not using your time wisely.*

4. **The sheets are always wet when you arrive at your client's house. You suggest to his wife that external drainage be used. She likes the idea. How do you go about starting it?**

   a. *You go the pharmacy, buy the setup, and put it on.*

   b. *You call your supervisor to discuss this, and she requests an order for it from the doctor.*

   c. *You tell the wife to get the setup and put it on, herself.*

   d. *You put the client in diapers and rubber pants until the doctor calls back.*

5. **Your client does not change his ostomy bag until you arrive at the house every other day.**

   a. *This is fine as long as it is on well and his skin is not red.*

   b. *You tell him he has to change it every day even though you are not there to help him.*

   c. *You stop by every day even though your agency doesn't know.*

   d. *You call your supervisor and discuss this with her.*

CHAPTER 19

Common Diseases You Will See

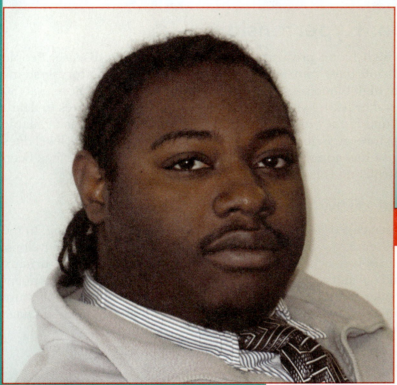

CASE STUDY

Mr. Martinez has just been told he has diabetes. He is a salesman in a small store and fears that his employer will not understand that he has to eat frequent meals. His family is supportive and interested in changing their lifestyle if necessary to treat his disease, but he refuses to discuss it. His children have checked out several library books and have printed a great deal of information from the Internet. They are sure that Mr. Martinez will be able to continue working and his life will be as full and as enjoyable as before he was diagnosed. Mr. Martinez is not as confident.

Keep the case study in mind as you read the chapter. After you have read the chapter, answer the Explore and Apply questions at the end of the chapter that relate to the case study.

Hypertension

OBJECTIVES

What You Will Learn to Do

1. Discuss the most common signs and symptoms of hypertension.

2. Discuss your role in caring for clients with hypertension.

Introduction: Hypertension

hypertension
high blood pressure

Hypertension, or high blood pressure, is a treatable chronic disease. People who have hypertension have more stress placed on their circulatory systems than people without high blood pressure. Latest estimates are that more than 50 million Americans suffer from hypertension. Hypertension contributes to death from heart disease and kidney disease. Treatment for hypertension is available but must be kept up forever. Bringing blood pressure to an acceptable level does not mean the disease has gone away; it only means that the disease has been brought under control, and this control must be continued.

HOW DO PEOPLE KNOW THEY HAVE HYPERTENSION?

Hypertension has been called "the silent killer" because it gives no warning. In the early stages of this disease, there often are no symptoms. As the disease develops, people may complain of headaches, vision changes, or problems with their urinary output. If they would consult a physician at this point in their disease, permanent damage to a vital organ could be avoided. Some people with high blood pressure do not seek help until they have severe problems. By that time, permanent damage to vital organs is common. You have a higher risk of hypertension if you:

- Have a family history of hypertension, heart disease, or kidney disease
- Smoke cigarettes
- Are overweight
- Use a lot of salt in your diet
- Are African-American
- Eat a large amount of saturated fats

CAUSES AND TREATMENT OF HYPERTENSION

Many conditions seem to cause hypertension, and some causes are still unknown. Research scientists are investigating diet, heredity, birth control pills, kidney infections, and chemicals as possible causes of this chronic disease. An individualized treatment plan is developed by a physician after a thorough medical examination. Treatment may consist of a combination of diet, medication, and exercise.

Your Role as a Homemaker/Home Health Aide

Follow the plan of care for your client. Support your client in complying with his medication plan, diet, and exercise. Report to your supervisor any deviation from the care plan.

Assist the client with incorporating his treatment into his usual daily routine. Because he will always be on some treatment for this disease, it is important that the treatment become a regular part of his day.

Listen to your client. If he has questions about hypertension and/or his treatment, answer him honestly. If you do not know the answer, call your supervisor and be sure that the client receives his answers.

Be observant for possible side effects from the medication. Depending on the drug and the client, side effects range from a stuffy nose to muscle cramps, weakness, nightmares, and impotence. Careful observations and objective, timely reporting of these and other symptoms will result in a treatment plan the client can live with the rest of his life. If the client starts taking any medications, including nonprescription drugs, report this to your supervisor.

SECTION 2

Heart Attack/Myocardial Infarction

OBJECTIVES

What You Will Learn to Do

1. Define *myocardial infarction*.
2. Define *atherosclerosis*.
3. List the common symptoms of a heart attack.
4. Discuss three kinds of pacemakers.
5. Discuss the homemaker/home health aide's role in caring for a client recovering from a myocardial infarction.

Introduction: Myocardial Infarction

Heart attack is a general term that describes sudden damage to the heart. There are many medical reasons people have heart attacks, but they all have the same results—a decrease in the blood supply to the heart eventually leads to heart muscle damage and possibly permanent tissue death.

The word *infarct* means "death of tissue due to lack of blood." The word *myocardial* refers to heart muscle. So a **myocardial infarction**, or **MI**, is really the death of part of the heart due to a blockage in a blood vessel. If the blood vessel involved is a small one and only a small amount of heart muscle is affected, this may be called a minor or small heart attack. If the blood vessel involved is a large one and a large portion of the heart is damaged, it is often called a massive heart attack. The ultimate recovery of the injured heart depends on the location of the MI within the heart; presence of atherosclerosis; age, sex, and the health history of the individual.

ARTERIOSCLEROSIS

Arteriosclerosis is hardening of arteries and leads to a decrease in the blood supply to body tissue due to a thickening of vessel walls (Figure 19.1 ■). **Atherosclerosis** is a form of arteriosclerosis that takes place in several steps:

- A fatty streak develops in the vessel.
- A fibrous plaque develops on top of the fatty streak. Depending on the size of this plaque, the vessel remains open or becomes completely obstructed.
- Sometimes, a clot develops in the same spot as the fibrous plaque.

heart attack
general term referring to damage to the heart; a myocardial infarction

myocardial infarction (MI)
death of a part of the heart due to blockage in a blood vessel

arteriosclerosis
hardening of the arteries due to thickening of the blood vessel walls

atherosclerosis
increased formation of fatty deposits and fibrous plaques, resulting in decrease of the lumen of the blood vessel

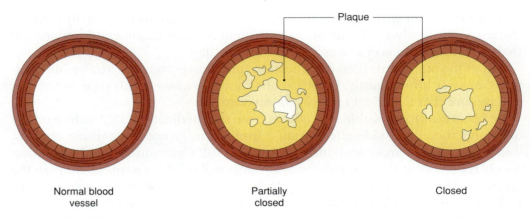

Normal blood vessel

Partially closed

Closed

FIGURE 19.1 ■ Elimination of plaque-forming foods from the diet should begin in early childhood.

If atherosclerosis is discovered and treated after the first stage, the condition is reversible. However, once a vessel is completely blocked by plaque, it usually remains that way.

SIGNS AND SYMPTOMS OF A HEART ATTACK

The following signs and symptoms may appear in your client or in a member of the family. Call for emergency help immediately and keep the client quiet and warm until help arrives.

- Chest pain that may or may not radiate to the arm or jaw
- Wet, clammy skin
- Weak and/or rapid pulse rate
- Pale color
- Low blood pressure
- Shortness of breath
- Nausea

The single best way to prevent or minimize permanent damage to the heart is to get help at a hospital as soon as possible. Every minute is important!

Your Role as a Homemaker/Home Health Aide

After hospitalization, your client will return with an individualized plan of care based on:

- The type of heart attack he had
- His recovery up to that point
- His home situation
- His prognosis

Allow him as large a part in his care as his activity level permits. The plan of care you will receive from your supervisor will include instructions about:

- Activity restrictions
- Diet restrictions
- Medications
- Emotional support

While giving care to a person with a cardiac disability, every caregiver balances the desire to allow the client to be a self-sufficient person and the need to restrict his activity level. Continual discussion with your supervisor as to your client's condition will assist you in making correct decisions.

A client usually receives an exercise regime. If your client is unable to progress with the exercise or tries to advance too quickly, report this to your supervisor.

After a heart attack, a person may become a "cardiac cripple." He is so afraid of another heart attack that he does not exert himself at all or take any part in his care. He even removes himself from family relationships. Everything he does is blamed on his heart attack and his fear of another one.

The opposite of this is a total disregard for one's condition. The client denies any disability. He does not follow any suggestions from his physician, take his medication, or adhere to his diet. Report this behavior to your supervisor.

A client often is concerned about how his heart attack will affect his sexual activities. A client usually will return to a full sexual life; however, a discussion on this topic is best handled by the client's physician or nurse, who knows what the client has already been told. Do not give the client any opinions or folktales, but rather say, "I know you are concerned about this, and I will tell the nurse. She will get you the information you want."

A family member may need help in dealing with the stress of lifestyle changes and fear caused by cardiac disease. Suggest that any family member who needs help or expresses these fears seek the assistance of a support group or his own physician.

PACEMAKERS

A **pacemaker** is an electrical device placed either in the left or right upper chest under the skin (Figure 19.2 ■). The job of this device is to regulate the heart rhythm. A pacemaker can be temporary or permanent. There are three types of pacemakers:

pacemaker
electrical device used to stimulate the heart

1. *Fixed-rate.* Stimulation rate is fixed usually between 60 and 70 beats per minute. This is used only if the heart is totally dependent on electrical stimulation and is only used temporarily. It is rarely seen in the home.
2. *Synchronous.* Stimulation occurs after a predetermined lack of the heart's own activity. This type is not seen often in the home.
3. *Demand.* When the heartbeat falls below a predetermined rate, the pacemaker takes over. This is the most common type.

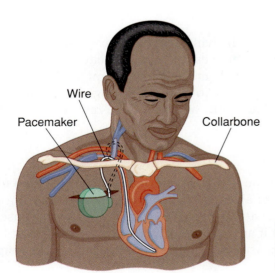

FIGURE 19.2 ■
Pacemakers permit people to live normal productive lives with only a few restrictions.

Care of a Pacemaker

It is helpful to know what type of pacemaker your client has. It is also important to know at what rate it is set. There are several guidelines to keep in mind when you have a client with a pacemaker.

- Electrical appliances may be used around pacemakers.
- Microwave ovens should not be used around pacemakers. Some clients have difficulties being around lawn mowers and cellular telephones.
- If your client has hiccups, report this immediately. This could be an indication that the electrical wires are out of place.
- If your client's pulse is below the preset level of the pacemaker, report it immediately.
- Report pain or discoloration near the pacemaker.
- Detecting devices in airports should be avoided.
- Report any complaints of dizziness, **edema** (swelling), shortness of breath, or irregular heart beat.
- When moving, lifting, or assisting a client who has a pacemaker, support him without putting pressure under his arms.
- Batteries have to be replaced from time to time. The physician decides when this is to be done. It varies from client to client.
- Assist your client with his telephone monitoring procedure. Be sure he understands it so that he can do it when you are no longer in the house.

edema
abnormal swelling of a part of the body caused by fluid collecting in that area

---

SECTION 3

Angina

OBJECTIVES

What You Will Learn to Do

1. Define angina and list its major causes and risk factors.
2. Discuss treatments for angina.
3. Discuss your role as a homemaker/home health aide when caring for a patient with angina.

Introduction: Angina

angina
brief, temporary chest pain resulting from a decrease in oxygen to the heart

Angina is a brief, temporary pain or heaviness in the chest that results from lack of oxygen to the heart. Usually after resting and medication, the client no longer experiences discomfort. An episode may be brought on by stress or physical activity. Angina differs from person to person. Changes in your client's angina signal a change in his cardiac status and should be reported to your supervisor immediately.

CAUSES OF ANGINA

Angina is caused by narrowing of the coronary arteries that bring oxygen to the heart. As these vessels narrow, the amount of oxygen decreases, causing pain and discomfort. This is not a heart attack or myocardial infarction because it is a temporary condition. However, if angina is allowed to continue without treatment, the sufferer could have a heart attack, and sustain permanent damage to the heart.

You have a higher risk of angina if you:

- Have high blood pressure
- Have high blood cholesterol
- Smoke cigarettes
- Are overweight
- Have high stress levels

TREATMENT

There is no sure cure for angina. Most people with the disease, however, learn to live productive and meaningful lives. The aim of all treatment is to increase the flow of blood and oxygen to the heart. This is accomplished in several ways.

- *Medication.* The physician will prescribe a regime of medication to help the client and decrease his pain. The medication will be individualized for his particular condition and should not be altered without consulting the doctor.
- *Control of risk factors.* The client may be put on a weight-reducing diet, told to decrease his use of cigarettes, and advised to decrease his stress. These alterations in lifestyle are difficult, and the client and his family will need a great deal of encouragement and support to reach the goal.
- *Surgery.* If this treatment has been recommended by a physician and your client or his family have questions, report this to your supervisor immediately so that questions can be answered.

Your Role as a Homemaker/Home Health Aide

Your role is to help the client and his family maintain the regime set up for him. Remember, activity levels, diets, and medications are individualized and should not be compared to other clients' or changed without medical consultation.

By providing support to your client and his family as he tries to alter his lifestyle and decrease his risk factors, you will be giving him the care he needs. Point out the achievements he has made and the progress he hopes to make in the near future. Do not dwell on his failures. It is usual for a client who is trying to make changes in his lifestyle to slip back into old patterns from time to time. Do not be judgmental, but rather encourage him to return to the more healthy activities.

Be alert to stress in the family. Sometimes when there is change in the family function, the other members, not the client, will exhibit stress. If you notice such family discord, report it to your supervisor.

SECTION 4

Diabetes

OBJECTIVES

What You Will Learn to Do

1. Define *diabetes*.
2. Recognize the signs and symptoms of diabetes.
3. Recognize the signs and symptoms of too much insulin and not enough insulin.
4. Discuss the role of the homemaker/home health aide in caring for a diabetic client.

Introduction: Diabetes

When the body cannot change **carbohydrates** (sugars and starches) into energy because of an imbalance of **insulin**, the result is the chronic disease known as **diabetes mellitus**. The pancreas usually produces insulin on a feedback mechanism. When the body needs insulin following a meal or when extra energy is needed, the pancreas is alerted and it pumps extra insulin into the bloodstream. If, however, the body needs insulin and none is produced, starches and sugars cannot be converted into energy and absorbed by the cells. Sugar remains in the bloodstream and is eventually excreted in the urine as waste.

SIGNS AND SYMPTOMS OF DIABETES MELLITUS

- Fatigue, tiredness
- Loss of weight
- Sores heal poorly and slowly
- High blood sugar
- Sugar in the urine
- Frequent and large amounts of urine
- Excessive thirst
- Poor vision
- Inflammation of the vagina

There are two types of diabetes. Type I results in the person having to take insulin. In Type II diabetes, the pancreas produces some insulin, but not enough for normal body function. In this type of diabetes, the person may take oral medications or just regulate his diet. Because a diabetic has a regulated amount of insulin in his body, his food intake must be regulated also. If the amount of food is greater than the amount of insulin available, there will be too much unmetabolized sugar left in the blood. If the amount of insulin is greater than the amount of food available, there will not be any carbohydrates for the insulin to metabolize, and this will cause other problems.

Diabetes can be controlled, but never cured. A diabetic must maintain a special diet and must sometimes take medication by mouth or insulin by injection forever. A person with diabetes can live a full and productive life if he keeps to a diet and a medication schedule. Diagnosis of this disease can be made only by a physician following laboratory tests.

DIABETIC COMA AND INSULIN SHOCK

Be alert for signs and symptoms of **diabetic coma** and **insulin shock** or **insulin reaction**, and follow the emergency procedure for your client.

Signs and Symptoms of Diabetic Coma (Hyperglycemia/High-Blood-Sugar Diabetic Ketoacidosis)

Diabetic coma (**ketoacidosis**) occurs when the blood has too many carbohydrates and not enough insulin to metabolize it. The symptoms include:

- Air hunger; heavy, labored breathing; increased respiration
- Loss of appetite
- Dulled senses
- Nausea and/or vomiting
- Weakness

carbohydrate
one of the basic food elements necessary for the body to function properly; includes all sugars and starches

insulin
hormone produced by the pancreas that is needed for the metabolism of sugars and starches

diabetes mellitus
condition that develops when the body cannot change sugar into energy

diabetic coma
hyperglycemia: an excess of circulating sugar in the blood

insulin shock or insulin reaction
hypoglycemia caused by too much insulin in the blood

ketoacidosis
a condition characterized by a large amount of ketone bodies in the urine

- Abdominal pains or discomfort
- Generalized aches
- Increased thirst and parched tongue
- Sweet or fruity odor of the breath
- Flushed dry skin
- Increased urination
- Soft eyeballs
- Upon examination: large amounts of sugar and ketones in the urine and high blood sugar

Signs and Symptoms of Insulin Shock (Hypoglycemia/ Low-Blood-Sugar Insulin Reaction)

Insulin shock, or insulin reaction, occurs when a person's blood has more insulin than the amount of carbohydrates available for metabolism. The symptoms include:

- Excessive sweating, perspiration
- Faintness, dizziness, weakness
- Hunger
- Irritability, personality change, nervousness
- Numbness of tongue and lips
- Inability to awaken, coma, unconsciousness, stupor
- Headache
- Tremors, trembling
- Blurred or impaired vision
- Upon examination: low blood sugar and no sugar in the urine

Your Role as a Homemaker/Home Health Aide

Your role is to help the client and his family learn to live with this disease and the routine of medication and diet. Point out the positive aspects of the client's situation. Help the family adapt the prescribed diet to its lifestyle. If this diet seems difficult, report to your supervisor. She will get in touch with the nutritionist, who will try to adapt the diet to the family's needs.

Assist your client with his medication, but never give him an injection or oral medication. Insulin is always taken by injection, not by mouth. Insulin should be kept in a cool place, away from heat and strong light. Notify your supervisor if the client does not keep to his medication schedule or has any reaction to his medication.

You may be asked to test the client's urine for sugar and acetone. Be sure that you ask your supervisor when to call her with the results. If possible, the client may do this procedure under your supervision.

A diabetic may have difficulty with his feet. Observe nails and toes for infection or pressure areas. Report these immediately. Do not cut toenails or fingernails. This procedure should be done by a podiatrist or a family member who has been specially trained.

As you care for the client, notice the condition of his skin. Is it dry, is it flaky, Do you see bruises and any bruises healing? Because a diabetic has a harder time healing than a nondiabetic, it is important to prevent bruises and pressure areas. If the skin is dry, lubricate it. Dry skin often itches, and a client who scratches himself could injure the skin, causing bruises or infection.

SECTION 5

Cerebrovascular Accident

OBJECTIVES

What You Will Learn to Do

1. Describe a CVA.
2. List several causes of a CVA.
3. Discuss your role as a homemaker/home health aide when caring for a client who has had a CVA.

Introduction: Cerebrovascular Accident

cerebrovascular accident (CVA)
death of brain tissue caused by a blood vessel blockage within the brain

stroke
cerebrovascular accident

The term **cerebrovascular accident (CVA)** has three important parts:

1. *Cerebro:* having to do with the brain
2. *Vascular:* having to do with the blood vessels
3. *Accident:* something unpredictable and unexpected

A CVA (or **stroke**/"brain attack"), the third leading cause of death in the United States, occurs when the blood supply to a part of the brain is stopped by a blocked blood vessel. When blood flow stops, the tissue dies. Because each part of the brain controls a different function, the result of a CVA depends on which blood vessel is blocked and which brain center is destroyed.

It is important to remember that the results of the CVA may be paralysis, loss of speech, or loss of vision, but that the cause of the problem is disruption of nerve impulse transmission from brain tissue damage.

collateral circulation
circulation taken over by smaller blood vessels after obstruction of larger ones

In some brains, when a blood vessel is blocked, the surrounding blood vessels take over to supply the injured part of the brain. This is called **collateral circulation**. In this case, the damage may not be as great as if there were no collateral circulation.

The speech center of the brain is on the left side, so if the CVA occurs on that side, speech may be affected. If the CVA occurs on the right side, varying degrees of muscle weakness may be the result (Figure 19.3 ■).

CAUSES OF A CVA

There are four main causes of a CVA:

clot
semisolid mass of blood

embolus
a clot carried by the circulatory system from its place of formation to another site, usually causing an obstruction

1. A blood **clot** can form elsewhere in the body, travel to the brain, and lodge in a small vessel. This is called an **embolus** (Figure 19.4a ■).

Motor Area

Sensory Area

Pain,
Temperature
Touch,
Pressure
Position,
Body image

FIGURE 19.3 ■
Every part of the brain governs a specific function.

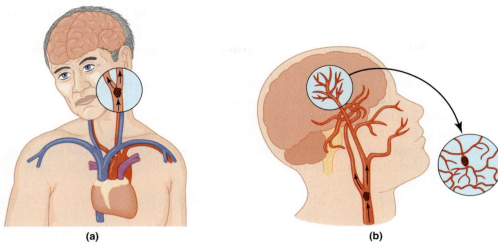

FIGURE 19.4 ■ (a) An embolus can form anywhere and travel to the brain. (b) A hemorrhage can take place in any part of the brain.

2. A blood clot can form in the brain itself and remain there. This is called a **thrombus**.
3. **Plaque** can accumulate in the blood vessels and eventually close them.
4. A blood vessel can burst, causing a **hemorrhage**. This is most common in people who have hypertension (Figure 19.4b ■).

Your Role as a Homemaker/Home Health Aide

It is important to remember that when you meet the client, he will be in a stable condition. However, his condition may change, so be alert. Caring for a person recovering from a CVA is a team effort. You are the team member who will spend the most time with the client. Your careful, objective observations of the client are important to his eventual recovery.

It is impossible to predict when a body part function will return following a CVA. Do not promise! Do not compare one client with another! People who have suffered a CVA resulting in severe speech and/or motor loss have been known to live 30 or 40 years with tender care from their families.

Follow the principles of good personal care and the instructions of the physical, occupational, and speech therapists. These therapists will plan an individualized program for your client. You will play an important part in seeing that he and the family follow this routine. The care will be planned with the following in mind:

■ Prevention of complications due to decreased mobility
■ The need for proper nutrition
■ Safety
■ Emotional aspects of the chronic condition for both the client and his family

After you have received the care plan from the therapists, it will be your responsibility to make these plans part of the client's routine throughout the day so that the client does not tire. Having many things to relearn is emotionally

thrombus
blood clot that remains at its site of formation

plaque
fatty deposits within the blood vessels attached to the vessel walls

hemorrhage
excessive bleeding

painful and at times frustrating. Just think how you would feel if you had to re-learn the alphabet or how to walk.

- Always encourage the client. Point out the positive aspects of his progress.
- Use simple instructions in words familiar to the client and his family. Speak slowly and clearly while looking at the client. Do not use baby talk.
- Always show patience and understanding.
- Do only the exercises you have been told to do. If you have a question, call the appropriate therapist.
- Assist the client with his medication. Work out a system with your supervisor so that the client and his family can keep track of which medications have been taken.
- If visitors tire your client, tactfully suggest that they leave so that your client can rest.
- Listen to the client and his family. Discuss your conversations with your supervisor. A client and his family may benefit from a mental health clinician or psychiatric nurse to help them cope with the changes in the family.

SECTION 6

Arthritis

OBJECTIVES

What You Will Learn to Do

1. Define *arthritis*, and tell how it affects people.
2. List the four most common types of arthritis.
3. Discuss your role as a homemaker/home health aide in caring for clients with arthritis.

Introduction: Arthritis

arthritis
disease characterized by inflammation and destruction of the joints

Arthritis means inflammation and destruction of joints. At times, there may be other symptoms. The shoulders, ankles, elbows, wrists, fingers, and toes are the most common joints affected by this disease. Arthritis or inflammation can be due to an allergy, an injury, or an infection. Some causes of arthritis cannot be determined—it just appears. Everyone seems to have a different reaction to this disease.

There are more than 100 types of arthritis, but we will only discuss the four most common ones.

osteoarthritis
the most common type of arthritis

Osteoarthritis: This is the most common type. It is thought that after continual use, the joints and their linings just wear out and become thin (Figure 19.5 ■). The bony surfaces become thick and develop little spurs that cause

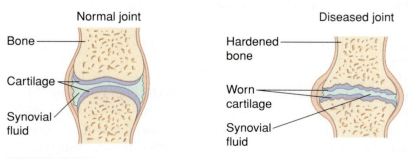

FIGURE 19.5 ■ Osteoarthritis causes a deterioration in the joints.

pain and inflammation every time the joint moves. Then the bones rub against each other, and causing pain and inflammation. This type of arthritis is most common among the elderly.

Rheumatoid arthritis: This is a crippling, chronic disease. All connective tissue may be affected (Figure 19.6 ■). If the disease starts in the joints, connective tissue in other organs may eventually be affected. This type of arthritis usually starts in young adulthood or childhood. Three times more women than men have this type of arthritis.

Gout: This disease is most common among men. Uric acid crystals build up in the blood and lodge in the joints, causing inflammation and pain. This can be sudden and painful. Any joint can be affected.

Ankylosing spondylitis: This disease, more common in men than in women, may start in childhood and almost always before the age of 35. It is an arthritic disease that attacks only the spine and/or the shoulders and hips. Following treatment, persons with the disease usually remain stiff but can function and lead normal lives.

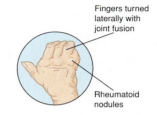

Fingers turned laterally with joint fusion

Rheumatoid nodules

FIGURE 19.6 ■ Rheumatoid arthritis causes joints to become deformed.

rheumatoid arthritis
crippling chronic disease of the joints

gout
the buildup of uric acid crystals in the blood and joints

ankylosing spondylitis
an arthritis-type disease that affects the spine and/or shoulders and hips

Your Role as a Homemaker/Home Health Aide

Remember, arthritis is a chronic disease. That means the client will have it forever. Help him to establish a safe and efficient routine for daily care and that decreases muscle stress and fatigue.

Exercise and rest are important parts of the client's plan of care. Follow the exercise routine. Do not change it unless you have discussed the change with your supervisor. If you notice that your client's response to the exercises has changed, report it.

A client may try unconventional methods of treating his arthritis. Do not assist in these treatments, and make your supervisor aware of them. It is not your role to judge these treatments; just report their existence.

Assist the client with his medication and treatment plan. Each client is treated differently. Treatment may include diet, weight reduction, rest, and exercise. An occupational therapist and physical therapist may also be involved with this client.

Listen to the client. He may have many feelings about this disease, and he may require emotional counseling from a mental health clinician or psychiatric nurse. Discuss your conversations in the home with your supervisor so that she can make the decision whether to call these professionals.

SECTION 7

Cancer

OBJECTIVES

What You Will Learn to Do

1. Define cancer.

2. Become familiar with possible causes of cancer.

3. Become familiar with your role in caring for clients with cancer.

Introduction: Cancer

Cancer, or a **malignancy**, is a tumor made up of cells that have changed from normal ones to abnormal ones. This change can happen in any organ, at any time, and at any age. As the abnormal cells reproduce and multiply, they destroy the normal tissue and usually form a tumor. The course of the disease depends on many factors:

- Location of the tumor
- Type of tumor
- When the cancer was discovered
- Type of treatment available
- General health of the client

CAUSES AND SYMPTOMS OF CANCER

There is no proven cause of cancer, but many possible causes are being investigated (Figure 19.7 ■). Although a change in the way your body functions may mean many things (not necessarily cancer), eight changes, usually called early warning signs of cancer, should be reported to a doctor immediately (Figure 19.8 ■).

The spread of cancer cells from one area to another is called **metastasis**. This does not always occur when there is cancer in the body, but it may. The first site of the cancer is called the **primary site**, and the place it metastasizes to is called the **secondary site**.

The only way a tumor is known to be malignant (cancerous) or **benign** (not malignant) is by taking a small piece of it and examining it under a microscope. This is called a **biopsy**. It is usually done in the operating room in the hospital.

TREATMENT

Treatment varies from client to client. The client may undergo surgery, radiation, chemotherapy, or a combination. The choice of treatment is usually made by the doctor after discussion with the client and his family.

Sometimes, a family will choose not to tell the client he has cancer. Even though you may not agree with this decision, you must go along with it. It is not your place to give the client his diagnosis. Discuss this situation with your

malignancy
cancer

metastasis
the spreading of cancer within the body

primary site
place of the original cancerous lesion

secondary site
place in the body in which cancerous cells are found other than at the primary site

benign
nonmalignant

biopsy
examination of tissue taken from the body

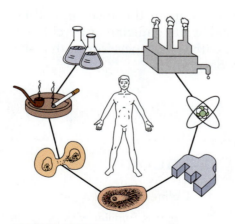

FIGURE 19.7 ■ Cancer may be caused by a combination of these elements and by elements not yet identified.

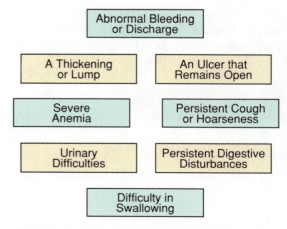

Abnormal Bleeding or Discharge

A Thickening or Lump

An Ulcer that Remains Open

Severe Anemia

Persistent Cough or Hoarseness

Urinary Difficulties

Persistent Digestive Disturbances

Difficulty in Swallowing

FIGURE 19.8 ■ Any of the warning signs of cancer should be investigated immediately.

supervisor so that you will know what to tell the client if he asks you. Do not lie to the client and tell him he will be better unless this is what the family and doctor have decided to tell him.

Your Role as a Homemaker/Home Health Aide

Your role is to give the client the best care you can. This includes both physical and emotional support. If the client is terminally ill, you and the supervisor will make a plan of care to meet his specific needs. A person is usually said to be terminally ill when there is little or no hope for recovering from the disease.

Cancer is not contagious. Encourage family members to visit the client and be supportive. Follow the principles of good personal care. Follow the instructions of the therapists within the limits of the client. Discuss with the therapists your responsibilities for exercises. Encourage the client to take part in his care.

If the client wishes to talk, let him. If he does not seem to be able to talk to you, ask him if you can call the nurse or someone else. Many people live for many years with cancer. Do not give the client false hope, but do not assume he will die unless you have been told this. Help family members deal with this diagnosis by letting them take part in the client's care if they wish. Encourage them to talk to someone who can help them accept this diagnosis.

SECTION 8

Alzheimer's Disease

OBJECTIVES

What You Will Learn to Do

1. Define Alzheimer's disease.
2. Recognize several of the behaviors exhibited by Alzheimer's sufferers.
3. Discuss the effect of Alzheimer's disease upon the family.
4. Discuss your role in caring for these clients.

Introduction: Alzheimer's Disease

Alzheimer's disease is the major cause of mental deterioration in people. It is the diagnosis of more than 50 percent of the nursing home residents of this country. Most of the victims of this disease, however, receive treatment and care in their homes. This disease is chronic, progressive, and ultimately renders the client totally dependent on others. There is no known cure.

Alzheimer's disease
a form of irreversible mental deterioration

BEHAVIOR OF CLIENTS WITH ALZHEIMER'S DISEASE

You may see a client in any one of three stages of this disease. If you care for a client for a long time, you will see him progress from one stage to the next.

Stage I

At this beginning stage, before and even after diagnosis, a person may be able to cover up his memory loss; decreased speech; and even his emotional agitation, depression, or apathy. During this stage, a person may sense that something is changing and, rather than be embarrassed, simply withdraw from his familiar activities. Family members may not recognize the pattern of this deterioration, may not admit to it, or may think all older people are forgetful and withdrawn. Family members may label the client careless or disinterested.

Stage II

During this period, extending over many years, the client's memory progressively worsens. He may stop speaking, wander, and repeat movements in a meaningless way. The client becomes less involved in his care and less a contributing member of the family. He may put all types of things in his mouth. His appetite may increase, and his activity may be in the form of continual pacing in small areas. The client starts to need 24-hour supervision.

Stage III

This is the terminal stage. It is a time when families must give continual supervision to the client. His appetite may decrease, and he must be coaxed to eat and drink. The client may become unresponsive. At this point, an exhausted family often seeks to institutionalize the client.

Your Role as a Homemaker/Home Health Aide

You are an important part of the care of this client and the relief of the family. Follow the care plan carefully. The maintenance of a routine is one way to ease the care of the client. If you feel the need to change the plan of care, be sure to discuss it with the family and your supervisor. Your continued support is important for the family of an Alzheimer's victim. Be on time and be conscientious about coming to work. A change of personnel is a disrupting factor in these households.

- Be alert for the safety of the client. Remember, he is unable to remember your instructions so you must be aware of his activities and movements.
- Provide a quiet, unstressed environment.
- Maintain the personal hygiene of the client. Careful washing of the perineal area will prevent skin breakdown. Frequent cleaning of the teeth will decrease mouth odor and improve general appearance.
- Maintain a toileting routine. If the client is incontinent and can no longer participate in his personal hygiene, discuss with your supervisor the use of various appliances.
- Offer small nutritious meals. Frequent sips of water will decrease the chance for dehydration.
- Monitor the client's sleep habits and report if they are markedly disturbed or they change.
- Be supportive of family members who care for the client. Encourage them to leave the house when you are there. Encourage them to seek relief and enjoyment while you are available to care for the client.
- Be alert to family tension. Report this to your supervisor, who will discuss with the family the appropriate counseling or support groups.
- Do not be judgmental or compare the care one family gives to the way another family cares for their relative.
- Be alert to your feelings. If you find you cannot continue caring for the client, discuss your feelings with your supervisor so that relief can be arranged.

SECTION 9

Chronic Obstructive Pulmonary Disease

OBJECTIVES

What You Will Learn to Do

1. State what chronic obstructive pulmonary disease is.
2. Describe behaviors exhibited by clients who have this disease.
3. Describe the effect of this disease on families.
4. Discuss your role as a homemaker/home health aide in caring for a client with COPD.

Introduction: Chronic Obstructive Pulmonary Disease

Chronic obstructive pulmonary disease (COPD) refers to all diseases that cause irreversible damage to the lungs over a period of time. This condition is one of the leading causes of death in the United States. People with a diagnosis of asthma and emphysema are often said to have COPD. This means that their lungs cannot expand; remove oxygen from air breathed in; or expel waste products such as carbon dioxide. These clients also find it difficult to perform activities that require exertion of any kind. Eating and speaking are difficult, and exercise is often impossible. Most of these clients are susceptible to infection, due to the pooling of pulmonary secretions in their lungs. When the levels of carbon dioxide and other gases are incorrect, these clients exhibit unusual behavior and cannot make decisions or be left alone. When the blood gases are corrected, this behavior disappears.

Clients with COPD also suffer from a change in body image. They must learn to live with machines as constant companions because they depend on oxygen equipment and suction equipment to help them breathe. Some clients may have tracheostomy tubes, IVs, or even feeding tubes.

chronic obstructive pulmonary disease (COPD)
refers to diseases that cause permanent damage to lung tissue, including emphysema, asthma, and chronic bronchitis

EFFECTS ON THE FAMILY

As the client demands more and more care, the family function changes. The primary caregiver becomes isolated from friends because the client's care takes up so much time. Family members become socially isolated and depressed and often suffer from sensory deprivation. Relationships with friends change because the client often is too tired, or even unable, to speak. Visitors may stop coming, and family members often find themselves without any outside activities.

While all this is occurring, families must often become accustomed to a change in finances and a change in the work status of the client.

Your Role as a Homemaker/Home Health Aide

Your presence in a home where your client has COPD is a most important one. You will assist the primary caregiver to provide a break in his or her routine. Encourage the caregiver to go out and tend to personal needs while you are in the house. Assure both client and family that you will adhere to the routine they have established and will not make changes without discussing them with your supervisor and the client. This respite for the caregiver often enables him or her to continue the care for the rest of the day and possibly into the night.

Encourage the client to adhere to his medication schedule. Report any change in behavior. No change is too small. If you report changes as soon as they occur, your supervisor can change the plan of care to meet the client's changing needs. Often, you will be the first person to see a change in behavior, which will mean that the client's blood gases are incorrect.

Try to interest the client in eating nutritious, small meals. Because eating is a chore for this client and his taste buds often are less sensitive than yours, every bit of food should be nutritious and tasty. Fluids may or may not be restricted. Be sure to check. Prepare foods the client likes. This is not the time to introduce new foods.

Expose the client to activities to occupy his time (Figure 19.9 ■). If the client has no hobbies, discuss with him and his family what type of activities he might enjoy. Then keep on trying each one. Do not be discouraged. The client and the family will appreciate your concern and interest, and you will eventually find an activity that will please the client. For example, if the client liked to play sports but is no longer able to participate in games, be sure to have him listen to the radio when ball games are on or make him comfortable so he can look at TV. Plan your schedule around these important times in his day. Many of the clients you care for will be using oxygen therapy. This is not necessarily a problem, except that many of the people who have COPD also smoke. Although the client and family are taught that oxygen cannot run when there is an open flame or someone is smoking in the area, the clients may often forget. Be firm, but polite. Tell the client and the family that oxygen and smoking is a dangerous combination and that you will have to report this situation. In addition, discuss with your supervisor how she wants you to act. Does she want you to remove the matches and cigarettes?

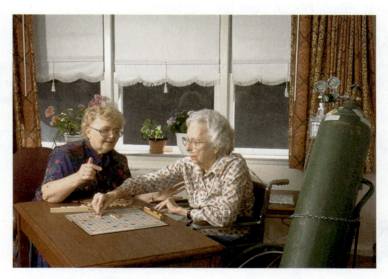

FIGURE 19.9 ■ Make a special effort to include clients in normal family activities.

Neurological Disorders

OBJECTIVES	
What You Will Learn to Do	**1.** Discuss the signs and symptoms of Parkinson's disease, multiple sclerosis, and amyotrophic lateral sclerosis.
	2. Discuss the role of the homemaker/home health aide in caring for clients with neurological disorders.

Introduction: Common Neurological Diseases

Three neurological diseases you will see in the home setting are Parkinson's disease, multiple sclerosis (MS), and amyotrophic lateral sclerosis (ALS). Clients who have these diseases usually remain in the home setting, using adaptive aids. Some remain at home until they die. Although the diseases are different, there are many similarities in the care of these clients. All three diseases result in the need for assistance with care, attention to safety, and support for clients and their families. As these diseases progress, clients require a great deal of personal care and protection. Their ability to respond to changes and slight infections becomes progressively less.

CAUSES OF THE THREE DISEASES

Parkinson's disease is a progressive disease that affects the part of the brain controlling movement and balance. The first signs are usually tremors of the hands or legs, difficulty walking, and slowness of movement. Other symptoms may be changes in vision, drooling, difficulty swallowing, and inability to control bowel and bladder function. The cause of the disease is unknown, but clients respond to drug therapy that replaces certain chemicals they seem to be lacking. People with this disease often work many years after the diagnosis. Drugs must be carefully and continuously regulated. Side effects from the drugs often occur many years after the therapy has started. Sometimes, clients may appear to be getting better and conclude that they no longer need the medication or may change their routines. This is a great mistake and should be reported to their physicians immediately.

Multiple sclerosis is a progressive disease that affects the transmission of impulses through the central nervous system. The first signs are usually fatigue, emotional changes, and difficulty with speech. This disease affects young adults with young families who are in the first stages of their careers. The people who have this disease often work for many years if they are protected from infection and have a safe environment. Medications help some people, but no one medication has been found useful for all clients. The cause is unknown, and the course of the disease varies.

Amyotrophic lateral sclerosis is a progressive disease that degenerates the neurons. The cause is unknown, and most clients die within 3 years of diagnosis. Many of these clients choose to stay at home. They need assistance with all aspects of personal care and maintenance of a safe environment.

Your Role as a Homemaker/Home Health Aide

Treatment is prescribed by a physician. Support the clients and their families as they follow the regime. Most clients find it important to follow the same routine every day. This may seem difficult for people who like variety, but these clients find the same routine comforting. They know what to expect. They know how it will affect them. Assist them as they incorporate the regimes into their daily lives. If you have suggestions for change, discuss them with the clients and their families. Do not change the routine without first telling everyone involved. Areas of concern are:

- *Medication.* It must be taken as prescribed and should not be stopped unless the client's physicians are notified. Report clients' reactions to medication. Be sure to report the slightest changes as they may indicate that dosage changes are necessary.
- *Regular exercise.* This can take the form of active or passive exercise. It could be walking, swimming, or riding a bike. Exercises should be supervised and done regularly. Report fatigue or pain. Be alert to safety needs during exercise. Clients who tire easily should have several short exercise periods rather than one long one. Do not alter the exercise routines without discussing the changes with your supervisor.
- *Nutritional intake.* Small meals high in nutrients and fiber are important. Swallowing liquids may be difficult, so monitor fluid intake. Safety is important. Be sure foods are an acceptable temperature and not too hot. Pieces of food should be small enough to chew easily. Report bowel and bladder changes.
- *Support.* Encourage your client to be as independent as possible. Encourage family members to pursue their own interests. There are many local support groups for clients and families. Discuss the possibility of referrals with your supervisor. Allow all family members time to express their feelings. Do not be judgmental. Support the family members in their roles. Be alert to changes in roles. Family members, as well as clients, often need to voice their feelings of frustration, fear, and fatigue. Listen attentively. Offer to put them in touch with professional counselors if they wish. Discussing feelings can be helpful to both the clients and the caregivers.

SECTION 11

Tuberculosis

OBJECTIVES

What You Will Learn to Do

1. Describe the causes of tuberculosis.
2. Describe three common misconceptions about the disease.
3. Describe the most common treatments for this disease.
4. Discuss your role as a homemaker/home health aide in caring for a client with tuberculosis.

Introduction: Tuberculosis

Tuberculosis (TB) is a disease caused by a bacteria. It is spread not by animals, but by people, when they laugh, cough, sneeze, or speak to one another. Coughing or sneezing into a tissue or a handkerchief is one way to decrease the spread of the disease. The other way is to wash hands frequently and not touch hands to eyes, nose, or mouth.

The disease is known all over the world. It was once thought that the disease was only seen in poor people and was unknown in the United States. This is untrue. Today the disease is seen in all countries and in people in all living conditions. People are more at risk, however, when living in crowded, poorly ventilated conditions; when malnourished; and when in poor health.

Some people have TB infection. This mean the bacteria is in their body, but it is inactive and cannot be spread or cause harm. Medication is often prescribed for these people to prevent the germs from becoming active.

SIGNS AND SYMPTOMS

There are many signs and symptoms of this disease. Any combination of them could mean that a person has active tuberculosis. These should be brought to the attention of a doctor immediately. A person may be embarrassed to know he has the disease, and this fear prevents him from seeking medical help. Postponing medical help may result in the person getting worse and spreading the disease to people with whom he comes in contact.

Any of the following symptoms should be brought to the attention of a doctor, clinic, or emergency room immediately.

- Weight loss, loss of appetite
- Feeling sick, weak, or tired
- Fever
- Sweating, especially during the night
- Chest pain
- Coughing
- Coughing up blood
- Unexplained pain in any body part

HOW IS TUBERCULOSIS DIAGNOSED?

The diagnosis of tuberculosis, active or inactive, can only be made by a physician after a skin test, an X-ray, and/or a sputum sample is taken. Any hospital, clinic, or health department can assist with finding a place to have these tests done quickly and inexpensively.

Usually, once the diagnosis of tuberculosis is made, close contacts of the infected person are also tested. It is important that all contacts be tested, including those who are family members, live in the same house, or are close by.

TREATMENT FOR TUBERCULOSIS

Medication is always prescribed and is taken for a long time. It is important that the medication be taken exactly as it is prescribed. If not, the disease may not be cured and may return. Often, more than one medication is given. Other activities, such as physical exercise, diet, and breathing exercises, may also be part of the regime.

When the medication is first started, the client is usually hospitalized and isolated to decrease contact with others. As soon as the disease is under control, the client can go home and be around others without fear of infecting them.

Your Role as a Homemaker/Home Health Aide

You are important in maintaining a routine in the house, in encouraging the client to maintain the regime set up by the physician, and in teaching the family the truth about this disease. A nourishing diet is important. If the medication causes the client to have a decreased appetite, encourage small frequent meals rather than a few large ones. Encourage adequate fluid intake. This should include water, juice, and nourishing soups.

Some family members may be afraid they will catch the client's disease and therefore isolate or ignore him. Explain to them that once the disease is under treatment, the chance of contracting the disease is past. The family may make the client feel guilty or even ashamed he has contracted tuberculosis. If this should happen, contact your supervisor and request written information that you can share with the family.

SECTION 12

AIDS (Acquired Immune Deficiency Syndrome)

OBJECTIVES

What You Will Learn to Do

1. Describe three common misconceptions about the disease.
2. Describe the most common treatments for this disease.
3. Discuss your role as a homemaker/home health aide in caring for a client with AIDS.

Introduction: Aids

AIDS is a virus spread through contact of blood and body fluids. It cannot be transmitted by holding hands, by giving blood, or by being near someone who has the disease. There is no evidence that AIDS can be spread from sharing the same equipment or bathroom. You will not get sick if you sit next to someone who has any form of AIDS. The virus is not spread by food or sharing a kitchen. It is only transmitted by contact with blood, seminal fluid, or vaginal fluid in the mouth, rectum, vagina, penis, or open wound on the body.

Often, a person has a form of this disease and does not know it. Therefore, it is always important to practice Standard Precautions with all clients. There are several forms of this infection. Only a physician can diagnose the disease. Anyone who thinks he has been exposed to AIDS should go to a physician, a hospital, or health department immediately. Although a person may not appear to have the disease, if he is infected in any form, he can transmit it to another person.

RISK FACTORS

You are at risk of giving, getting, or having AIDS if:

- You are an IV drug user who shares needles.
- You received blood or blood products before 1978.
- You have several sexual partners and do not use condoms.
- You do not know your sexual partners well.
- Any of your sexual partners have had "unprotected" sex since 1978.

FORMS OF AIDS

There are three forms of AIDS:

1. ***AIDS carrier.*** The only sign of the disease in these people may be a positive blood test. Some carriers never show active signs of the disease. Some carriers remain healthy for many years and then gradually show signs and symptoms. There is no way to predict which course the disease will take. The carriers can, however, transmit the disease.
2. ***AIDS-related conditions.*** Some people may be healthy for years after the first positive blood test and then show related symptoms. Whether they have mild or severe symptoms, they can transmit the disease.
3. ***AIDS.*** The disease may appear years after the first positive blood test and years after AIDS-related conditions have appeared and been treated. When this happens, the immune system is compromised and the body is no longer able to protect itself against infection. Death occurs.

Your Role as a Homemaker/Home Health Aide

You will be asked to demonstrate standard precautions while caring for the AIDS clients just as you would when caring for other clients. Use these precautions only when necessary so that neither the clients nor their families think you are afraid of catching the disease. AIDS clients often are lonely. Family and friends often do not want to spend time with them, touch them, or hold their hands. Your demonstration that this activity is without danger will help decrease needless fears and myths.

AIDS clients often take medication and have set routines to conserve strength and maintain their muscle tone. Assist the clients with these and maintain routines comfortable for the families and the clients. If family members are unavailable to assist the clients when you are not there, discuss with your supervisor the availability of support groups or community volunteers. Make these suggestions carefully so the clients know that you are concerned but not trying to get somebody else to assume the care.

Report all changes in behavior, pain tolerance, activity tolerance, and skin integrity. Often, AIDS clients have difficulty breathing, so be alert to possible changes in their ability to breathe or speak. Protect the clients from friends and neighbors who may have slight colds or infections. If you believe any visitor is not 100 percent healthy, suggest the guest return at another time or speak to your client on the telephone.

Should you have any questions about the disease or the safest way to care for the client, discuss these openly with your supervisor to increase your knowledge and decrease your fears.

CHAPTER REVIEW

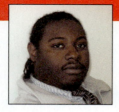

Case Study

Review the case study that appears on the first page of the chapter. Answer two sets of questions about the case study contained in the Explore and Apply sections below.

EXPLORE

1. Do you believe that Mr. Martinez will be able to live a productive and meaningful life? Why do you think that way?

2. Think about how you would react to the news that you have a chronic illness. What activities would it affect? What changes in your life would you be forced to make?

APPLY

1. Mr. Martinez shows you a liquid which he has gotten from a local herbalist. He says it will cure his diabetes and improve his sex life. How do you react? Do you think that herbalists and non-Western medicines can help cure diseases?

2. Mr. Martinez refuses to follow the prescribed diet and includes no exercise in his day. He seldom walks and seems to be gaining weight. You are concerned that Mr. Martinez is developing complications of diabetes. What do you tell him? Can a client develop a second and third chronic disease if he does not take care of his first chronic disease? What do you tell the client and his family?

Certification Exam Review Questions

Choose the best answer for each question or statement.

1. **Hypertension is called the silent killer because**

   a. *children contract it and cannot tell anyone.*

   b. *it may have no symptoms that people notice until it is too late.*

   c. *no one likes to talk about it.*

   d. *it is not a silent killer.*

2. **Heart attacks are**

   a. *all preventable.*

   b. *never preventable.*

   c. *always fatal.*

   d. *all different and must be treated immediately.*

3. **Tuberculosis**

   a. *is always fatal.*

   b. *is a great shame because it indicates that you are poor.*

   c. *is curable.*

   d. *only attacks the weak and the young.*

4. **Alzheimer's disease**

   a. *appears only after age 65.*

   b. *is curable if noticed soon enough.*

   c. *is a normal part of aging.*

   d. *is not a normal part of aging.*

5. **A cerebrovascular accident**

   a. *is also called a stroke.*

   b. *never results in some sort of paralysis.*

   c. *never results in some speech difficulty.*

   d. *is always preventable.*

CHAPTER 20

Emergency Procedures

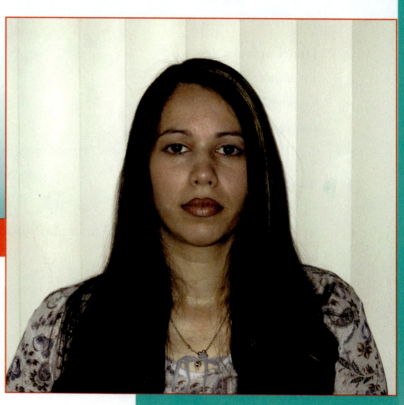

CASE STUDY

Mrs. Soledad has worked all her life as a seamstress. She sews both for her employer and her family and enjoys the creativity and the praise she receives. She is now faced with arthritis in her hands and her hips. Some days she is unable to thread a needle or cut a pattern. Mrs. Soledad, an outgoing and talkative woman, has become much quieter and has started keeping to herself at lunch. She no longer brings food to share or talks about her family. Her employer has mentioned that Mrs. Soledad's work, although still perfect, seems to take longer to complete. Her coworkers notice that at times she rubs her hands and finds it difficult to get up from the chairs.

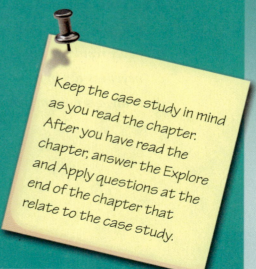

Keep the case study in mind as you read the chapter. After you have read the chapter, answer the Explore and Apply questions at the end of the chapter that relate to the case study.

Emergency Essentials

OBJECTIVES

What You Will Learn to Do

1. Define *emergency*.
2. Define *first aid*.
3. Discuss the steps to take in an emergency.

Introduction: Agency Policies

This chapter covers the essentials of emergency procedures in the home. You and your instructor may want to refer to the many other texts on emergency care for further detail.

Emergencies are situations that call for immediate action. **First aid** is the action taken to assist people who suffer injuries or sudden illnesses until more appropriate help arrives.

Every agency has an emergency procedure. It includes a plan of whom to call during what emergency. Specific information includes telephone numbers of fire, police, and rescue squads. It is your responsibility to be familiar with this plan and these telephone numbers. In many places, the emergency number is 911. In some places, however, the number is different. Do not assume you know the appropriate emergency number for your client. ASK!

As you make a decision about giving first aid, remember that the person is a whole unit and will react physically and emotionally to the emergency situation.

If you are faced with a situation in which nobody can help you or go for help, take care of the person and stay until help arrives. If you face an emergency situation in which more than one person needs help, you will have to review the whole situation to decide whom to help first.

emergency
a sudden unexpected crisis, injury, or illness

first aid
emergency treatment given for injury or illness before regular medical treatment is available

STEPS TO BE TAKEN IN AN EMERGENCY

Before you take any action, you must know the following:

- What is the problem or emergency?
- What must be done?
- What are *you* capable of doing?
- Can the person be moved?

Determine the problem or emergency by asking the person, family members, or bystanders what happened or what is wrong. Decide what must be done based on your training and the policies of your agency. Know what you are capable of doing. For example, if you must lift or move a person, be sure that you can do so without injuring yourself. If the person can be moved, move him or her to safe, firm ground away from danger of electrical shock, fire, or explosion. Moving an injured person may cause further injury such as increased blood loss, increased pain, and/or paralysis. Do not move the person unless he or she is in great danger of further injury. Remember, you should do this without causing serious injury to yourself.

Do not leave a person who needs help. Have someone else call for additional help. If the person does not need immediate help to maintain life, your responsibility is to prevent additional injury and to provide comfort and security until medical help arrives. Keep the person warm, comfortable, and safe. If she is on the floor, leave her there until medical help arrives.

A severely injured person is treated according to common first-aid priorities (Figure 20.1 ■) by properly trained people.

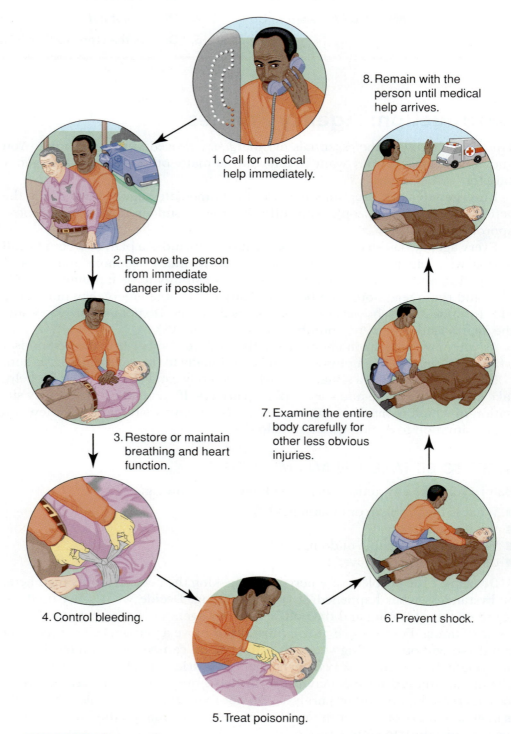

1. Call for medical help immediately.

2. Remove the person from immediate danger if possible.

3. Restore or maintain breathing and heart function.

4. Control bleeding.

5. Treat poisoning.

6. Prevent shock.

7. Examine the entire body carefully for other less obvious injuries.

8. Remain with the person until medical help arrives.

FIGURE 20.1 ■ In an emergency, it is important to follow common first-aid practices to ensure the safety of the person until medical help arrives. Move the person only if there is immediate danger and you see no possible serious injuries.

SECTION 2

Restoring Breathing

OBJECTIVES

What You Will Learn to Do

1. Demonstrate the proper techniques for dislodging a foreign body in the airway.

2. Demonstrate the proper techniques for mouth-to-mouth resuscitation.

3. Demonstrate the proper techniques for dislodging a foreign body in the airway of infants.

Introduction: Restore or Maintain Breathing Function

Heart function and breathing function are related. When oxygen to the lungs is cut off, oxygen to the brain also decreases. When this happens, cells that control heart function die and the heart becomes weak. As a homemaker/home health aide, you will be concerned only with restoring an open airway and restoring breathing.

You should carry a pocket face shield so that if you perform artificial breathing, you will be protected.

When an object blocks air from getting into a person's lungs, it must be removed or the person will choke to death (Figure 20.2 ■).

OBSTRUCTED AIRWAYS

A person's airway can be **obstructed** (blocked) by:

obstructed
blocked

■ Foreign matter in the mouth, throat, or windpipe, such as food, vomitus, blood, or a foreign object

■ Unconsciousness, leading to relaxed muscles and the tongue falling back into the throat and blocking the airway

A person can have either a partial or a complete airway obstruction. Partial airway obstruction: Some air passes to and from the lungs, but the conditions

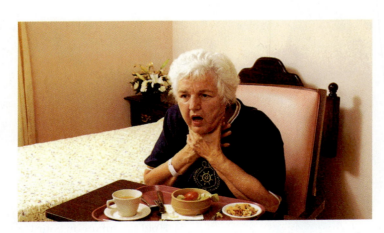

FIGURE 20.2 ■ A blocked airway can threaten life and must be treated immediately.

must be improved. Snoring sounds, weak coughs, gurgling, or crowing sounds are signs of this. Also, if the lips, nails, tongue, and skin have a dark or bluish color, a partial obstruction might be the cause. *Do not interfere with the person if he is able to breath, cough, or speak.* Just call for help.

Complete airway obstruction: No air passes to and from the lungs. The person may be conscious or unconscious. The conscious person will be unable to speak or cough and may clutch his throat. He will become unconscious if the situation is not remedied. The unconscious person will have no chest movement.

Children Less than One Year Old

Children and infants are treated differently than adults when they have difficulty breathing. *If the child or infant is breathing, speaking, or coughing, do not help, but call for assistance immediately* as you have been instructed by your agency. If the child or infant has had an infection, a high fever, or has taken medication and is having difficulty breathing, call for help immediately.

If the child or infant is unable to speak or cry and is conscious, act quickly to relieve the obstruction. Use a combination of back blows and chest thrusts on an infant. Do not use abdominal thrusts on an infant, as this action can damage his underdeveloped organs. Back blows are quick, forceful blows between the shoulder blades used to dislodge objects from an infant; chest thrusts are similar to the compressions given in CPR. Do not use back blows on a child. Perform abdominal thrusts on a child similar to the way they are performed on adults.

For the infant:

- Call out for help.
- Turn the infant face down on your forearm and support his head in your hand. Rest your arm on your thigh for support and keep the infant's head lower than his body (Figure 20.3 ■).
- Deliver up to five back blows forcefully between the shoulder blades with the heel of one hand.
- Sandwich the infant between your arms and turn the infant over as you continue to support his head in your hands. Again, support him on your thigh.

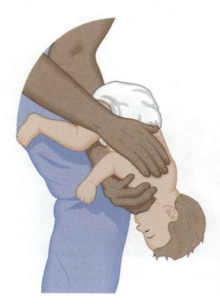

FIGURE 20.3 ■
Hold the infant on your leg while sitting so that head and body are supported.

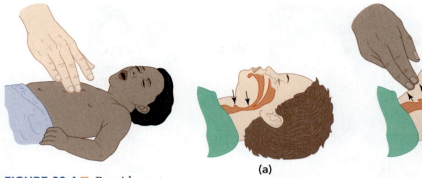

FIGURE 20.4 ■ Provide up to five quick downward chest thrusts with two fingers in the same location as for chest compressions.

FIGURE 20.5 ■ Open the airway and attempt rescue breathing.

(a)   (b)

■ Provide up to five quick downward chest thrusts with two fingers in the same location as for chest compressions (the lower third of the sternum, approximately one finger-width below the nipple line). Again, support him on your thigh. (Figure 20.4 ■).

■ Check the mouth. If you see the foreign object, use your little finger in a hooking motion to remove it. If you do not see it, do not sweep the mouth.

■ Open the airway and attempt rescue breathing. If no air enters, reposition the head and attempt to breathe again. If the airway is still obstructed, repeat these steps until the airway is clear (Figure 20.5 ■ a and b).

Abdominal Thrust

Manual thrusts are a series of quick movements to the upper abdominal area or chest area to force the obstruction to move. An **abdominal thrust**, also called the **Heimlich maneuver**, is used when the person cannot breathe, cough, or speak. Talk to the person as you are doing this. Tell him you are going to do the Heimlich maneuver to help him breathe easier. Do not use the Heimlich maneuver on pregnant women, infants, or small children.

When the person is sitting or standing and conscious:

■ Stand behind the person and wrap your arms around his waist.

■ Put the thumb side of your hand on the abdomen between the navel and the end of the breastbone (sternum).

■ Grasp this hand with the other hand and press it into the abdomen with a quick upward movement (Figure 20.6 ■).

■ Repeat and continue the thrusts until the object is expelled. Each thrust should be separate and distinct.

When the person is lying down and unconscious:

■ Position the person on his back. Open his airway and attempt to ventilate. If no air enters, reposition his head and attempt to ventilate again. If unsuccessful, perform the following steps.

■ Kneel astride the person at hip level.

■ Put the heel of your hand on his abdomen between the navel and the end of the breastbone (Figure 20.7 ■).

■ Put your other hand on top of this hand.

■ Rock forward and push your hands upward. Repeat five times.

■ Open the mouth and look for the object. If you see it, sweep it with one finger using a hooking motion. If you do not see it, do not sweep the mouth.

manual thrust
a quick movement of the hands to remove an obstruction of the airway

abdominal thrust
quick movement in the abdomen to remove a foreign body from the airway

Heimlich maneuver
a system developed by Heimlich to remove a foreign body from the airway

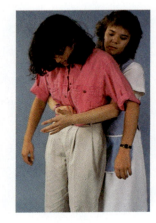

FIGURE 20.6 ■ The Heimlich maneuver

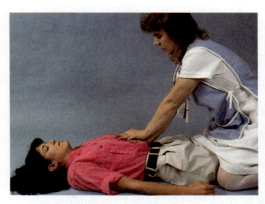

FIGURE 20.7 ■ Place the heel of your hand just above the lowest end of the breastbone.

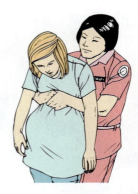

FIGURE 20.8 ■ On large persons or pregnant women, use the chest thrust to dislodge any obstructions.

■ Attempt to ventilate. If unsuccessful, reposition the head and attempt to ventilate again.
■ If unsuccessful, repeat sequence of abdominal thrusts, look for objects, use finger sweeps if you see it, attempt to ventilate, reposition and repeat the steps until the airway is clear.

Chest Thrust

The chest thrust is a useful procedure when the person with an obstruction is large and your arms will not reach around her abdomen but will reach around her chest. It is also used when the person is pregnant (Figure 20.8 ■).

When the person is standing or sitting and conscious:

■ Put your arms around the person's chest.
■ Put the thumb side of your fist on his breastbone (sternum) just above the lower end.
■ Grasp this hand with your other one and push quickly directly backward.
■ Repeat until airway is clear.

When the person is lying down and unconscious:

■ Position the person on her back. Open her airway and attempt to ventilate. If no air enters, reposition her head and attempt to ventilate again. If unsuccessful, perform the following steps.
■ Kneel beside her close to her chest.
■ Place the heel of your hand two fingers above the lowest end of the breastbone.
■ Put your other hand on top of this hand, and lean forward. As you do so, exert quick pushing pressure (Figure 20.9 ■).
■ Give five chest thrusts.
■ Open her mouth and look for the object. If you see it, sweep it clear of the mouth. If you do not see it, do not sweep.
■ Attempt to ventilate. If unsuccessful, reposition her head and attempt to ventilate again.
■ If unsuccessful, repeat the steps until the obstruction is dislodged.

Finger Sweeps

A finger sweep of the mouth will remove an object that you can see. Do not use this technique unless you can *clearly see the object* (Figure 20.10 ■).

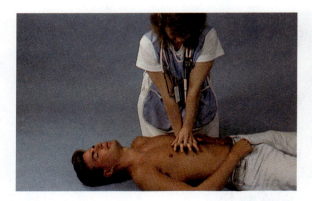

FIGURE 20.9 ■ Put one hand on top of your other hand, and lean forward. As you do so, exert quick pushing pressure.

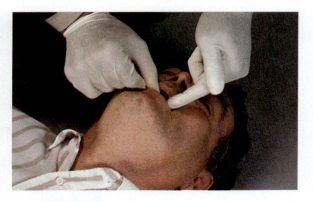

FIGURE 20.10 ■ Using your finger to remove an object visible in another's mouth is sometimes referred to as a finger sweep.

Rescue Breathing

Rescue breathing is the exchange of air between you and an unconscious nonbreathing person or a person who loses consciousness while you are trying to dislodge an obstruction. You must dislodge the obstruction first or you will not be able to ventilate the person.

To provide rescue breathing, perform the following steps:

- Check for response. If there is no response, call or send someone for medical assistance (Figure 20.11 ■).
- Open your mouth and take a deep breath. (Always use a barrier device or mouth shield when giving mouth-to-mouth ventilation.)
- Blow into the one-way valve on the barrier device and watch for the chest to rise. Give two initial breaths, about 1½ to 2 seconds per breath (Figure 20.12 ■).

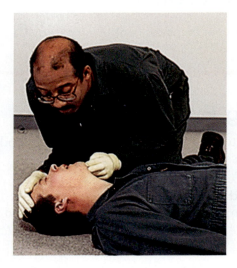

FIGURE 20.11 ■ Check for response. If there is no response, call or send someone for medical assistance.

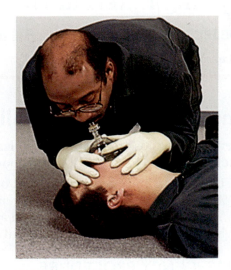

FIGURE 20.12 ■ Blow into the one-way valve on the barrier device and watch for the chest to rise. Give two initial breaths, about 1½ to 2 seconds per breath.

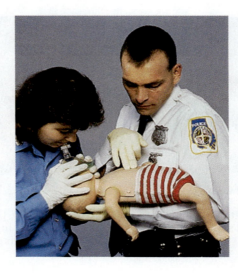

FIGURE 20.13 ■
Be sure not to hyperextend
the neck when ventilating
infants.

- Remove your mouth and allow him to exhale passively. You should be able to see the chest fall. The air will escape through a vent in the one-way valve so you do not have to remove the device.
- Check his pulse.
- If the airway is unobstructed and there is no pulse, continue mouth to mask resuscitation until medical help or someone who is qualified to administer CPR arrives. Give 10 to 12 breaths per minute.
- Ventilating infants and small children: Deliver two slow initial breaths (1½ to 2 seconds per breath) with sufficient volume to make the chest rise. Then give a breath every 3 seconds. Do not hyperextend the neck (Figure 20.13 ■).

SECTION 3

Stopping External Heavy Bleeding

OBJECTIVE
What You Will Learn to Do

1. Demonstrate the proper steps for controlling external bleeding.

Introduction: Controlling External Bleeding

hemorrhage
excessive bleeding

Severe blood loss or **hemorrhage** leads to several serious effects on the body, including shock (see Section 5). Blood loss causes:

- Damage to body cells due to lack of circulating oxygen
- A drop in blood pressure so oxygen and nutrients do not reach tissues
- The heart pumping too fast in an attempt to circulate the remaining blood, but each heart beat is less forceful

EMERGENCY PROCEDURE

external
outside the body

External blood loss (bleeding outside the body) can come from an artery, a vein, or a capillary. Each of these must be controlled in the same way.

- Apply direct pressure over the wound (Figure 20.14 ■). Use any clean cloth. Keep pressure for 10 to 30 minutes while someone else calls for help. If the

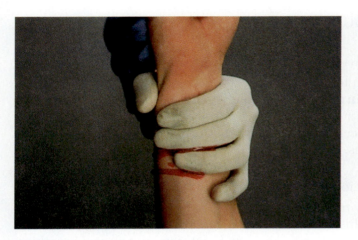

FIGURE 20.14 ■ Apply direct pressure to the wound.

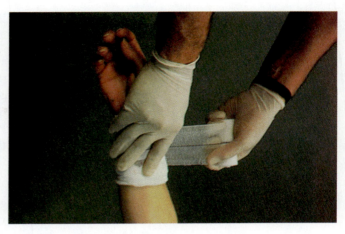

FIGURE 20.15 ■ Cover the wound with a clean dry cloth held in place with a bandage and elevate the limb, if possible.

dressing becomes saturated with blood, put another one on top of it. Do not remove the saturated dressing.
■ If possible, elevate the limb to decrease the blood supply (Figure 20.15 ■).
■ Remain with the person until help arrives.

SECTION 4

Poisoning

OBJECTIVES

What You Will Learn to Do

1. List the four kinds of poisoning.
2. Discuss first aid for a victim of poisoning.

Introduction: Poisoning

A **poison** is any substance to which the body has a bad reaction. What is poisonous to one person may not be to another. Quick action and careful observation are necessary if poisoning or an overdose of medication is suspected.

poison
substance causing illness or death when ingested

■ Look for a container that might have held the poison. Do not follow antidotes on the bottle. Call the poison control center.
■ Check in and around the mouth for chemical burns.
■ Check the breath for odors.
■ Gather as much information as possible about this incident before you act.
  A person can be poisoned by:
  a. Swallowing a poison
  b. Inhaling a poison through his mouth and nose
  c. Injecting himself or being injected (drugs, insect bites) with it
  d. Absorbing it through his skin

EMERGENCY PROCEDURE

Swallowed Poisons

If the person is conscious and does not have convulsions:

- Do not cause the person to vomit until you check with the poison control center. Some poisons burn tissue and would cause more damage as the person vomited.
- Call the poison control center with as much information as you have. Follow their instructions.
- Save any vomitus.

If the person is unconscious:

- Do not give anything by mouth.
- Position the person on his side. If he or she vomits, it will drain out.
- Maintain a clear airway. If the person stops breathing, give rescue breathing with a barrier device.
- Call for help and remain with the person until someone arrives.

Inhaled Poisons

Chemicals and gases can poison people and cause various reactions, such as irritation of eyes, throat, and/or skin; difficulty seeing, hearing, and/or speaking; hallucinations; fatigue; and/or collapse.

- If you can move the person to a safe area away from the poison, do so, but do not expose yourself to a hazardous environment.
- Send someone for help. Ventilate the area, if possible.
- Loosen tight clothing around the neck.
- Call the poison control center.
- Keep the person warm and comfortable.
- Rescue breathing may be necessary if the person stops breathing. See *Section 2* on how to restore breathing.

Injected Poisons

- Insect bites can cause allergic reactions. If the person experiences difficulty breathing, tingling, swelling, and/or redness in the area of the bite, call for assistance immediately.
- If you suspect that someone has had a drug overdose, call for help. Do not leave the person alone, and be alert for changes in condition.

Absorbed Poisons

- Some chemicals react violently with water. Powders should be brushed off.
- Call the poison control center.
- Poison ivy and related plants can cause irritation and rashes. Wash the area with clear water and not soap. Report the incident to your supervisor.

SECTION 5

Shock

OBJECTIVES

What You Will Learn to Do

1. Define shock.
2. Demonstrate first aid for a shock victim.

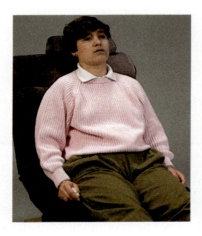

FIGURE 20.16 ■
Shock is the failure of the
heart and vascular system to
pump enough blood to all
parts of the body.

Introduction: Shock

Shock is the failure of the heart and vascular system to pump enough blood to all parts of the body. There may be many causes for this, such as loss of blood or heart damage, but the result is the same (Figure 20.16 ■).

shock
state of collapse resulting
from reduced blood
volume and pressure
usually caused by severe
injury or emotional
reaction

SIGNS AND SYMPTOMS OF SHOCK

■ Eyes are dull and pupils wide.
■ Face is pale; may be bluish in color. (Lips and nail beds will be dusky blue.)
■ Person may be nauseated.
■ Respirations are shallow, irregular, and labored.
■ Pulse is rapid and weak.
■ Skin is cold and clammy.
■ Person is restless.
■ Person is weak and may collapse.

EMERGENCY PROCEDURE

■ Send someone for help. Talk to the person and make her comfortable until help arrives.
■ Position the person with her head lower than her legs. Keep her warm. Blood loss makes a person cold, so cover her. If you cannot move the person because of injury, keep her warm until help arrives (Figure 20.17 ■).

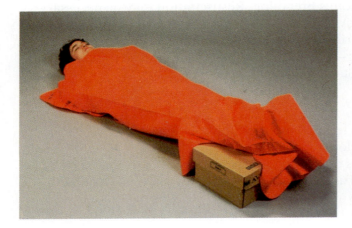

FIGURE 20.17 ■
Keep a shock victim warm.
Blood loss makes a person
cold, so cover him.

Burns

OBJECTIVE 1. Demonstrate first aid for a victim of a burn.

What You Will Learn to Do

Introduction: Burns

burn

injury to tissues caused by exposure to heat or to substances that simulate the sensation of heat

A **burn** is tissue damage caused by excessive heat regardless of the source. The heat may come from fire, electricity, chemicals, the sun, or steam. Any source of burns can cause damage to the skin and sometimes to various organs. By acting quickly and correctly, you can stop the burning process and prevent further injury.

A burn is labeled a "superficial burn," meaning the least severe burn, a "partial thickness burn," which causes blistering and destruction of underlying tissue; or a "full thickness burn," which indicates near-destruction of the body part.

Complications from burns are many. They include infection, shock, pain, loss of body heat and fluid, swelling of breathing passages, and death. All treatment for burns is aimed at preventing complications and speeding up the healing process.

EMERGENCY PROCEDURE

Small Burn Areas (Superficial—Reddening of Skin)
- Put the body part in cool water, if possible. Let it remain there for 2 to 5 minutes. Do not put ice on the burn.
- Cover the area with a sterile or clean cloth.
- Continue to put cool water over the dressing.
- Get medical help. Stay until someone arrives.

Larger, Deeper Burn Areas (Partial Thickness—Blistering; Full Thickness—Charring)
- Stop the burning, if necessary, by dowsing with cool water.
- Check to see if the person is breathing. Resuscitation may be necessary.
- Keep the person's airway open.
- Cover the area with sterile or clean dry cloth or sheet.
- Do not wet the dressing—it will chill the person and cause shock.
- Call for medical help. Stay until someone arrives.

Chemical Burns
- Flush with water for at least 20 minutes.
- Wrap area with clean cloth or sheet.
- If the person complains of burning, flush again.
- For lime burns, first brush away most of the powder, then flush with water.
- Call for medical help.

SECTION 7

Heart Attack

OBJECTIVES

What You Will Learn to Do

1. Define a heart attack.
2. List the signs and symptoms of a heart attack.
3. Demonstrate the proper first aid for a heart attack victim.

Introduction: Heart Attack—Myocardial Infarction—Chest Pain

The heart is a muscle that has its own blood supply. Any damage to the blood supply may lead to damage to the heart muscle. This is a **heart attack** or **myocardial infarction**. Therefore, anyone who has any type of chest pain should seek medical attention immediately! Most heart attacks do not necessarily follow unusual physical activity but may occur during sleep or after eating.

heart attack
layman's term referring to damage to the heart; a myocardial infarction

myocardial infarction
death of a part of the heart due to blockage in a blood vessel

INDICATIONS OF A HEART ATTACK

Symptoms of a heart attack are:

- Pain like a vise or a belt around the chest that may radiate to the jaw, neck, or inner left arm.
- Wet, clammy skin
- Perspiration
- Pulse rate is rapid and weak
- Color is pale
- Generalized weakness
- Low blood pressure
- Shortness of breath
- Nausea
- Respirations are shallow and difficult

EMERGENCY PROCEDURE

- If the person is unconscious, check for breathing response. If there is no response, call for help.
- Begin rescue breathing, with a barrier device (if possible), if the person has had a cardiac arrest. Cardiac arrest occurs when the heart has stopped beating and there is no breathing.
- If conscious, help the person into a comfortable position. Loosen his clothing if it is tight. If he wants to walk around, tell him it is important to rest and remain quiet.
- Reassure him. Continue to talk to him. Tell him what you are doing. If he asks you if he is having a heart attack, tell him that this could be many things, but it is safest to treat it as though it were a heart attack.
- Do not give him anything to eat or drink.
- If he stops breathing, start rescue breathing with barrier device.

Stroke/Cerebrovascular Accident

OBJECTIVES

What You Will Learn to Do

1. List the signs and symptoms of a CVA.
2. Demonstrate the proper emergency care for a victim of a CVA.

Introduction: Cerebrovascular Accident

stroke
cerebrovascular accident

cerebrovascular accident (CVA)
a blockage of a blood vessel within the brain leading to death of brain tissue

When a blood vessel to the brain is damaged and a part of the brain no longer has its own blood supply, it dies. This occurrence is called a **stroke**, "brain attack," **cerebrovascular accident**, or **CVA**, as discussed in Chapter 19. If you suspect that a person is having a CVA, treat him as though he were.

SIGNS AND SYMPTOMS

- Headache
- Difficulty with speech or vision
- Change in state of consciousness or orientation
- Paralysis in an extremity or one side of the face
- Seizure
- Difficulty breathing
- Unequal size of pupils
- Weakness on one side of the body or inability to use an arm or leg
- Uncontrolled drooling
- Loss of bowel or bladder control

EMERGENCY PROCEDURE

- Call for help.
- Provide ventilation, if needed.
- If the person is conscious, assist her into a comfortable, safe position. Position paralyzed extremities in proper body alignment.
- Be sure that the person can control her saliva. If she is lying down, position her on her side for drainage.
- Do not give her anything to eat or drink.
- Remain with her and reassure her that help is coming.

Bioterrorism, Terrorism, Natural Disasters

OBJECTIVES

What You Will Learn to Do

1. Become familiar with differences between terrorism, bioterrorism, and natural disasters.
2. Identify and learn your agency's policies for response to each one of these occurrences.

Introduction: Bioterrorism, Terrorism, Natural Disasters

In recent years, awareness has been increasing regarding the possibility of both terrorism and bioterrorism. **Bioterrorism** is the use of a biological substance to hurt, cause fear, infect, or kill. **Terrorism** is the use of random force or weapons to cause hurt, fear, or death. Unfortunately these may occur at any time or any place. Although we do not live our lives in a state of fear, we should be aware of such possibilities.

- If you see any package that you do not believe is either appropriate or in the appropriate place, do not touch it. Call the local authorities immediately!
- Do not transport any package for anyone you do not know.
- If you are asked to go into a home and you are afraid, for whatever reason, discuss this with you supervisor immediately.
- If someone threatens you, leave the area as soon as possible and call the authorities.

Natural disasters are unstoppable occurrences in nature such as floods, fires, volcanoes or power outages. Sometimes we get warnings that these things will happen and sometimes they happen without warning.

- Heed a warning whether it comes on the radio or television or you receive a telephone call. Act as the warning dictates.
- Call the authorities if you are in doubt as to what to do.

EMERGENCY PROCEDURES

- Know your agency's policies pertaining to response to bioterrorism, terrorism, and natural disasters.
- Be familiar with the telephone numbers for local authorities in case of emergency.
- Be familiar with all the exits and entrances to the home in which you are working.
- Always try to leave an area under siege. Do not stay to watch what happens.
- Follow the directions of the agency in charge of the disaster.
- It is always a good idea to have a small disaster kit available, including bottled water, candles, matches, flashlight, and portable radio.

bioterrorism
the use of a biological substance to hurt, cause fear, infect, or kill

terrorism
the use of random force or weapons to cause hurt, fear or death

natural disasters
unstoppable occurrences in nature such as floods, volcanoes, or power outages

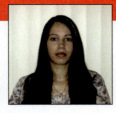

Case Study

Review the case study that appears on the first page of the chapter. Answer two sets of questions about the case study contained in the Explore and Apply sections below.

EXPLORE

1. You often meet Mrs. Soledad, who shares with you that she does not feel well, has some weakness in one arm, and is short of breath. Remembering that she is not your client, how do you respond when she tells you this information? What do you do with this information?

2. What are your main concerns about Mrs. Soledad? Do you have these concerns for people in your family? What will you do?

APPLY

1. Your client is independent. When you arrive one morning, you find her in the kitchen with a towel wrapped around her hand, which is bloody. The client states that she was cutting an orange and the knife slipped. She says it will heal soon and asks you not to call your supervisor or the rescue squad. What do you do? Why?

2. Discuss your feelings about giving rescue breathing. Review your agency policy as to when it is done and when it might not be done.

Certification Exam Review Questions

Choose the best answer for each question or statement.

1. **An emergency is**
   a. an occurrence that is not a complete surprise.
   b. an occurrence that calls for immediate action.
   c. an occurrence in which you have to call for help.
   d. always a reason to call an ambulance.

2. **If your client is bleeding, you should**
   a. put the area in cold water if you are able.
   b. cover the area with a clean cloth and apply pressure, elevating the area if possible.
   c. give the client his pain pills so he will be more comfortable.
   d. call the doctor.

3. **You suspect that your client's grandchild has drunk a liquid that was under the kitchen sink. The child appears fine. You should**
   a. tell his mother when she comes back.
   b. call the poison control center immediately.
   c. call your supervisor.
   d. call the pediatrician.

4. **Your client was cooking oatmeal this morning and caught her bathrobe sleeve on fire. She is sitting in the kitchen when you arrive with her arm wrapped in a kitchen towel. You should**
   a. remove the towel and peel away the sleeve material on her arm.
   b. call 911.
   c. call her physician.
   d. bring her pain pills because she is crying.

5. **Your client is suddenly weak and complaining of pain in his chest and arm. You should**
   a. put him to bed and bring him hot tea.
   b. have him sit down and take deep breaths.
   c. put your client in a safe place and immediately call 911.
   d. take your client's temperature and blood pressure and report this to your supervisor.

Abbreviations

abd.	Abdomen		liq, liq.	Liquid
ac, Ac	Before meals		LPN, L.P.N.	Licensed practical nurse
ad lib	As desired, if the client so desires		LVN, L.V.N.	Licensed vocational nurse
			MD, M.D.	Medical doctor
ADL	Activities of daily living		ml	Milliliter
A.M., a.m., am	Morning		O_2	Oxygen
Amt.	Amount		OB, O.B.	Obstetrics
AP	Antepartum, before delivery		OOB, O.O.B.	Out of bed
@	At		OPD, O.P.D.	Outpatient department
B&B, b&b	Bowel and bladder training		ortho	Orthopedics
bid, B.I.D., b.i.d.	Twice a day		OT, O.T.	Occupational therapy, or oral temperature
BM, B.M., bm, b.m.	Bowel movement, feces, stool			
B.P., BP	Blood pressure		oz	Ounce
BR, br, B.R., b.r.	Bedrest		pc	After meals
BRP, B.R.P., brp	Bathroom privileges		Ped, Peds	Pediatrics
BSC, bsc	Bedside commode		P.M., p.m., pm, PM	Afternoon
C°	Centigrade or Celsius degree		po	By mouth
c, c̄	With		p, p̄	After
Ca	Cancer		PP	Postpartum (after delivery)
Cath.	Catheter		prn, p.r.n.	Whenever necessary, when required
CBC, C.B.C.	Complete blood count			
mL	Cubic centimeter		Pt, pt.	Patient, pint
C/i, c/o	Complains of		PT, P.T.	Physical therapy
CO_2	Carbon dioxide		q	Every
CVA, C.V.A.	Cerebrovascular accident or stroke		qd	Every day
			qh	Every hour
CPR, C.P.R.	Cardiopulmonary resuscitation		q2h	Every 2 hours
			q3h	Every 3 hours
dc, d/c	Discontinue		q4h	Every 4 hours
drsg.	Dressing		nightly	Every night at bedtime
Dr., Dr	Doctor		qam, q am, q.a.m.	Every morning
DX	Diagnosis		qs	Quantity sufficient: as much as required
ECG, EKG	Electrocardiogram			
EEG, E.E.G.	Electroencephalogram		qt.	Quart
EENT, E.E.N.T.	Eyes, ears, nose, and throat		r, R	Rectal temperature
F°	Fahrenheit degree		RN, R.N.	Registered nurse
FF, F.F.	Force fluids		rom, R.O.M.	Range of motion
ft.	Foot		R_x	Prescription or treatment ordered by a physician
Fx	Fractured bone			
gal.	Gallon		s, s̄	Without
GI, G.I.	Gastrointestinal		SOB	Shortness of breath
gt.	One drop		one-half, ½	One-half
gtt.	Two or more drops		stat	At once, immediately
GU, G.U.	Genitourinary		S&A, S.&A.	Sugar and acetone test
Gyn.	Gynecology		S&K, S.&K.	Sugar and ketone test
H_2O	Water or aqua		tid. T.I.D.	Three times a day
hr	Hour		TPR	Temperature, pulse respiration
HS, hs	Bedtime or hour of sleep			
ht.	Height		Ung.	Ointment
in. or in	Inch		V.D.	Venereal disease
I&O or I.&O.	Intake and output		V.S., VS	Vital signs
irr.	Irregular		WBC, W.B.C.	White blood count
L	Liter		w/c	Wheelchair
lb	Pound		wt.	Weight

Appendix A

Answer Key for Certification Review Questions

CHAPTER 1
1. D
2. A
3. B
4. C
5. B

CHAPTER 2
1. A
2. B
3. D
4. B
5. C

CHAPTER 3
1. D
2. C
3. C
4. A
5. D

CHAPTER 4
1. C
2. A
3. B
4. C
5. C

CHAPTER 5
1. D
2. C
3. D
4. C
5. B

CHAPTER 6
1. C
2. B
3. A
4. B
5. B

CHAPTER 7
1. A
2. A
3. B
4. B
5. D

CHAPTER 8
1. B
2. D
3. D
4. C
5. C

CHAPTER 9
1. B
2. D
3. A
4. B
5. C

CHAPTER 10
1. C
2. A
3. D
4. B
5. B

CHAPTER 11
1. C
2. C
3. C
4. B
5. C

CHAPTER 12
1. A
2. B
3. D
4. C
5. B

21 Dehydration

22 Intake

23 Output

24 Vomitus

25 Specimen

26 Clean-Catch Diastolic Pressure

27 Catheter

28 Ureterostomy

29 Seizures

30 Hypertension

31 Myocardial Infarction

32. Angina

33.) Diabetes Mellitus

34.) Shock

35. Cerebrovascular Accident

36. Bony Prominences

37. Decubitus ulcer

38. Shearing

39. Incontinence   INCONTINENCE

40. Urinal

41. Commode

42. Perineal Care

43. Perineum

44. Rehabilitation

45.) Expressive Aphasia

46.) Receptive Aphasia

47. Functional Limitation

48 Pulse

49 Respirations

50 Systolic Pressure

CHAPTER 13
1. B
2. C
3. A
4. C
5. A

CHAPTER 14
1. B
2. D
3. D
4. D
5. C

CHAPTER 15
1. D
2. C
3. B
4. B
5. A

CHAPTER 16
1. B
2. C
3. C
4. D
5. B

CHAPTER 17
1. C
2. A
3. D
4. A
5. C

CHAPTER 18
1. C
2. B
3. A
4. B
5. A

CHAPTER 19
1. B
2. D
3. C
4. D
5. A

CHAPTER 20
1. B
2. B
3. B
4. B
5. C

Appendix B

Additional Recipes

CHICKEN/TURKEY SAUSAGE WITH ONIONS, PEPPERS, AND MUSHROOMS

Prep time: 15 minutes
Cook time: 40 minutes

3–4 servings

Ingredients

1 pound chicken or turkey sausage
1 tablespoon vegetable oil
1 cup chopped onion
½ cup chopped green pepper
½ cup sliced mushrooms

¼ teaspoon chopped parsley
½ teaspoon chopped basil
½ teaspoon chopped oregano
1½ cup tomato sauce

Instructions

1. Cut the sausage into bite-size pieces.
2. Heat the oil in a skillet.
3. Brown the sausage about 10 minutes.
4. Add the onion, green pepper, and mushroom. Cook about 10 minutes.
5. Add the spices and tomato sauce. Cook additional 10–15 minutes or until the meat is cooked thoroughly.

Nutrient Content

Calories 275
Protein 18 g
23% calories from protein
Carbohydrates g
Fat 20 g

58% calories from fat
Cholesterol 0 mg
Sodium 1557 mg
Dietary fiber 2 g

Adaptations for Physical Limitations

• Adjust the consistency to the client's swallowing ability by cutting the sausage into small pieces or pureeing the food once it has completed the cooking process. Add liquid or a thickening agent if necessary.

Substitutions

• Add *Parmesan cheese* when serving.
• Add hot red pepper flakes when serving.
• Use *tomato sauce with no added salt.*
• Use *veal, lamb,* or *pork sausage.*

Source: Capron, Mary Ellen; Zucker, Elana. *Ultimate Cooking Companion for At-home Caregivers,* 1st Edition, © 2003 pp. 62, 108, 116, 135, 163, 176, 239. Reprinted by permission of Pearson Education, Inc., Upper Saddle River, NJ.

PASTA WITH HERBS AND CHEESE

Prep time: 4 minutes   *2 servings*
Cook time: 10 minutes

Ingredients

4 ounces pasta   1 tablespoon chives
6 ounces whole milk ricotta cheese   1 clove garlic
1 teaspoon oregano   2 tablespoons olive oil

Instructions

1. Fill a medium saucepan with water. Bring to a boil.
2. Put pasta into boiling water. Cover and bring back to a boil. Uncover.
3. Let boil until pasta is done to the preference of the client.
4. Drain. Do not rinse.
5. Meanwhile, mix together cheese, chives, oregano, and garlic.
6. Combine the pasta, cheese, and olive oil.
7. Warm and serve.

Nutrient Content

Calories 486   48% calories from fat
Protein 17 g   Cholesterol 41 mg
14% calories from protein   Sodium 77 mg
Carbohydrates 48 g   Dietary fiber 2 g
Fat 26 g

Adaptations for Physical Limitations

- Adjust the consistency to the client's swallowing ability by cutting the pasta into small pieces or pureeing in a blender. Add liquid to desired consistency.

Substitutions

- Vary the ***cheese*** used to include small-curd cottage cheese, Parmesan, Jarlsberg, and cheddar.
- Add ½ cup cooked ***vegetables*** before serving.
- Add small ***meatballs*** or cup of cut up cooked ***chicken.***

Source: Capron, Mary Ellen; Zucker, Elana. *Ultimate Cooking Companion for At-home Caregivers,* 1st Edition, © 2003 pp. 62, 108, 116, 135, 163, 176, 239. Reprinted by permission of Pearson Education, Inc., Upper Saddle River, NJ.

RICE MEXICAN STYLE

Prep time: 10 minutes
Cook time: 35 minutes

4 servings

Ingredients

1 teaspoon minced garlic
1 cup minced onion
½ cup minced green pepper
1 cup cooked crushed tomatoes

½ teaspoon paprika
1 cup long-grain rice
2 cups chicken broth
Vegetable oil spray

Instructions

1. Spray a saucepan with vegetable oil spray.
2. Heat the saucepan and cook the onions and garlic until the onions are clear.
3. Add the rice and stir until the rice becomes toasted and brown.
4. Add the green pepper, tomatoes, and chicken broth. Cover and cook until the liquid is absorbed.
5. Add the paprika and serve.

Nutrient Content

Calories 214
Protein 5 g
10% calories from protein
Carbohydrates 44 g
Fat 1 g

6% calories from fat
Cholesterol 0 mg
Sodium 614 mg
Dietary fiber 2 g

Adaptations for Physical Limitations

• Adjust the consistency to the swallowing ability of the client by mashing the rice.

Substitutions

• Add red pepper flakes before serving.

Source: Capron, Mary Ellen; Zucker, Elana. *Ultimate Cooking Companion for At-home Caregivers,* 1st Edition, © 2003 pp. 62, 108, 116, 135, 163, 176, 239. Reprinted by permission of Pearson Education, Inc., Upper Saddle River, NJ.

CHILI

Prep time: 20 minutes *4 servings*
Cook time: 40 minutes

Ingredients

1 cup cooked kidney beans
1 tablespoon vegetable oil
1 cup onion, chopped
1 clove minced garlic or ½ teaspoon garlic
  powder
12 ounces (¾ pound) lean ground beef

1 tablespoon oregano
3 tablespoons chili seasoning powder
¼ teaspoon black pepper
¼ teaspoon ground cumin
1½ cups tomato sauce—no salt added
1½ tablespoons cider vinegar

Instructions

1. Heat the kidney beans according to the package. Do not add salt.
2. Heat oil in deep pot or skillet over medium heat.
3. Add the onion and garlic, and sauté until soft.
4. Add the beef. Stir with a fork to break up the meat as it continues to brown.
5. Stir in seasoning, tomatoes, and vinegar.
6. Add the beans and mix well.
7. Reduce heat to low and cook covered for additional 30 minutes, stirring occasionally.

Nutrient Content

Calories 368
Protein 20 g
23% calories from protein
Carbohydrates 22 g
Fat 21 g

53% calories from fat
Cholesterol 64 mg
Sodium 245 mg
Dietary fiber 7 g

Adaptations for Physical Limitations

• Adjust the consistency to the client's swallowing ability by cutting the meat into small
  pieces or pureeing the food once it has completed the cooking process. Add liquid or a
  thickening agent if necessary.

Substitutions

• Use any combination of ground meat *(turkey, chicken, veal, pork)*.
• Drain excess fat from meat prior to adding seasonings and tomatoes.
• Use any cooked *beans* in place of or in addition to kidney beans.
• Serve with *grated cheese* on top.

Source: Capron, Mary Ellen; Zucker, Elana. *Ultimate Cooking Companion for At-home Caregivers,*
1st Edition, © 2003 pp. 62, 108, 116, 135, 163, 176, 239. Reprinted by permission of Pearson
Education, Inc., Upper Saddle River, NJ.

YOGURT SMOOTHIE

Prep time: 5 minutes   *3 servings*

Ingredients

1½ cups low-fat vanilla yogurt   ¾ cup frozen peaches
1 small banana   1 cup frozen whole strawberries
1 tablespoon orange juice concentrate   3 ice cubes

Instructions

1. Place all ingredients in a blender and cover.
2. Blend at high speed for 30 seconds or until smooth.
3. Pour into glass.
4. Serve immediately.

Nutrient Content

Calories 202   9% calories from fat
Protein 8 g   Cholesterol 7.5 mg
14% calories from protein   Sodium 92 mg
Carbohydrates 40 g   Dietary fiber 3.5 g
Fat 2 g

Adaptations for Physical Limitations

• Adjust the consistency to the client's swallowing ability by blending longer or adding
  additional liquid or thickening agent.

Substitutions

• Use any kind of *vanilla yogurt*.
• Serve with *whipped topping* if desired.

Source: Capron, Mary Ellen; Zucker, Elana. *Ultimate Cooking Companion for At-home Caregivers,*
1st Edition, © 2003 pp. 62, 108, 116, 135, 163, 176, 239. Reprinted by permission of Pearson
Education, Inc., Upper Saddle River, NJ.

Glossary

A glossary is a list of words and their definitions. All new words used in this book are defined here. Many of the words are familiar to you, but they may have been used in this book with new health-related meanings. These words are included here, too. The boldface numeral in parentheses, for example **(5)**, indicates the chapter in which the term is defined.

abdominal thrust   quick movement in the abdomen to remove a foreign body from the airway **(20)**

abduction   to move an arm or leg away from the center of the body **(7)**

abuse   any act that causes another harm; using a substance to excess **(5)**

abusive   insulting or mistreating **(3)**

acetone   a chemical found in urine **(18)**

activity tolerance   the most activity the client will be able to do **(11)**

acute   state of illness that comes on suddenly and may be of short duration **(3)**

adduction   to move an arm or leg toward the center of the body **(7)**

administer   to give a client medication without his assistance **(18)**

advanced directive for health care/living wills
legal documents that describe a person's health-care wishes, to be used when they can no longer make the choices for themselves **(6)**

airborne transmission   transfer of pathogens via evaporated droplets or dust particles moving through the air **(8)**

age-competent   caregiver is knowledgeable about needs of specific age group **(1)**

aging process   changes in the body caused by growing older **(4)**

aging   to grow older **(4)**

align   to put the body into its proper anatomical position **(11)**

alveoli   microscopic air sacs in the lungs where oxygen passes into the blood in exchange for waste products **(7)**

Alzheimer's disease   a form of irreversible mental deterioration **(19)**

ambulate   to walk **(14)**

anatomy   the study of the structure of the body **(7)**

aneroid   one type of sphygmomanometer **(15)**

angina   brief, temporary chest pain resulting from a decrease in oxygen to the heart **(19)**

ankylosing spondylitis   an arthritis-type disease that affects the spine and/or shoulders and hips **(19)**

antagonistic groups   groups having opposing actions; for example, muscles that flex the upper arm act in opposition to the muscles that extend it **(7)**

anus   opening of the rectum onto the body surface **(7)**

aorta   major artery that carries blood away from the heart **(7)**

apical   refers to the apex of the heart **(15)**

appendix   slender growth attached to the large intestine **(7)**

arteries   blood vessels that carry blood away from the heart **(7)**

arteriosclerosis   hardening of the arteries due to thickening of the blood vessel walls **(19)**

arthritis   disease characterized by inflammation and destruction of the joints **(19)**

asepsis   the process of creating an environment free of disease-causing organisms **(8)**

aspiration   when food or fluid is taken into the lungs **(7)**

atherosclerosis   increased formation of fatty deposits and fibrous plaques, resulting in decrease of the lumen of the blood vessel **(19)**

atria   the two upper chambers of the heart **(7)**

aura   sensation before an epileptic seizure **(18)**

aural   pertaining to the ear **(15)**

autonomic nervous system   part of the nervous system that carries messages without conscious thought **(7)**

bacteria   microorganisms that may or may not be pathogens **(8)**

base of support   part of the body that bears the most weight **(11)**

bed cradle   frame placed over a body area to hold bed covers away from a body part **(9)**

bedpan   container into which a person defecates or urinates while in bed **(13)**

bedsores   decubiti **(12)**

benign   nonmalignant **(19)**

bile   substance needed for digestion that is secreted by the liver and stored in the gallbladder **(7)**

biopsy   examination of tissue taken from the body **(19)**

bioterrorism   the use of a biological substance to hurt, cause fear, infect, or kill **(20)**

bladder   membranous sac that serves as a container within the body, such as the urinary bladder, which holds urine **(7)**

blood   fluid that circulates through the heart, arteries, veins and capillaries; carries nourishment and oxygen to the tissues and takes away waste matter and carbon dioxide **(7)**

blood pressure cuff   another term for sphygmomanometer **(15)**

blood pressure   force of blood on the inner walls of blood vessels as it flows through them **(15)**

blood vessels   the tubes that carry the blood throughout the body **(7)**

blood-borne pathogens   disease-causing entities transmitted through contact with blood **(8)**

body alignment   arrangement of the body in a straight line, placing of body parts in correct anatomical position **(11)**

body language   gestures that function as a form of communication **(2)**

body mechanics   proper use of the human body to do work and to avoid injury and strain **(11)**

bony prominences   areas of the body where the bones are close to the skin surface and subject to decubiti **(12)**

brain   main organ of the central nervous system, found in skull **(7)**

bronchi   two main branches of the bronchial tree that lead to the lungs **(7)**

burn   injury to tissues caused by exposure to heat or to substances that simulate the sensation of heat **(20)**

burp   the release of air from the stomach through the mouth **(5)**

bursa   sac of fluid within a joint capsule that provides lubrication for joint movement **(7)**

calibration   graduations on a measuring instrument **(16)**

calories   unit for measuring the energy produced when food is oxidized in the body **(10)**

capillaries   minute blood vessels that connect arteries to the veins **(7)**

carbohydrate   one of the basic food elements necessary for the body to function properly; includes all sugars and starches **(19)**

cartilage   tough connective tissue that holds bones together **(7)**

carrier   a person who has a disease that can be transmitted to others but who displays no signs or symptoms of the disease **(8)**

case manager   coordinator of care for the client with all caregivers **(1)**

cast   rigid dressing molded to the body to give support and proper alignment **(18)**

catheter   a tube used to remove body fluids from a cavity **(7) (16) (18)**

causative agent   the pathogen responsible for the disease **(8)**

cell   basic unit of living matter **(7)**

center of gravity   point at which, when held, you will have the greatest control over an object **(11)**

central venous lines   intravenous lines surgically placed, in large veins of the body **(18)**

cerebrovascular accident   a blockage of a blood vessel within the brain leading to death of brain tissue **(14) (19) (20)**

chain of infection   the process by which an infection is transmitted to and develops in a host **(8)**

chemotherapy   the regime of taking drugs to treat a malignancy **(10) (12)**

Cheyne-Stokes   a type of noisy breathing alternating with periods of no breathing; usually precedes death **(7)**

Cheyne-Stokes respiration   a type of noisy breathing alternating with periods of no breathing; usually precedes death **(6) (15)**

chronic obstructive pulmonary disease   refers to diseases that cause permanent damage to lung tissue, including emphysema, asthma, and chronic bronchitis **(19)**

chronic   state of disease that lasts a long time **(3)**

circulatory system   organs of the body concerned with circulation **(7)**

circumcision   removal of the foreskin of the penis by a surgical procedure **(5)**

clean   uncontaminated by harmful microorganisms **(8)**

clean-catch   urine specimen captured directly by the client into a sterile container, following the careful cleansing of the urinary meatus and surrounding area **(17)**

clot   semisolid mass of blood **(19)**

collateral circulation   circulation taken over by smaller blood vessels after larger ones have been obstructed **(19)**

colon   large bowel **(7)**

colostomy   surgical procedure that creates an artificial opening through the abdominal wall into a part of the large bowel through which feces can leave the body. Can be temporary or permanent **(18)**

commode   a portable frame, with pan or pail, into which a client urinates and/or defecates **(13)**

communicable   spread from one person to another **(8)**

communication   exchange of information **(2)**

congenital anomaly   a deviation from the normal, present at birth **(5)**

constipation   having hard, difficult-to-expel bowel movements **(5)**

contagious   readily transmitted by direct or indirect contact **(3)**

continuous infusion   uninterrupted: without a stop **(18)**

contract   become smaller **(7)**

contracture   a permanent muscle shortening often resulting in loss of function **(7)**

contraindication   condition that forbids the use of a particular treatment or drug **(9)**

coronary   pertaining to the heart **(7)**

corporate compliance   when organizations deliver care according to state and federal laws and regulations **(1)**

credential   a letter or certificate indicating that a right or privilege has been attained or that a position of authority may be exercised **(1)**

cross-infection   infection by a new or different microorganism from a visitor or health team member **(8)**

cubic centimeter   a unit of measure used in the metric system **(16)**

culture   the collective shared thoughts, values, beliefs, and behaviors of a group **(2)**

culturally competent   to have a basic understanding of the clients' culture and function within their family and the greater community **(3)**

customer   a person receiving a service from another person for a payment **(1)**

customer satisfaction   meeting patient's expectations thus leaving them content **(1)**

cystitis   inflammation of the bladder **(7)**

daily ability level   the capability of the client to perform an activity on a given day **(11)**

daily living skills   those tasks done each day to meet a person's basic needs **(14)**

decubitus ulcer   bedsore; open wound that occurs from lack of blood supply to an area usually located on a bony prominence **(9) (12)**

defecate   to have a bowel movement **(13)**

defense mechanism   a thought used unconsciously to protect oneself against painful or unpleasant feelings **(3)**

dehydration   condition in which the body has less than normal amount of fluid **(16)**

delegation   the act of assigning tasks to others **(1)**

dementia   loss of mental powers **(4)**

denial   refusal to believe or accept reality **(3)**

dentures   false teeth **(13)**

depression   low spirits that may or may not cause a change of activity **(3)**

dermis   the skin in general; specifically, the second layer of skin **(7)**

developmental disability   any condition that interferes with the normal development of a person **(5)**

diabetes mellitus   condition that develops when the body cannot change sugar into energy **(19)**

diabetic coma   hyperglycemia: an excess of circulating sugar in the blood **(19)**

diaphragm   muscular partition between the chest cavity and the abdominal cavity **(7)**

diarrhea   abnormally frequent discharge of liquid fecal matter **(5)**

diastolic pressure   the pressure in the blood vessels measured when the heart is relaxed **(15)**

digestion   the act of converting food into energy the body can use **(7)**

digestive system   the group of organs responsible for converting food into energy for the body **(7)**

digital thermometer   a thermometer with temperature readout **(15)**

dilate   expand; grow bigger **(7)**

direct contact   body surface to body surface transfer of pathogen **(8)**

dirty   contaminated by harmful microorganisms **(8)**

disability   partial or complete loss of the use of a part or parts of the body **(3)**

disc   round piece of cartilage between the vertebrae **(7)**

discipline   a system of rules **(5)**

disinfection   process of destroying most disease-causing organisms **(8)**

dominant   stronger half of a pair **(14)**

do not resuscitate (DNR) order   a legal document that states a person's wishes for attempt to reverse death when his or her heart stops beating **(6)**

double-bagging   technique of putting contaminated material into two plastic bags for protection **(8)**

drainage   discharge from a sore, wound, or body part **(18)**

draw sheet   small sheet made of plastic, rubber, or cotton placed across the middle of the bed to cover and protect the bottom sheet and assist in moving the client **(9)**

dressing   bandage for an external wound **(18)**

droplet transmission   transfer of pathogens via droplets propelled through the air by coughing, talking, or sneezing **(8)**

duct   passage for fluids **(7)**

duodenum   first part of the small intestine **(7)**

earmold   an impression of the ear used with a hearing aid **(14)**

edema   abnormal swelling of a part of the body caused by fluid collecting in that area **(16) (19)**

ejaculate   to discharge fluid suddenly, especially the discharge of semen from the male urethra **(7)**

ejaculatory ducts   part of the male reproductive system **(7)**

embolus   a clot carried by the circulatory system from its place of formation to another site, usually causing an obstruction **(19)**

emergency   a sudden unexpected crisis, injury, or illness **(20)**

emesis   vomitus **(16)**

endocrine glands   ductless glands in the body that secrete hormones into the blood **(7)**

endometrium   lining of the uterus **(7)**

epidermis   outermost layer of skin **(7)**

epididymides   organs attached to the testes **(7)**

epiglottis   a flap of tissue located in the back of the throat that covers the larynx while swallowing **(7)**

esophagus   muscular tube for the passage of food, extending from the back of the throat (pharynx), down through the chest and diaphragm, and into the stomach **(7)**

ethics   system of moral behavior and beliefs **(1)**

ethnic diversity   a variety of religions, cultures, and races living within an area **(2)**

evaporation   to pass off as vapor, as water evaporating into the air **(7)**

exhale   to breathe out air in respiration **(7)**

expressive aphasia   difficulty communicating in writing and orally **(14)**

extend   straighten an arm or leg **(7)**

external   outside the body **(20)**

fallopian tubes   also called the oviducts, through which an egg travels from the ovary to the uterus **(7)**

family dynamics   the ways in which family members interact with each other **(3)**

feces   solid waste material discharged from the body through the rectum and anus **(7)**

feedback mechanism   process whereby the output of a system is fed back into the system (input) to change the way the system works or what it produces (output) **(7)**

fertile   the period of the month when a woman is able to conceive **(7)**

fetus   developing infant in the uterus, after the first 2 months **(5)**

first aid   emergency treatment given for injury or illness before regular medical treatment is available **(20)**

flammable   substance that will burn quickly **(9)**

flex   to bend **(7)**

flexion   bending of a joint **(7)**

fluid balance   the relationship of intake fluid with excreted fluid output **(16)**

fluid intake liquid taken into the body **(16)**

fluid output liquid excreted by the body **(16)**

food groups the division of nutrients into four categories of dairy products, vegetables and fruits, meat and fish, and bread and cereal products **(10)**

foot drop a contraction of the foot due to a shortening of the muscles in the calf of the leg; the foot falls forward and cannot be held in proper position **(9)**

footboard a flat piece of wood or cardboard placed at the end of the bed, under the covers so that the client can rest his feet flatly against it and so that covers do not touch the client's toes **(9)**

force fluids extra fluids taken in according to doctor's orders **(16)**

fracture break **(7)**

functional usable **(11)**

functional limitations the inability to perform a task due to the deficit of a body part **(14)**

gallbladder a reservoir that holds bile secreted by the liver **(7)**

geriatrics knowledge and care of persons over 65 **(4)**

glucose sugar **(7)**

gout the buildup of uric acid crystals in the blood and joints **(19)**

grand mal seizure type of epileptic seizure **(18)**

guarding belt device placed around the waist, used to assist a client during ambulation **(14)**

health-care proxy a person designated to make health-care–related decisions when a person can no longer do so **(6)**

hearing aid mechanical device used to help a person perceive sounds **(14)**

heart attack general term referring to damage to the heart; a myocardial infarction **(19) (20)**

heart four-chambered, hollow, muscular organ in the chest cavity, pointing slightly to the left, that pumps blood throughout the body **(7)**

Heimlich maneuver a system developed by Henry J. Heimlich to remove a foreign body from the airway **(20)**

hemiplegic one who is paralyzed on one side of the body **(14)**

hemorrhage excessive bleeding **(19) (20)**

hemorrhoid swollen vein near the anus **(7)**

hormones protein substance secreted by an endocrine gland directly into the blood **(7)**

hospice program of care that allows a dying client to remain at home and die at home while receiving professionally supervised care **(6)**

host the place where an infection develops **(8)**

hyperalimentation process of giving nutrients directly into the blood stream **(18)**

hypertension high blood pressure **(15) (19)**

hypotension low blood pressure **(15)**

hysterectomy removal of the uterus **(7)**

ileostomy surgical procedure that makes an artificial opening through the abdominal wall into the ileum, though which waste is discharged **(18)**

illness deviation from the healthy state **(3)**

improvise to make do with the tools or equipment at hand; to use an item for a task for which it was not originally designed **(9)**

incontinence the inability to control one's bowel movements or urination **(12) (16)**

indirect transmission contact with a contaminated object and transfer of pathogen **(8)**

inflammation reaction of the tissues to disease or injury; usually involves pain, heat, redness, and swelling of the body part **(7)**

inflexible unbending, rigid **(13)**

inhale to breathe in air in respiration **(7)**

insulin hormone produced by the pancreas needed for the metabolism of sugars and starches **(19)**

insulin shock or insulin reaction hypoglycemia due to too much insulin in the blood **(19)**

intake all substances ingested by the body, sometimes refers only to fluid consumed **(16)**

intermittent infusion alternating; stopping and beginning again **(18)**

intravenous therapy giving of fluids or medication directly into the vein **(18)**

involuntary action taken without conscious input **(7)**

involved body part undergoing therapy or part of a disease process **(11)**

irrigate cleanse or wash with water or fluid **(18)**

job description written document listing the parts of employment, such as the tasks for which one is responsible **(1)**

joint part of the body where two bones come together and there is movement **(7)**

ketoacidosis a condition characterized by a large amount of ketone bodies in the urine **(19)**

ketones chemical compounds sometimes found in urine **(18)**

kidney organ lying in the upper posterior portion of the abdomen that removes wastes from the bloodstream and discharges them in the form of urine **(7)**

labored difficult **(15)**

large intestine the last section of colon starting at the end of the small intestine and ending at the rectum **(7)**

larynx area of the throat containing the vocal cords **(7)**

ligament a tough band of tissue connecting bone to bone **(7)**

liver body's largest organ located in the upper right quadrant of the abdominal cavity, which helps process waste products **(7)**

living will see *advanced directive* **(6)**

lungs primary organs of breathing **(8)**

lymph clear, colorless fluid carried by an independent system of vessels that returns the fluid to the heart **(7)**

lymph nodes organs of lymph tissue **(7)**

malignancy cancer **(19)**

manual thrust a quick movement of the hands to remove an obstruction of the airway **(20)**

meatus opening of the urethra to the outside of the body **(7)**

mechanical lift machine used to lift a client from one place to another **(14)**

medication substance or preparation used in treating a disease **(18)**

menopause period of life in the female usually between the ages of 45 and 50 when menstruation stops; change of life **(7)**

menstruation cyclical discharge of blood from the uterus **(7)**

mental disability the temporary or permanent disruption of a person's ability to function satisfactorily in society **(3)**

mental health the ability to function satisfactorily in a society; a sense of well being **(3)**

mercury one type of sphygmomanometer **(15)**

metastasis the spreading of cancer within the body **(19)**

metric system a method of measuring temperature, length, and volume of fluid based on the decimal system **(16)**

microorganism living body so small it can be seen only through a microscope **(8)**

mitered corner folding the bedding at the corners when making a bed so that the sheet is tightly stretched with no wrinkles **(9)**

muscular system group of organs that allow the body to move **(7)**

myocardial infarction death of a part of the heart due to blockage in a blood vessel **(7) (19) (20)**

natural disasters unstoppable occurrences in nature such as floods, fires, volcanoes **(20)**

need a lack of something **(3)**

nerve bundle of neurons held together with connective tissue; nerves go to all parts of the body from the central nervous system, that is, from the brain and spinal cord **(7)**

nerve impulse regular wave of negative electrical impulses that transmit information along a neuron from one part of the body to another **(7)**

nervous system system that controls all body functions **(7)**

neuron cell that is part of all nerves **(7)**

nonfunctional having no use; not usable **(11)**

nonjudgmental accepting communication without stating a personal opinion **(2)**

nonsterile not subjected to the sterilizing process and therefore possibly having pathogens **(18)**

nosocomial infection an infection acquired while in a health-care facility **(8)**

nutrients food substances required by the body to repair, maintain, and grow new cells **(7) (10)**

nutrition that which nourishes; food **(10)**

objective reporting reporting exactly what you observe **(2)**

observation gathering information about a client **(2)**

obstructed blocked **(20)**

occupational therapist trained person who assists people with performing their daily living tasks **(14)**

oral hygiene cleanliness of the mouth **(13)**

organ several types of tissues grouped together to perform a certain function **(7)**

organism living thing **(8)**

osteoarthritis the most common type of arthritis **(19)**

ostomy artificially created opening through the abdominal wall that provides a way for the intestinal organs to discharge waste products **(18)**

output material discharged from the body, may refer only to fluids **(16)**

ovaries organs in the female that produce mature eggs and the primary female sex hormones, estrogen and progesterone **(7)**

ovulation period of time in which the ovum is pushed out from the surface of the ovary and usually picked up by the oviduct **(7)**

ovum egg **(7)**

oxygen a colorless, odorless gas making up about one-fifth of the air we breathe. It is essential for life **(18)**

pacemaker electrical device used to stimulate the heart **(19)**

palliative care a multidisciplinary approach to managing care of dying people who continue to accept curative medical intervention **(6)**

pancreas an organ producing both digestive juices and hormones **(7)**

pathogen disease-causing microorganism **(8)**

penis male sexual organ; urine is also ejected through the penis **(7)**

perineal care cleansing of the perineal area **(13)**

perineum area between the anus and the external genital organs **(13)**

peripheral line intravenous lines in place in the upper extremities **(18)**

peristalsis movement of the intestines that pushes food along to the next part of the digestive system **(7)**

perspiration body moisture given off during physical activity **(7)**

petit mal seizure type of epileptic seizure **(18)**

pharynx area behind the nasal cavities, mouth, and larynx that opens into them and the esophagus **(7)**

physiology study of the functions of body tissues and organs **(7)**

pigment substance that gives the skin color **(7)**

placenta oval, spongy structure in the uterus from which the unborn baby receives its nourishment. Sometimes called afterbirth, the placenta is discharged from the mother's body soon after childbirth **(5)**

plaque fatty deposits within the blood vessels attached to the vessel walls **(19)**

plasma liquid portion of blood **(7)**

poison substance causing illness or death when ingested **(20)**

pore opening to the outside of the skin **(7)**

portal of entry the method by which the pathogen enters the new host **(8)**

portal of exit the place where the pathogen leaves the host **(8)**

postmortem after death **(6)**

prepuce foreskin of the penis, often removed in a procedure called a circumcision **(5)**

pressure sore decubitus **(12)**

primary site place of the original cancerous lesion **(19)**

principal care person person in charge of the client's care **(1)**

priority giving one thing more importance than another **(14)**

prioritize to organize or schedule, usually listing the most important task first and the least important item last **(1)**

prostate gland male gland behind the outlet of the urinary bladder **(7)**

protective barriers equipment to protect you from splashes, spills, droplets, or other sources of contamination **(8)**

protein one of the nutrients necessary to all animal life **(10)**

protocol rules directing the actions of specific people **(1)**

pull sheet a sheet or piece of cloth placed under the client and used by the caretaker to facilitate moving the client in the bed **(11)**

pulling braid a device used to assist a person in moving and/or sitting up in bed **(14)**

pulmonary refers to the lungs **(7)**

pulse rhythmic expansion and contractions of the arteries caused by the beating of the heart **(15)**

punishment action performed as the result of wrongdoing **(5)**

pus a waste product of inflammation **(7)**

radiation therapy the use of X-rays to treat a tumor or a condition **(10) (12)**

range-of-motion (ROM) exercises exercises that take a body part through its entire ability to move **(14)**

reagent a substance used to measure or detect another substance **(18)**

reality orientation a technique to orient people to their surroundings **(4)**

receptive aphasia inability to understand stimuli due to a deficiency within the brain **(14)**

rectum lower 8 to 10 inches of the colon **(7)**

regulated medical waste waste products that require special disposal by law **(8)**

rehabilitation process by which people who have been disabled by injury or sickness are helped to recover as many as possible of their original abilities and live with the remaining disabilities **(14)**

reinfection to become ill again with the same microorganism **(8)**

respiration process of breathing; inhaling and exhaling air **(15)**

responsibilities tasks one must execute and for which one is held accountable **(1)**

restraint a device prescribed by a physician to confine a client and prevent injury to that client or others **(9)**

rheumatoid arthritis crippling chronic disease of the joints **(19)**

role one's function, place within a group of people **(1)**

route of transmission the method by which the pathogen goes from the reservoir to the new host **(8)**

safety razor razor provided with a guard to prevent cutting the skin **(13)**

saliva secretion of the salivary glands into the mouth; moistens food and is necessary for digestion **(7)**

scrotum pouch below the penis that contains the testicles **(7)**

secondary site place in the body in which cancerous cells are found other than at the primary site **(19)**

seizure convulsions or involuntary muscular contractions and relaxations **(18)**

self-inoculation infecting oneself with one's own organisms **(8)**

semen the fluid of ejaculation **(7)**

seminal ducts and vesicles small glands in the male near the prostate and urethra where semen is stored before it is discharged **(7)**

sense organs groups of tissue that make it possible for us to be aware of the outside world through sight, hearing, smell, taste, and touch **(7)**

shearing the action of skin being moved in one direction while underlying tissue and/or bone is moved in another direction **(12)**

shock state of collapse resulting from reduced blood volume and pressure usually caused by severe injury or emotional reaction **(20)**

sitz bath bath in which the client sits in a specially designed chair or tub with his hips and buttocks in water **(18)**

skeletal system bones of the body that give the body shape and protection **(7)**

skin the largest organ in the body whose functions include protection from infection, temperature regulation, and removal of waste products **(7)**

small intestine the digestive tract between the stomach and the large intestine **(7)**

smooth muscle appears smooth under a microscope; usually associated with involuntary actions **(7)**

specimen samples of bodily products collected and sent to a laboratory for examination **(17)**

sperm male reproductive cell **(7)**

spermatic ducts tubes containing sperm **(7)**

sphincter ring-like muscle that controls the opening and closing of a body opening **(7)**

sphygmomanometer apparatus for measuring blood pressure of which there are two types, mercury or aneroid; blood pressure cuff **(15)**

spinal cord one of the main organs of the nervous system; carries messages from the brain to other parts of the body and from parts of the body back to the brain; located inside the spine (backbone) **(7)**

spleen abdominal organ **(7)**

spontaneous combustion process of catching fire as a result of the heat of burning chemicals **(9)**

spore microorganism that has formed a hard shell around itself for protection. It can only be destroyed by sterilization **(8)**

sprain to twist a ligament or muscle without dislocating the bones **(7)**

stabilizes returns to normal **(7)**

standard precautions those routine activities recommended to protect health-care workers from contamination with blood and all body fluids (except sweat) **(8)**

static electricity electrical discharges in the air **(9)**

sterilization process of destroying all microorganisms including spores **(8)**

stethoscope instrument that allows one to listen to various sounds in the human body **(15)**

stimulus activity that causes the body to respond **(7)**

stoma artificially made opening connecting a body passage with the outside **(18)**

stomach part of the digestive tract between the esophagus (food pipe) and the duodenum **(7)**

stool solid waste material discharged from the body through the rectum and anus. Other names include "feces," "excreta," "excrement," "B.M.," and "fecal matter" **(5) (17)**

straight drainage method of collecting urine from a Foley catheter into a closed container **(18)**

stretch receptors nerve cells that relay messages to the brain as the organ enlarges **(7)**

striated muscle appears lined under a microscope; usually associated with voluntary action **(7)**

stroke cerebrovascular accident **(19) (20)**

subjective reporting giving your opinion about what you have observed **(2)**

substance abuse the use of anything, usually alcohol or drugs, to excess and to the detriment of the person **(3)**

support systems arrangements that aid and comfort a person **(3)**

susceptible host a host that possesses optimal conditions in which the pathogen can live **(8)**

system group of organs acting together to carry out one or more body functions **(7)**

systolic pressure force with which blood is pumped when the heart contracts **(15)**

tact knowing the proper thing to say; a sensitive skill in dealing with people **(2)**

temperature measurement of the amount of heat in the body at a given time. The normal body temperature is 98.6°F (37°C) **(15)**

tendon tough cord of connective tissue that binds muscles to bony parts **(7)**

terrorism the use of random force or weapons to cause hurt, fear, or death **(20)**

testes pair of reproductive organs in the male that lie in the scrotum hanging from the perineal area, dorsal to the penis **(7)**

testosterone a male hormone **(7)**

therapeutic an act that helps in the treatment of disease or discomfort **(10)**

thermometer instrument used for measuring temperature **(15)**

thrombus blood clot that remains at its site of formation **(19)**

thymus ductless gland, part of the lymphatic system, located in the chest cavity just above the heart **(7)**

tissue group of cells of the same type **(7)**

toxin toxic substance **(7) (8)**

trachea organ of the respiratory system located in the throat area, commonly called the windpipe **(7)**

transmission-based precautions additional isolation precautions that become part of the patient's plan of care if a diagnosis of a specific pathogen is made **(8)**

tubules small tubes **(7)**

umbilical cord long, flexible, round organ that carries nourishment from the mother to the baby. It connects the umbilicus of the unborn baby in the mother's uterus to the placenta **(5)**

umbilicus small depression on the abdomen that marks the place where the umbilical cord was originally attached to the fetus; belly button **(5)**

uninvolved body part not affected by the disease process or injury **(11)**

unit pricing a system of showing the cost of food items in terms of common measurements such as ounces or pounds **(10)**

ureterostomy an incision through the abdominal wall into the ureters resulting in drainage to the outside of the body **(18)**

ureters tubes leading from the kidneys to the urinary bladder **(7)**

urethra the tube-like structure carrying urine from the bladder to the outside of the body **(7)**

urinal container into which male clients can urinate; women use female urinals **(13)**

urinary system organs that work together to produce urine **(7)**

urine liquid waste manufactured in the kidneys and discharged from the urinary bladder **(7)**

uterus expandable female reproductive organ in which an embryo grows and is nourished until gestation is complete **(7)**

vagina the birth canal leading from the cervix to the outside **(7)**

varicose vein abnormal swelling of a vein **(7)**

vas deferens tubes carrying sperm from the testicles to the glands where they are stored in preparation for ejaculation **(7)**

veins blood vessels that carry blood to the heart **(7)**

ventricles lower two chambers of the heart **(7)**

vertebrae bones of the spinal column **(7)**

vertebral column backbone **(7)**

villi tiny fingerlike projections in the lining of the small intestines into which the end products of digestion are absorbed and distributed through the bloodstream **(7)**

vital signs temperature, pulse, respiration, and blood pressure **(15)**

voiding/urinating passing water **(7)**

voluntary muscles moved consciously **(7)**

vomitus vomited material emesis **(16)**

Index